Imaging for Reconstructive Microsurgery

Joon Pio Hong • Bernard T. Lee
Akitatsu Hayashi • Giuseppe Visconti
Editors

Imaging for Reconstructive Microsurgery

Springer

Editors
Joon Pio Hong
Department of Plastic Surgery
Asan Medical Center
Seoul, Korea (Republic of)

Akitatsu Hayashi
Lymphedema Center
Kameda Medical Center
Kamogawa City, Chiba, Japan

Bernard T. Lee
Division of Plastic Surgery
Department of Surgery
Beth Israel Deaconess Medical Center
Harvard Medical School
Boston, MA, USA

Giuseppe Visconti
Unit of Plastic Surgery
Fondazione Policlinico Gemelli IRCCS
Università Cattolica del Sacro Cuore
Rome, Italy

ISBN 978-981-97-7277-3 ISBN 978-981-97-7278-0 (eBook)
https://doi.org/10.1007/978-981-97-7278-0

This Springer imprint is published by the registered company Springer Nature Singapore Pte Ltd.
The registered company address is: 152 Beach Road, #21-01/04 Gateway East, Singapore 189721, Singapore

Foreword

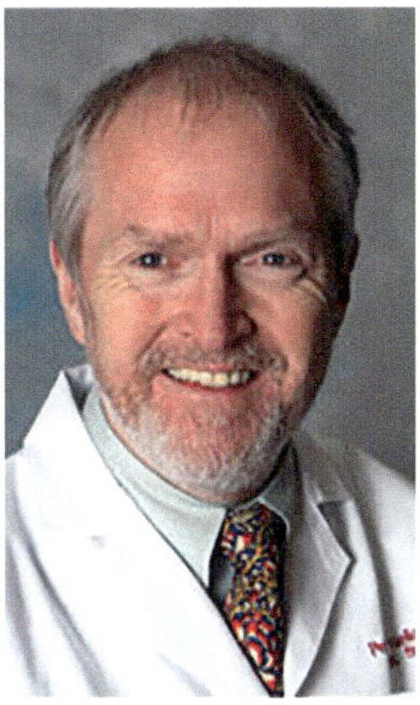

When I started my training in Plastic Surgery, imaging was not something that was considered relevant to Plastic Surgery. The only modality available at that time was X-ray and its only application was in the diagnosis of fractures. So it was relevant to the practice of traumatic hand and facial surgery albeit in a very limited way. Yet here we have a textbook devoted to imaging, in multiple modalities, all relevant to plastic surgery. Not only are these techniques germane to the discipline, they are essential to the successful practice of the specialty in the twentieth century. Prof. Hong describes imaging in his introductory chapter as "The ultimate game-changer in reconstructive microsurgery." While I fully agree with this, I would argue that its application is much more than to reconstructive microsurgery. Imaging is relevant to everything we do in Plastic Surgery.

Knowing what the modalities are and understanding how they work is important but doesn't help with understanding how these techniques are applied nor how the results are interpreted and utilized. In order to obviate this difficulty, the editors have categorized imaging by arranging the content in sections. Focused explanations of the various modalities and techniques introduce each imaging procedure. This section is followed by how these techniques are then applied in flap surgery as well as lymphatic surgery.

Ian Taylor, through his careful lead-oxide injections and meticulous anatomic dissections gave us a roadmap of the blood supply of the integument and an understanding of the anatomy of the lymphatic system. Use of the various imaging modalities in this book allows the surgeon to see this anatomy in greater detail than has ever been possible in the past. The reader will appreciate how this not only expands the horizons of our specialty but increases safety by allowing the surgeon to plan procedures accurately.

This book is extremely valuable to Plastic Surgeons but especially to any specialty involved in reconstructive microsurgery as well as those practicing lymphatic surgery. The editors are to be congratulated on compiling such a comprehensive volume.

University of Washington
Seattle, WA, USA

Peter C. Neligan

Preface

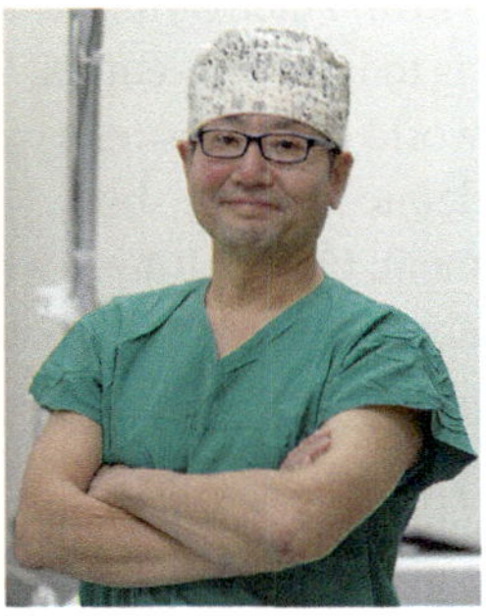

As a reconstructive surgeon, I was fortunate and privileged to witness the incredible advancements and evolution that have been made in the field of microsurgery during those three decades. Microsurgery gives the surgeon the ability to reconstruct what is missing, to regain function, and to help physiologically recover. Microsurgery entails delicate surgical procedures on small structures such as blood vessels, nerves, and lymphatic vessels opening new avenues to solve problems that were unsolvable before. One of the key elements in propelling the evolution of microsurgery was our ability to image what lies beneath the skin. The understanding of anatomy and physiology is not only in the preoperative phase but now throughout the entire process of reconstruction it has also allowed us to go further, faster, and most of all better.

This book serves as a comprehensive guide that explores the vital role of imaging techniques in the field of reconstructive microsurgery. With the rapid advancements in medical imaging technology, the ability to visualize anatomical structures with unprecedented detail and to understand the physiology has revolutionized the way reconstructive surgeons plan, perform, and follow-up for complex procedures.

In this book, we have gathered a diverse group of experts in the field, and I personally want to thank all the authors who have shared their knowledge, experiences, and insights into the various imaging techniques used in reconstructive microsurgery. Most of all, I want to thank my co-editors, Akitatsu Hayashi, Bernard T. Lee, and Giuseppe Visconti. Without their enthusiasm and curiosity to make reconstructive surgery predictable and easier, this book would not have come to life. Most of all, the friendship and camaraderie were able to spread the importance of this subject through meetings (Imaging in reconstructive microsurgery, IRM meetings) and publications.

I hope that this book will serve as a comprehensive reference, guiding other microsurgeons to navigate the waters of reconstructive surgery and inspire further advancements in this exciting field. We are fortunate to be living in the age of rapid technological development and by embracing and leveraging the power of imaging technology; we can further contribute to the field of reconstructive microsurgery and continue to find solutions for challenges that were not solvable before.

I want to express my sincere gratitude to God who has led me in every step of the journey and my late father Soon Young Hong who has taught me to do the right thing. My partners Prof. Peter Hyunsuk Suh and John Pak who have made this team into what it is today. My mentors, Prof. Yoon Kyu Chung who showed me the wonderful world of microsurgery, KyungSuk Koh who was a role model to what an academic surgeon should be, Jason Yoon who taught me about business management, Chris Attinger who showed me what we can do to help patients with diabetic foot, Scott Levin and Marco Innocent who taught me about the orthoplastic concept, David Chang who was a confidant through my journal and Geoffrey Hallock who is the definition of a true scholar, they all have immense impact in my journey and I am indebted to them. Finally, my family and beloved friends are the source to push on and without them this journey would be meaningless. Thank you.

Let the journey into the world of imaging for reconstructive microsurgery begin!

Seoul, Republic of Korea Joon Pio Hong

The original version of this book was inadvertently published with wrong photos of the editors in the Preface. The above mentioned corrections have been included in the revised publication.

Preface

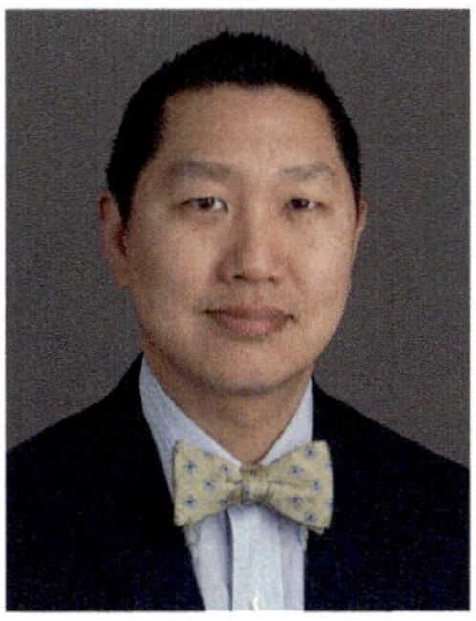

As plastic and reconstructive surgeons, we continue to work to improve clinical outcomes and provide the highest quality care for our patients. The rapid advancements in imaging technology have transformed the field of microsurgery. Identifying blood supply and perforating vessels prior to surgery is making difficult surgery more reliable. Visualizing nerves and lymphatics with higher resolution imaging has allowed surgeons to minimize issues with patient-to-patient variability.

This textbook consolidates the current state of the field of imaging in reconstructive microsurgery. It serves as a launch point for our readers to develop an understanding of how imaging technology can augment their practice. For surgeons looking to incorporate new technology, the key is to identify the benefits of the specific imaging modality and what information one hopes to obtain with its use.

I want to thank the co-editors, Profs. JP Hong, Akitatsu Hayashi, and Giuseppe Visconti for their vision and work on this project. I am eternally grateful to my mentors in plastic surgery, Drs. Berish Strauch, Joseph Upton III, Robert Goldwyn, and Sumner Slavin. Finally, I would like to express my gratitude towards my family, especially my wife Britt, for supporting me throughout my career as an academic microsurgeon.

Boston, MA, USA   Bernard T. Lee

Preface

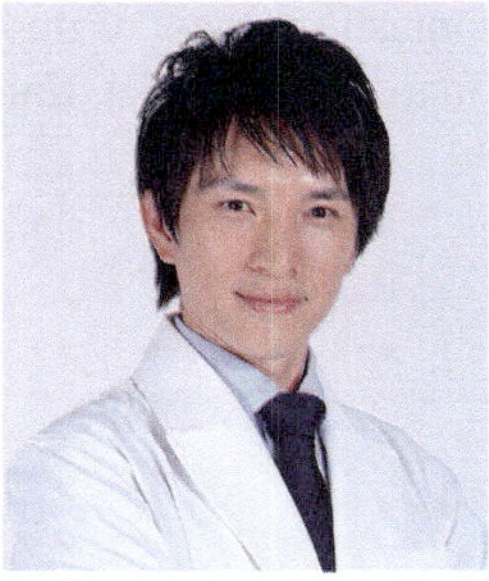

Currently, we are in the era of supermicrosurgery and perforator flap reconstruction, in which microsurgeons preserve major vessels, decreased operative time, initial debulking of the flap, and increased flexibility for the reconstructive surgeons. As these reconstructions frequently utilize vessels that are smaller than a single millimeter, understanding of perforator anatomy and the location of small vessels preoperatively is essential. Recently, the introduction of new or updated modalities for the imaging of lymphatic vessels, capillary perforators, and intradermal plexus has responded to the previously unmet need for a submillimeter resolution imaging of small anatomy and superficial tissue layers. In this viewpoint, imaging modalities are closely related to the field of reconstructive microsurgery.

By always doubting whether the current imaging exams are the best, we will be able to develop more efficient exams which leads to more effective microsurgery. It could develop new imaging techniques, or it may just modify conventional techniques. There are many wonderful technologies in the world that are buried without knowing how to use them. I believe that those imaging modalities will guide us to the future of microsurgery and supermicrosurgery. And I hope that this book will be the beginning of your new journey and challenge for the better outcome.

I am especially honored to collaborate with such an inspiring group of colleagues and, in particular, to have had the privilege to work so closely with my esteemed coeditor, Prof. Joon Pio Hong, Prof. Bernard T. Lee, and Dr. Giuseppe Visconti. We have brought enormous passion to applying imaging techniques for microsurgery for a long time through IRM meetings and publications. Without their enthusiasm and passion to create a better world of reconstructive microsurgery, this book would not have come to fruition.

I want to express my sincere gratitude to my late father Dr. Tamamine Hayashi who inspired me to become a doctor and my mentors Prof. Isao Koshima who showed me the wonderful world of supermicrosurgery, Prof. Eisuke Fukuma who has supported and watched over my work and challenge with warm eyes, Dr. Takumi Yamamoto and Dr. Hidehiko Yoshimatsu who have been a role model to what an academic microsurgeon should be, and Ms. Mayumi Handa who has supported my imaging studies for a long time with conviction. Finally, thank you to my family for supporting me throughout the years, and thank you to each child who has let me their foster father.

I believe this textbook would be a keystone to open new frontier for all ambitious reconstructive microsurgeon. Once you master these imaging techniques, you can enjoy the fantastic voyage of micro- and supermicrosurgery more. I promise it brings you to the next level. Enjoy micro-imaging and Bon Voyage!!!

Kamogawa, Japan Akitatsu Hayashi

Preface

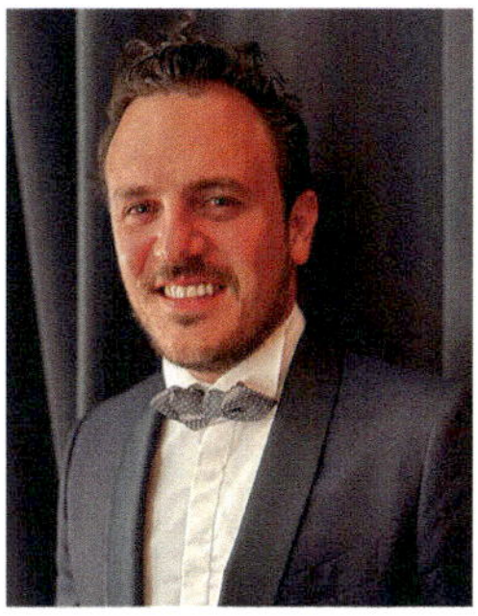

In the last three decades, reconstructive surgery has known a progressive and hyperbolic growth in terms of microvascular anatomical and physiological knowledge that nowadays allows very sophisticated reconstructions with reduced morbidity, improved function and cosmetic outcomes. The technical and knowledge improvements allowed to extend the application of reconstructive procedures to very complex cases, including diabetic foot and limb salvage that were not common indications before. In the last decade, a further revolution has been represented by lymphatic micro- and supermicrosurgery, and nowadays the very large population of patients affected by lymphatic diseases have finally the possibility to treat their disease that was before neglected.

All these fast advancements were possible also thanks to the use of imaging technologies. They were initially conceived to provide a general micro-anatomical knowledge before surgery, but nowadays they can be used to drive the surgery and the decision-making process for indications, surgical planning and execution as well as for the postoperative care.

Nowadays, we are fortunate enough to be surrounded by very sophisticated technologies that provide us very detailed information, and in more and more cases we should take advantage of using also different technologies for the same surgery to offer to our patients the best reconstructive planning with the minimal morbidity and increased safety.

I feel fortunate enough to have been exposed to most of these technologies that I currently use in my clinical practice. In particular, I can say that ultrasound, both high-frequency and ultra-high frequency, has dramatically changed my practice in both flap and lymphatic surgery and nowadays I cannot image a surgery without using it. This short but intense journey is still ongoing as we can appreciate a continuous evolution in ultrasound use for reconstructive microsurgery from all over the world.

It is a privilege to have worked on this book with true leaders and friends like JP Hong, Bernard T. Lee and Akitatsu Hayashi who introduced me to the fantastic world of ultrasound. We had the honour to have among the world renowned Reconstructive Surgeons as contributors of this book.

Finally, I must thank my little Michele and Manuela as well as my family and friends for understanding the time that I have sacrificed for working on this and who are always ready to support me.

I truly hope that this book will not only serve as a guide for those who are interested in deepening their knowledge in imaging for reconstructive microsurgery but mostly this book can also be a true inspiration for the young generation of plastic surgeons to further evolve in our fantastic specialties for the hope and care of our patients.

Roma, Italy Giuseppe Visconti

Contents

Part III Section C. Application for reconstructive surgery – *will review all applicable modalities for these flaps, which is the most valuable modality*

Part IV Section D. Designing Perforator flaps

Part V Section E. application for lymphedema surgery - *will review all applicable modalities for these approaches, which is the most valuable modality?. It is talking about the algorithm of application imaging*

Part I

Introduction

Imaging: The Ultimate Game-Changer in Reconstructive Microsurgery

1

Joon Pio Hong

Over the years of reconstruction, the tools for diagnosis were limited for reconstructive microsurgeons. For decades, the main tools were the knowledge of anatomy, anecdotal experience, and most of all good judgment [1]. In the modern era, the angiogram and CT angiograms played a key role in providing critical information of the vascular status of the limb or the zone of injury [2, 3]. While the imaging was focused on understanding the overall circulation of the injury, imaging to evaluate the donor site was still difficult. With the introduction of handheld Doppler, it further brought understanding of recipient vessels, donor vessels like perforators and most of all, the simplicity allowed it to be used not only preoperatively but help intraoperative decision-making and postoperative monitoring [4–8]. The handheld Doppler opened the doors to freestyle flaps where the flap can be designed around any perforator [5, 9]. This revolutionized the reconstructive surgery approach and outcome reaching success rate as high as 90–99% [5, 10]. Despite entering the age where reconstructive microsurgery is now practiced routinely, microsurgeons continue the endeavor to make flap reconstruction easier, replicable, reliable, and efficient [1]. Thus, new diagnostic evaluation tools are constantly being introduced to this field. The introduction of thermography and indocyanine green angiography as new tools allows us to have a better understanding of flap surgery, which is even available on your mobile device [11–14]. However, all tools have their pros and cons. When considering the cost, imaging speed, learning curve, perforator imaging, flow physiology, and depth of tissue information, one must determine which imaging modalities are able to provide the best information [15] (Table 1.1). Of course, if the surgeon has the luxury to apply various and multiple imaging, it will provide you with more information that may lead to better understanding of the overall layout prior to and during the reconstruction. In the author's opinion, color duplex ultrasound (CDU) is the tool that is able to provide the most information with highest efficiency. Early reports of using CDU have shown it efficacy and precision in identifying various anatomical structures including perforators [8, 16–20]. Unfortunately, despite early reports, the CDU did not gain wide usage among reconstructive surgeons due to the lack of accessibility. These are the presently widely used and available imaging modalities for reconstructive surgeons [15]. A brief introduction will be made in this chapter, and the details will be covered by modality and approach in the following chapters.

J. P. Hong (✉)
Department of Plastic Surgery, Asan Medical Center
University of Ulsan, Seoul, South Korea
e-mail: joonphong@amc.seoul.kr

J. P. Hong et al. (eds.), *Imaging for Reconstructive Microsurgery*,
https://doi.org/10.1007/978-981-97-7278-0_1

Table 1.1 Summary of presently available noninvasive imaging modalities for reconstructive surgeons

	CTA	MRA	HHD	ICG	Thermogram	CDU
Cost	+++	++++	+	+	+	++
Imaging speed	++++	+	++++	+++	+++	+++
Learning curve			+	+	+	+++
Perforator imaging	++	++		++	+	++++
Flow physiology				+	+	++++
Depth of tissue information	++++	++++				+++

CTA computed tomography angiography, *MRA* magnetic resonance angiography, *HHD* handheld Doppler, *ICG* indocyanine green imaging, *CDU* color Doppler ultrasonography

1.1 Computed Tomography Angiography

Presently, there are several imaging tools available for reconstructive surgeons: angiograms, computed tomography angiography (CTA), magnetic resonance angiography (MRA), laser angiography, and duplex ultrasound [21, 22]. The majority of reconstructive surgeons routinely obtain CTA as a part of preoperative planning for DIEP (deep inferior epigastric perforator) flaps due to several reasons. The CTA is widely available in many centers, and it allows for a rapid imaging of perforators and visualization of vessels as small as 0.3 mm [23]. Therefore, it has become a gold standard for many reconstructive surgeons despite the use of intravenous iodinated contrast and risk of nephrotoxicity [22]. In addition, the CTA can visualize other conditions such as incidentaloma, metastatic diseases, and abdominal wall defects [24].

Several studies have found that the CTA has specificity and sensitivity close to 100%, can decrease operative time, and is associated with a lower risk of partial flap loss than other imaging modalities for breast reconstruction [25–28]. However, one of its pitfalls includes contamination of mapping from the veins. It is possible to mistake a large vein as an arterial perforator when the radiopaque artery and its radiolucent vena commitants run together [29–31].

1.2 Magnetic Resonance Angiography

Despite the wide popularity of CTA, some reconstructive surgeons prefer MRA to CTA due to radiation exposure from CTA. Furthermore, the gadolinium-based contrast agents are less likely to cause acute allergic reaction (0.07%) than radioactive agents (3%) [32, 33]. For the imaging quality, MRA has a specificity of 100% and a sensitivity of 91.3–100% in perforator mapping for breast reconstruction [34–36]. It provides a better imaging quality for intramuscular perforator than CTA due to its higher muscle to vessel contrast resolution [28, 37, 38].

While MRA offers advantage of no radiation exposure, the imaging typically takes longer, costs more, and is more likely to be impacted by motion artifacts. In addition, the smallest size of perforator visualized on the CTA is about 0.8 mm, which is bigger than that of CTA (0.3 mm) [21, 28, 37].

1.3 Handheld Dopplers (Doppler Ultrasonography)

The use of handheld Doppler for perforator mapping was performed in the 1990s, and it is routinely used by various surgical specialties as a means to locate and monitor vessels [39]. It comes as a portable unit, and the handheld units are often available in 8 and 10 MHz. Reconstructive surgeons typically use this type of Doppler to identify and confirm the perforator locations and monitor the flap postoperatively.

While ultrasound has advantages of low cost and no radiation, several studies show that CTA is superior to Doppler ultrasound in operative time and the rate of partial flap failure in DIEP breast reconstruction [27, 31]. In addition, disadvantages of ultrasound include steep-learning curve and operator dependency. Therefore, CTA has become the imaging of choice in various centers, and ultrasound is typically used as a means to confirm the CTA imaging, especially in DIEP breast reconstruction.

1.4 Color Doppler Ultrasonography

In the era of supermicrosurgery, the role of ultrasound has changed from an adjunct to primary imaging of the choice in reconstructive surgery such as supermicrosurgery and lymphedema surgery [40]. Because both types of procedure require a detailed preoperative planning of the perforators, especially in subcutaneous tissue for perforator-to-perforator anastomoses or lymphatic to superficial vein anastomoses, color Doppler ultrasonography (CDU) became a valuable tool.

1.5 ICG Imaging (Laser Angiography)

Laser angiography using indocyanine green (ICG) was first used by plastic surgeons in 1998, and it has been used as a vascular imaging tool to assess blood flow of flaps in the intraoperative or postoperative setting [41, 42]. ICG, a fluorescence agent, binds to plasma proteins and stays in the intravascular space when injected into patients. Laser angiography allows detailed visualization of tissue perfusion including skin, subcutaneous fat, muscle, and fascia and arterial and venous blood flows of perforators [43, 44]. With the real-time vascular imaging, plastic surgeons have been able to determine the patency of arterial and venous anastomoses and perforator perfusion zones without an exposure to ionizing radiation.

Despite its advantages, laser angiography has several drawbacks: high cost, machines that are often large, and learning curve on the interpretation of the perfusion information [43].

Now with improved technology and affordability, more surgeons are using various imaging modalities to assist preoperative, intraoperative, and postoperative decision-making process. The imaging is clearly becoming an important part in the reconstructive surgery field. However, there is clearly a lack of literature focused on reconstruction to address the reconstructive surgeon's needs. Now we are evolving from anatomy-based surgery into anatomy + physiology-based surgery. This allows the surgery to be efficient and to minimize complications. It is only with efficiently utilizing the imaging tools that we will be able to truly understand and continue to evolve in the field of microsurgical reconstruction.

References

1. Hong JP. The color duplex ultrasound: the reconstructive surgeon's stethoscope. J Reconstr Microsurg. 2022;38(3):169.
2. Kim JG, Lee SH. Comparison of the multidetector-row computed tomographic angiography axial and coronal planes' usefulness for detecting thoracodorsal artery perforators. Arch Plast Surg. 2012;39(4):354–9.
3. Kim EK, Kang BS, Hong JP. The distribution of the perforators in the anterolateral thigh and the utility of multidetector row computed tomography angiography in preoperative planning. Ann Plast Surg. 2010;65(2):155–60.
4. Nahabedian MY, Patel KM. Maximizing the use of the handheld Doppler in autologous breast reconstruction. Clin Plast Surg. 2011;38(2):213–8.
5. Chang CC, Wong CH, Wei FC. Free-style free flap. Injury. 2008;39(Suppl 3):S57–61.
6. Hallock GG. Prediction of nipple viability following reduction mammoplasty using laser Doppler flowmetry. Ann Plast Surg. 1992;29(5):457–60.
7. Hallock GG. Physiological studies using laser Doppler flowmetry to compare blood flow to the zones of the free TRAM flap. Ann Plast Surg. 2001;47(3):229–33.
8. Hallock GG. Evaluation of fasciocutaneous perforators using color duplex imaging. Plast Reconstr Surg. 1994;94(5):644–51.
9. Mardini S, Tsai FC, Wei FC. The thigh as a model for free style free flaps. Clin Plast Surg. 2003;30(3):473–80.
10. Hong JPJ, Song S, Suh HSP. Supermicrosurgery: principles and applications. J Surg Oncol. 2018;118(5):832–9.
11. Hallock GG. The use of smartphone thermography to more safely unmask and preserve circulation to keystone advancement flaps in the lower extremity. Injury. 2020;51(Suppl 4):S121–S5.
12. Pereira N, Hallock GG. Smartphone thermography for lower extremity local flap perforator mapping. J Reconstr Microsurg. 2021;37(1):59–66.
13. Cifuentes IJ, Dagnino BL, Salisbury MC, Perez ME, Ortega C, Maldonado D. Augmented reality

and dynamic infrared thermography for perforator mapping in the anterolateral thigh. Arch Plast Surg. 2018;45(3):284–8.
14. Suzuki Y, Shimizu Y, Kasai S, Yamazaki S, Takemaru M, Kitamura T, et al. Indocyanine green fluorescence videoangiography for reliable variations of supraclavicular artery flaps. Arch Plast Surg. 2019;46(4):318–23.
15. Cho MJ, Kwon JG, Pak CJ, Suh HP, Hong JP. The role of duplex ultrasound in microsurgical reconstruction: review and technical considerations. J Reconstr Microsurg. 2020;36(7):514–21.
16. Hallock GG. Color duplex imaging for identifying perforators prior to pretransfer expansion of fasciocutaneous free flaps. Ann Plast Surg. 1994;32(6):595–601.
17. Hallock GG. Doppler sonography and color duplex imaging for planning a perforator flap. Clin Plast Surg. 2003;30(3):347–57.
18. Hong JP, Hur J, Kim HB, Park CJ, Suh HP. The use of color duplex ultrasound for local perforator flaps in the extremity. J Reconstr Microsurg. 2022;38(3):233–7.
19. Hong JP, Kim HB, Park CJ, Suh HP. Using duplex ultrasound for recipient vessel selection. J Reconstr Microsurg. 2022;38(3):200–5.
20. Kehrer A, Sachanadani NS, da Silva NPB, Lonic D, Heidekrueger P, Taeger CD, et al. Step-by-step guide to ultrasound-based design of alt flaps by the microsurgeon—basic and advanced applications and device settings. J Plast Reconstr Aesthet Surg. 2020;73(6):1081–90.
21. Mohan AT, Saint-Cyr M. Advances in imaging technologies for planning breast reconstruction. Gland Surg. 2016;5(2):242–54.
22. Pratt GF, Rozen WM, Chubb D, Ashton MW, Alonso-Burgos A, Whitaker IS. Preoperative imaging for perforator flaps in reconstructive surgery: a systematic review of the evidence for current techniques. Ann Plast Surg. 2012;69(1):3–9.
23. Chae MP, Hunter-Smith DJ, Rozen WM. Comparative analysis of fluorescent angiography, computed tomographic angiography and magnetic resonance angiography for planning autologous breast reconstruction. Gland Surg. 2015;4(2):164–78.
24. Tong WM, Dixon R, Ekis H, Halvorson EG. The impact of preoperative CT angiography on breast reconstruction with abdominal perforator flaps. Ann Plast Surg. 2012;68(5):525–30.
25. Alonso-Burgos A, Garcia-Tutor E, Bastarrika G, Cano D, Martinez-Cuesta A, Pina LJ. Preoperative planning of deep inferior epigastric artery perforator flap reconstruction with multislice-CT angiography: imaging findings and initial experience. J Plast Reconstr Aesthet Surg. 2006;59(6):585–93.
26. Rosson GD, Williams CG, Fishman EK, Singh NK. 3D CT angiography of abdominal wall vascular perforators to plan DIEAP flaps. Microsurgery. 2007;27(8):641–6.
27. Wade RG, Watford J, Wormald JCR, Bramhall RJ, Figus A. Perforator mapping reduces the operative time of DIEP flap breast reconstruction: a systematic review and meta-analysis of preoperative ultrasound, computed tomography and magnetic resonance angiography. J Plast Reconstr Aesthet Surg. 2018;71(4):468–77.
28. Aubry S, Pauchot J, Kastler A, Laurent O, Tropet Y, Runge M. Preoperative imaging in the planning of deep inferior epigastric artery perforator flap surgery. Skelet Radiol. 2013;42(3):319–27.
29. Piorkowski JR, DeRosier LC, Nickerson P, Fix RJ. Preoperative computed tomography angiogram to predict patients with favorable anatomy for superficial inferior epigastric artery flap breast reconstruction. Ann Plast Surg. 2011;66(5):534–6.
30. Rozen WM, Ribuffo D, Atzeni M, Stella DL, Saba L, Guerra M, et al. Current state of the art in perforator flap imaging with computed tomographic angiography. Surg Radiol Anat SRA. 2009;31(8):631–9.
31. Rozen WM, Phillips TJ, Stella DL, Ashton MW. Preoperative CT angiography for DIEP flaps: 'must-have' lessons for the radiologist. J Plast Reconstr Aesthet Surg. 2009;62(12):e650–1.
32. Katayama H, Yamaguchi K, Kozuka T, Takashima T, Seez P, Matsuura K. Adverse reactions to ionic and nonionic contrast media. A report from the Japanese Committee on the Safety of Contrast Media. Radiology. 1990;175(3):621–8.
33. Dillman JR, Ellis JH, Cohan RH, Strouse PJ, Jan SC. Frequency and severity of acute allergic-like reactions to gadolinium-containing iv contrast media in children and adults. AJR Am J Roentgenol. 2007;189(6):1533–8.
34. Chernyak V, Rozenblit AM, Greenspun DT, Levine JL, Milikow DL, Chia FA, et al. Breast reconstruction with deep inferior epigastric artery perforator flap: 3.0-T gadolinium-enhanced MR imaging for preoperative localization of abdominal wall perforators. Radiology. 2009;250(2):417–24.
35. Greenspun D, Vasile J, Levine JL, Erhard H, Studinger R, Chernyak V, et al. Anatomic imaging of abdominal perforator flaps without ionizing radiation: seeing is believing with magnetic resonance imaging angiography. J Reconstr Microsurg. 2010;26(1):37–44.
36. Newman TM, Vasile J, Levine JL, Greenspun DT, Allen RJ, Chao MT, et al. Perforator flap magnetic resonance angiography for reconstructive breast surgery: a review of 25 deep inferior epigastric and gluteal perforator artery flap patients. J Magn Resonan Imaging JMRI. 2010;31(5):1176–84.
37. Rozen WM, Phillips TJ, Ashton MW, Stella DL, Gibson RN, Taylor GI. Preoperative imaging for DIEA perforator flaps: a comparative study of computed tomographic angiography and Doppler ultrasound. Plast Reconstr Surg. 2008;121(1):9–16.
38. Rozen WM, Stella DL, Bowden J, Taylor GI, Ashton MW. Advances in the pre-operative planning of deep inferior epigastric artery perforator flaps: magnetic resonance angiography. Microsurgery. 2009;29(2):119–23.
39. Chang BW, Luethke R, Berg WA, Hamper UM, Manson PN. Two-dimensional color Doppler imaging

for precision preoperative mapping and size determination of TRAM flap perforators. Plast Reconstr Surg. 1994;93(1):197–200.
40. Oni G, Chow W, Ramakrishnan V, Griffiths M. Plastic surgeon–led ultrasound. Plast Reconstr Surg. 2018;141(2):300e–9e.
41. Gurtner GC, Jones GE, Neligan PC, Newman MI, Phillips BT, Sacks JM, et al. Intraoperative laser angiography using the SPY system: review of the literature and recommendations for use. Ann Surg Innov Res. 2013;7(1):1.
42. Still J, Law E, Dawson J, Bracci S, Island T, Holtz J. Evaluation of the circulation of reconstructive flaps using laser-induced fluorescence of indocyanine green. Ann Plast Surg. 1999;42(3):266–74.
43. Phillips BT, Munabi NC, Roeder RA, Ascherman JA, Guo L, Zenn MR. The role of intraoperative perfusion assessment: what is the current state and how can i use it in my practice? Plast Reconstr Surg. 2016;137(2):731–41.
44. Liu DZ, Mathes DW, Zenn MR, Neligan PC. The application of indocyanine green fluorescence angiography in plastic surgery. J Reconstr Microsurg. 2011;27(6):355–64.

Part II

Section B. Modalities - *focused on technical aspects (how to use and interpret)*

2 What About Handheld Doppler?

Raphael Sinna, Christian Herlin,
and Benoit Chaput

2.1 Introduction

A few years ago, perforator flaps became a real game changer in the field of reconstructive surgery [1]. Harvesting reliable flaps around small vessels needed an accurate finding, before cutting the skin. Handheld Doppler (HHD) became then the first tool used in preoperative mapping. Furthermore, this device became even mandatory with the development of the freestyle flap concept [2–4].

Today, despite the development of other technologies, especially color Doppler, HHD remains the main everyday tool for a lot of surgeons: It is an easy, cheap, and reliable tool that is available widely [5]. But let us try to understand the place of this device in the increasing imaging armamentarium for plastic surgeon.

2.2 How It Works?

We believe that understanding the basic concept of the Doppler effect is mandatory to interpret the sound that we are listening to during the examination. In a continuous Doppler, there are two crystals at the level of the same sensor: one which emits a beam of ultrasound (US) in a continuous way and the other which receives the reflected signal, also in a continuous way. The apparatus compares the two frequencies F_e (emitted) and F_r (reflected) at the level of a demodulator to extract therefrom, continuously, the Doppler frequency (ΔF) that we are listening to (Fig. 2.1) (Video 2.1).

When the probe sends out and detects the reflected ultrasound on a nonmoving structure, F_e and F_r are the same: there is no Doppler effect ($\Delta F = 0$). When this same US hits a moving structure (like blood cells), the frequency of the reflected US will be modified. If the object is moving away, the frequency will decrease; if it is getting nearer, the frequency will increase. By chance ΔF is often between 50 Hz and 20 kHz, which is in the range of audible sound (Fig. 2.2).

This variation of frequencies (ΔF) can be calculated this way: $\Delta F = 2F_e V{\cdot}\cos\theta/c$ F_e is the initial frequency sent by the probe, V is the blood

Supplementary Information The online version contains supplementary material available at https://doi.org/10.1007/978-981-97-7278-0_2.

R. Sinna (✉)
Department of Plastic Reconstructive and Aesthetic Surgery, Amiens University Hospital, Amiens Cedex 1, France
e-mail: Sinna.raphael@chu-amiens.fr

C. Herlin
Department of Plastic Reconstructive and Aesthetic Surgery, Montpellier University Hospital, Montpellier, France

B. Chaput
Department of Plastic Reconstructive and Aesthetic Surgery, Toulouse University Hospital, Toulouse, France

J. P. Hong et al. (eds.), *Imaging for Reconstructive Microsurgery*,
https://doi.org/10.1007/978-981-97-7278-0_2

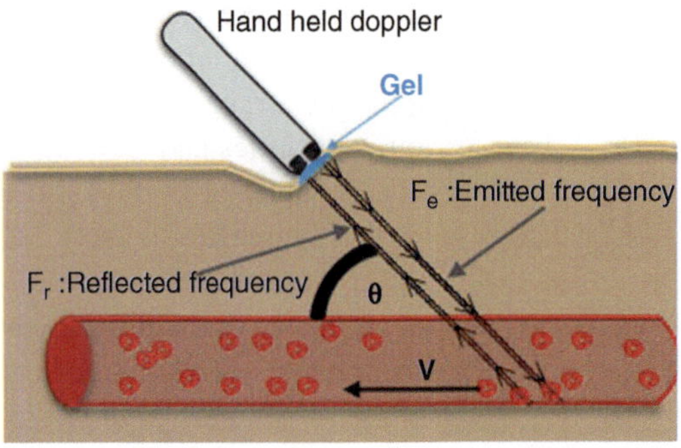

Fig. 2.1 The Doppler frequency depends on the emitted frequency (F_e), the reflected frequency (F_r), the blood flow speed (V), *the sound* wave travel time (C), and θ the angle between the probe and the studied vessel: $\Delta F = 2F_e V{\cdot}\cos\theta/c$

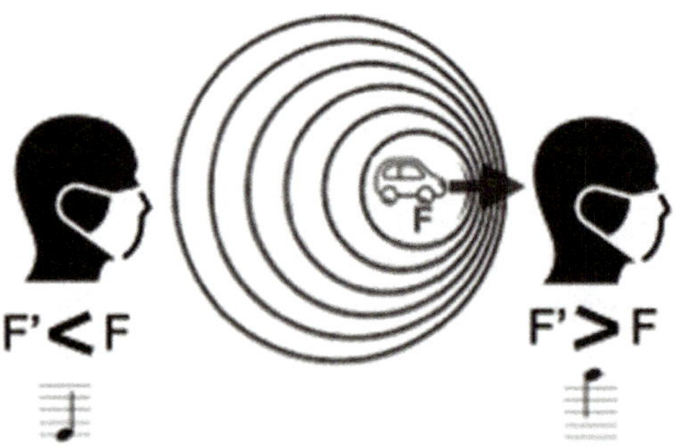

Fig. 2.2 With a moving structure, the reflected frequency will be modified. If the object is moving away, the frequency will decrease; if it is getting nearer, the frequency will increase

flow speed, *C is the sound* wave travel speed through tissue (1540 m/s), and θ is the angle between the probe and the studied vessel.

We can notice that when the angle θ (between the vessel and the probe) is equal to 90°, there will be no Doppler effect because cosinus 90 = 0. On the other hand, when the vessel is in the direction of the probe, like perforator vessels, the angle is equal to zero. In this situation, we have the best Doppler effect because cosinus 0 = 1.

2.3 What to Use?

Several frequency HDDs are available on the market. The penetration of ultrasound in the body will depend on the emitted frequency. Low frequencies have a good penetration but will be less accurate on low flow vessels. High frequencies will have a better sensitivity but will not be able to penetrate deep in the body. Therefore, a 2-MHz probe will detect deep flow and is especially used for fetal monitoring, and a 5-MHz probe will be used for deep vessel or when there is edema. Roukis [6] studied septocutaneous perforator of the plantar area using a 5-MHz probe. Unfortunately, in his study there is no evidence that the detected vessels were perforator and not more deep vessels.

Therefore, the two most commonly used frequencies are the 8 and 10 MHz. They have a peak sensitivity of only 20 and 15 mm deep, respectively [5].

Yu and Youssef [7] studied the locations of the anterolateral thigh flap perforators using an 8-MHz and a 10-MHz probe, compared to the intraoperative findings. The positive predictive value for the 8-MHz probe in detecting the perforator was 89%, while no false-negative results were found. For the 10-MHz probe, a positive predictive value of 94% and negative predictive value of 43% were found. They found that the 8-MHz probe was easier to use (faster detection of a perforator).

But they also noticed that the probabilities of correct detection of cutaneous perforator with both devices decrease with increasing body mass index (BMI). In the same idea, Shaw [8] found also more false-positive results in thin patients. Probably in this case the HHD was detecting muscular perforator that would be around 20 mm under the skin in thin patients. This points the fact that the frequency should be adapted. Therefore a 5 Mhz device will be more suitable in patients with high BMI and a 10-MHz device for thin patients.

During surgery, some acoustic Dopplers can be used sterile in case of doubt performing a patency test, for example. We have also used it to detect the level of a thrombus or the location of an arterial dissection. In practice, the use of this type of Doppler is relatively infrequent (Video 2.2).

2.4 How to Use It?

Most of the perforator clusters are now well known [9]. When HHD is used in preoperative mapping with "classical perforator flap," especially for free flaps, we believe that it is better to acquire a theoretical knowledge of perforator clusters to search in the correct anatomical area directly. Especially at the beginning, this will reduce the time for perforator localization. In the case of freestyle flaps or propeller flaps, the mindset is different because the perforator will be searched in the area that we need it to be (depending on the defect to be closed). In this case, preoperative planning will take more time.

The detection of perforators is initially done by placing the probe close to the skin without pressure, to search for different sounds in the area of interest. Perforator arteries often give a well-knocked and relatively loud sound, without having to apply excessive pressure to the skin with the probe (Video 2.1). Through the gel, you can even take the probe off the skin and continue to hear the perforator when the latter is truly perpendicular to the device.

When a positive signal is located, the probe should be moved in all directions to ensure that the signal stops in other directions, indicating that it is a perforator and not an axial vessel. This was well described by Stekelenburg et al. [10] in their article "What you hear is not always what you get." Particularly at the lower limbs, it is sometimes difficult to differentiate between the source vessel and the perforator vessels. At the level of the distal extremities, source vessels are more superficial, and in case of detection error, one can notice a sound not as "punchy" as with a perforator, over time, the experience of the operator can often recognize the difference. Therefore, we recommend always to use the same device to develop a specific ear for your device. Each device requires a learning curve to limit detection errors. That is why experience of the user is key to improve sensitivity and specificity with the HHD [11].

The "perforator compression test" described by Mun and Jeon (2006) is a good tool to help to distinguish between a perforator and a deep vessel [12]. The course of perforators is usually perpendicular to the skin surface, making perforators easily compressible and collapsible by an external force applied perpendicular to the surface of the skin. The loudness of the pulsating sound decreases with increasing pressure if the pulse originates from a perforator. Mun and Jeon reported 100% specificity in detecting perforators for their test. Since we adopted it, we have reduced our rate of perforator detection errors (Video 2.3).

Veins are sometimes pitfalls during perforator detection [13]. Indeed, the sound of the perforator arteries can be deported into the veins, sometimes even several centimeters away; this also represents a source of error and testifies of the high sensitivity and low specificity of HHD [14].

The sound of a vein is however identifiable with the HHD. It is a more breathy and relatively continuous sound, like the sound of "wind under the door" (Video 2.4). The saphenous vein, due to its substantial flow, is relatively easy to detect. It is thus possible to identify a superficial recipient vein (saphenous or other) to anastomose a free flap to it or to supercharge a pedicle flap.

2.5 Should We Still Use It?

The use of HHD in reconstructive surgery was described in the 1980s for postoperative free flap monitoring [15] (Video 2.5). Still today this device remains one of the most used devices for this indication. It can help salvaging a flap only on the variation of the signal before any cutaneous sign can be visible [16].

To make the monitoring easier for the team and because markers are not permanent, different tips can be done as using either an adhesive transparent film [17] or a stich [18] over the exact localization of the artery. Thus, after a relatively short learning period, the nurses but also the young residents will be able to monitor flaps even when they are too white (pale skin) or in patients with a difficult capillary refill time identification.

Intraoperative use of HHD was also described especially to identify the dominant vascular pedicle during intramuscular dissection, but it is not a common indication [19].

The HHD use in preoperative planning was directly correlated with the development of perforator flaps [1, 9, 7, 20]. Despite its convenience, we know that HHD Doppler is not the best device for perforator mapping especially when it is compared to more modern device [21].

In the literature, its reliability for perforator detection has shown a wide range of result. The best result found shows a positive predictive value rate between 82% and 94% [7, 22] where other studies were more humble and showed 52%, [23] 55% [10], and 69% [24]. This great difference can be explained by several points. The main bias was the diameter of the studied perforator. Probably the detection of the "classical perforator" (DIEP, ALT, etc.) is more easy because of its constancy and diameter compared to perforator of the elbow, for example, in case of freestyle flap [10]. The other point is the subcutaneous thickness of the studied area that can influence the reliability. This was pointed by Peirong et al. in their study showing the difference of specificity and sensitivity in the perforator detection when the frequency of the probe was not adapted to the subcutaneous tickness using two different frequency devices (8 MHz and 10 MHz) [7]. In his study on elbow perforators, this could be the reason why Stekelenburg [10] found that the false positives were 32% in axial vessels and 45% in intramuscular vessels.

Another point is the absence of spatial resolution. The received signal is not specific to a single depth, and the Doppler frequency measured is the resultant of all the Doppler frequencies extracted from the signal, average of the signals coming from all the vessels crossed by the wave which is also a source of error.

Frequently and especially on the lower limb, we associate the color Doppler sonography. The latter allows us to confirm the location of the perforator but also its orientation which can be slightly offset or oblique, particularly for posterior tibial artery perforator flap that remains a tricky propeller flap. Color Doppler sonography brings precision and provides information on the axis of the perforators. However, training in the use of HHD can greatly improve the detection performance of an operator and its use as a unique tool for preoperative diagnosis in most cases. For some authors, in the preoperative marking of specific flaps such as the anterolateral thigh flap, there is no advantage with color Doppler compared to acoustic Doppler [25]. Furthermore, the portability and low cost of these devices make them essential tools for humanitarian missions.

Apart from helping to locate perforator vessels, the HHD provides little information. Unlike the color Doppler, the HHD does not give the depth nor the caliber or the velocity of the perforators; it can nevertheless orient on the axis of the perforator. Ultimately, the size of the harvestable flap is a frequent question, but the acoustic Doppler does not provide any information about it.

2.6 Conclusion

HHD is widely used because it is cheap, portable, easy to use, and available everywhere. It proved its efficiency especially for postoperative management. Unfortunately, in preoperative planning, the lake of image of the detected vessels is the main drawback of this device especially compared to color Doppler. But in most of the cases especially with the "classical perforator flaps," HHD Doppler remains a good tool in planning the surgery (Table 2.1).

Probably the advantages of the HHD (cheap and portable) will not be enough to support its use in a few years' time. Indeed, we have now several ultra-portable color Doppler devices that are launched on the market. A few models can even be left in the white coat pocket just as the

Table 2.1 Comparison between handheld Doppler, conventional color Doppler, and ultraportable color Doppler

	Handheld Doppler	Conventional color Doppler	Portable color Doppler
Easy to use	+++	+	++
Portability	+++	+	++
Cheap	+++	+	++
Perforator visualization	0	+++	++
Operator dependent	++	++	++
Anatomy visualization	0	+++	++
Accurate pre-op mapping	+	+++	++

HHD. These modern color Dopplers are financially more affordable and very easy to use because most of the settings are already preset. So probably in a few years, "ultraportable color Doppler will be the new HHD."

References

1. Sinna R, Qassemyar Q, Pérignon D, Benhaim T, Robbe M. À propos des lambeaux perforants… 20 ans après. Ann Chir Plast Esthét. 2011;56:128–33.
2. Wallace CG, Kao H-K, Jeng S-F, Wei F-C. Free-style flaps: a further step forward for perforator flap surgery. Plast Reconstr Surg. 2009;124:e419–26.
3. Demirtas Y, Ozturk N, Kelahmetoglu O, Demir A. Pedicled perforator flaps. Ann Plast Surg. 2009;63:179–83.
4. Chang C-C, Wong C-H, Wei F-C. Free-style free flap. Injury. 2008;39:57–61.
5. Smit JM, Klein S, Werker PMN. An overview of methods for vascular mapping in the planning of free flaps. J Plast Reconstr Aesthet Surg. 2010;63:e674–82.
6. Roukis TS. The Doppler probe for planning septofasciocutaneous advancement flaps on the plantar aspect of the foot: anatomical study and clinical applications. J Foot Ankle Surg. 2000;39:270–90.
7. Yu P, Youssef A. Efficacy of the handheld Doppler in preoperative identification of the cutaneous perforators in the anterolateral thigh flap. Plast Reconstr Surg. 2006;118:928–33.
8. Shaw RJ, Batstone MD, Blackburn TK, Brown JS. Preoperative Doppler assessment of perforator anatomy in the anterolateral thigh flap. Br J Oral Maxillofac Surg. 2010;48:419–22.
9. Boucher F, Mojallal A. Atlas des artères perforantes de la peau du tronc et des membres—Guide dans la réalisation des lambeaux perforants. Ann Chir Plast Esthét. 2013;58:644–9.
10. Stekelenburg CM, et al. The hand held Doppler device for the detection of perforators in reconstructive surgery: what you hear is not always what you get. Burns. 2014;40:1702–6.
11. Chaput B, Bertheuil N, Gandolfi S, Grolleau JL, Herlin C. Perforator detection with a hand-held Doppler device: importance of the learning curve. Burns J Int Soc Burn Inj. 2015;41:197.
12. Mun G-H, Jeon B-J. An efficient method to increase specificity of acoustic Doppler sonography for planning a perforator flap: perforator compression test. Plast Reconstr Surg. 2006;118:296–7.
13. Hallock GG. Doppler sonography and color duplex imaging for planning a perforator flap. Clin Plast Surg. 2003;30:347–57.
14. Hallock GG. Attributes and shortcomings of acoustic Doppler sonography in identifying perforators for flaps from the lower extremity. J Reconstr Microsurg. 2009;25:377–81.
15. Solomon G, Yaremchuk M, Manson P. Doppler ultrasound surface monitoring of both arterial and venous flow in clinical free tissue transfers. J Reconstr Microsurg. 1986;3:39–41.
16. Bar-Meir E, Merali H, Yueh J, Tobias A, Lee B. Paradoxical venous Doppler signal: a sentinel sign of early venous congestion. J Reconstr Microsurg. 2008;24:255–7.
17. Smit JM, Whitaker IS, Acosta R. A simple adjunct to facilitate hand held Doppler perforator localisation following microsurgical breast reconstruction. J Plast Reconstr Aesthet Surg. 2008;61:1194.
18. Salgado CJ, Moran SL, Mardini S. Flap monitoring and patient management. Plast Reconstr Surg. 2009;124:e295–302.
19. Michelow BJ, Hartrampf CR, Bennett GK. TRAM flap safety optimized with intraoperative Doppler. Plast Reconstr Surg. 1990;86:143–6.
20. DellaCroce FJ, Sullivan SK. Application and refinement of the superior gluteal artery perforator free flap for bilateral simultaneous breast reconstruction. Plast Reconstr Surg. 2005;116:97–103.
21. Nassar AH, et al. Comparison of various modalities utilized for preoperative planning in microsurgical reconstructive surgery. J Reconstr Microsurg. 2022;38:170–80.
22. Jakubietz RG, et al. Propeller-Lappenplastiken: die Reliabilität der präoperativen, unidirektionalen Dopplersonografie. Handchir Mikrochir Plast Chir. 2011;43:76–80.
23. Ensat F, et al. Doppler-Sonografie und Farbdopplersonografie zur präoperativen Perforatordarstellung beim anterolateralen Oberschenkellappen. Handchir Mikrochir Plast Chir. 2011;43:71–5.
24. Giunta RE, Geisweid A, Feller AM. The value of preoperative Doppler sonography for planning free perforator flaps. Plast Reconstr Surg. 2000;105:2381–6.
25. Haribhakti VV, Thorat TS, Powle VR, Virarkar MK. Prospective study to analyse the efficiency of acoustic Doppler v/s colour duplex ultrasound in locating perforators for antero-lateral thigh flap in reconstructive head and neck surgery. J Plast Reconstr Aesthet Surg JPRAS. 2021;74:2026–33.

3 CTA Focused on Technical Aspects (How to Use and Interpret)

Jaume Masia, Cristhian D. Pomata,
and Juan A. Clavero Torrent

3.1 Introduction

Traditionally, microsurgical reconstruction has faced a significant challenge in preoperatively determining a suitable blood vessel to nourish the entire flap to be transferred. This difficulty was further compounded by the emergence of perforator flaps, due to their high anatomical diversity, including variations in the location and size of the perforator vessels, as well as in their course through the muscles and branching in the subcutaneous tissue.

Since the early days of microsurgery, handheld Doppler sonography has been used for the preoperative location of individual vessels. Despite being a convenient and inexpensive tool to investigate the position and flow of the perforator, it offers only limited information on perforator caliber and course and cannot distinguish perforating vessels from main axial vessels. Moreover, Doppler sonography may be too sensitive, detecting even minuscule vessels that may not be suitable to support flaps of medium or large dimensions. Furthermore, false positives in the location of the perforator can appear if the axial vessels run superficially, resulting in low specificity for this technique [1].

Color duplex ultrasound may offer more information on perforator caliber, flow direction, and velocity, allowing interpretation of its course or pattern. Unfortunately, this imaging technique also has some drawbacks, as it provides nonanatomical images, is time-consuming, and requires highly skilled and experienced scanning personnel with knowledge of perforator flap surgery. These substantial limitations have contributed to its relative underuse in microsurgical units [2].

In this context, the 1990s marked a golden period in vascular diagnosis and therapy, with the introduction of computed tomography angiography. Initially, scanning was spiral or helical with a single row of detectors. However, in the late 1990s, the development of multidetector computed tomography (MDCT) drastically changed the evaluation of vascular pathologies. MDCT had four detector rings capable of half-second gantry rotations, effectively multiplying the volume coverage per unit time by 8 at the same section thickness. Therefore, virtually all limits on longitudinal coverage disappeared. In addition, MDCT stood apart from other imaging modalities as a near-isotropic volumetric acquisition technique that allowed the reformation of Carte-

J. Masia (✉)
Plastic Surgery, Santa Creu i Sant Pau Hospital—Autonomous University of Barcelona, Barcelona, Spain

Clínica Planas, Barcelona, Spain
e-mail: jmasia@santpau.cat

C. D. Pomata
Clínica Planas, Barcelona, Spain

J. A. Clavero Torrent
Radiology Department, Clínica Creu Blanca, Barcelona, Spain

J. P. Hong et al. (eds.), *Imaging for Reconstructive Microsurgery*,
https://doi.org/10.1007/978-981-97-7278-0_3

sian planar and curved planar images as well as volume renderings [3].

At that time, MDCT had proven to be highly useful not only for evaluating the aorta and peripheral arteries but also as a promising noninvasive technique for detecting, visualizing, and characterizing stenotic coronary artery disease. In addition, it was able to evaluate the size of the lumen, the permeability, and the occlusion sites of the coronary vessels. From this application, the idea emerged of using MDCT in microsurgery as a more reliable method to precisely locate the most suitable vessels preoperatively [4–6].

Some reports on the use of preoperative MDCT angiography for planning microsurgical reconstruction date back to the early 2000s [7, 8]. The purpose was to examine major arteries in potential donor areas of the lower limb, as well as potential recipient sites in the head and neck, hip/thigh, and lower limb. However, independently, in 2002, Masià et al. [9] began utilizing MDCT with 16 detector rows to assess the vascular anatomy of the abdominal wall by focusing on the perforator visualization arose from this. The authors validated the technique in a study conducted in 2003 and published in 2006. For this purpose, they raised the flaps while simultaneously identifying and inspecting all perforators. When the MDCT results were compared with the intraoperative findings, no false-positive or false-negative results were obtained. Moreover, this technique also facilitated visualization of certain perforator variants, such as those with a paramuscular or extramuscular course [10], which were difficult to identify in the operating room without preoperative MDCT angiography. The authors also implemented a coordinate system that simplified the preoperative location of the perforator on the patient's abdominal skin.

This contribution was popularized as a valuable technique for studying the vascular anatomy of the perforators from various donor sites, identifying their size, location, and trajectory, to select the most suitable perforator for microsurgical reconstruction. Consequently, MDCT angiography became a widely accepted preoperative imaging method in the field of microsurgical reconstruction and is commonly employed in clinical practice [11–17].

In this chapter, we will describe the technical aspects of MDCT angiography, including image acquisition and interpretation, and the indications for the use of this imaging technique in preoperative planning of perforator flap surgeries.

3.2 Technical Aspects and Image Acquisition

MDCT angiography combines computer-analyzed X-ray images with a bolus of venous contrast medium to produce high-resolution reconstructions of vascular structures. The number of detector rows determines the speed of the scan and the level of detail that can be shown. Present multidetector MDCT scanners feature up to 320 detector rings, gantry rotation times as low as 270 ms, and, in some cases, two X-ray sources that use a lower radiation dose, enabling acquisition of submillimeter isotropic resolution over very large volumes in a matter of seconds [3].

Patients are positioned on an MDCT table exactly as they will be positioned for surgery. The entire scanning process is carried out while the patient receives an 80–100 mL bolus of non-ionic iodinated contrast medium with a concentration of 300 mg/mL. The contrast medium is mechanically injected at a rate of 4 mL/s through an 18-gauge intravenous catheter. The entire procedure takes less than 10 min and is therefore very well tolerated by the patient. The volumetric data acquired are then used to reconstruct images with a slice width of up to 0.5 mm. The resulting complete set of reconstructed images is automatically transferred to a computer workstation that generates reformatted images in multiple planes and 3D volume-rendered images. This system allows measurements to be taken so that different spatial planes can be automatically correlated. The data obtained can be conveniently stored on a compact disc or pen drive, which can be easily accessed and managed on a standard computer [18].

3.3 Image Analysis

The images obtained through MDCT angiography are usually analyzed by both the radiologist and the reconstructive surgeon who will harvest the flap. Several important parameters are assessed in these images, including (1) the source artery, (2) the location of the perforators, (3) the diameter of the perforators, (4) the trajectory of the perforators, (5) the perforators' side-branching and relationships with neighboring structures, (6) the thickness of the subcutaneous tissue, and (7) anomalies in the regional anatomical structures.

The axial view is the first and most crucial view to be analyzed. The assessment starts from the source vessel to then identify the origin of the perforators. The external diameter of the perforators is measured at the point where they pierce the fascia. Their course is then evaluated, determining whether the direction is medial or lateral and whether the trajectory is intramuscular, septal, or directly into the subcutaneous tissue. This view allows visualization of the perforators' branching and distribution within the subcutaneous tissue. Once the perforators are identified, they are marked with an arrow that will appear in all other views when that point is reached (Figs. 3.1a, 3.2a, b and 3.3a).

The sagittal view is the second view to be analyzed. It serves as a valuable reference to double-check the information obtained from the axial view and to complement the assessment by determining whether the direction of the perforators is superior or inferior. This view also aids in identifying the trajectory of the perforators and their relationship with adjacent anatomical structures, as well as the potential interconnections between the superficial and deep vascular system, if present (Figs. 3.1b, 3.2c, d and 3.3b, c).

The coronal view is the third view to be analyzed. Although the most crucial data have already been evaluated in the previous views, images from this perspective provide additional information on the trajectory of the perforators, offering clearer visualization of their course (i.e., lateral, medial, superior, inferior, or oblique), branching patterns, and connections with adjacent angiosomes. This view also allows clearer assessment of the relationships of the perforators with neighboring anatomic reference structures (Figs. 3.1c, 3.2e and 3.3d).

Lastly, a three-dimensional reconstruction of the assessed body region is undertaken to precisely locate the points on the skin surface where the best perforators enter the subcutaneous tissue (Figs. 3.1d, e, 3.2f, g and 3.3e).

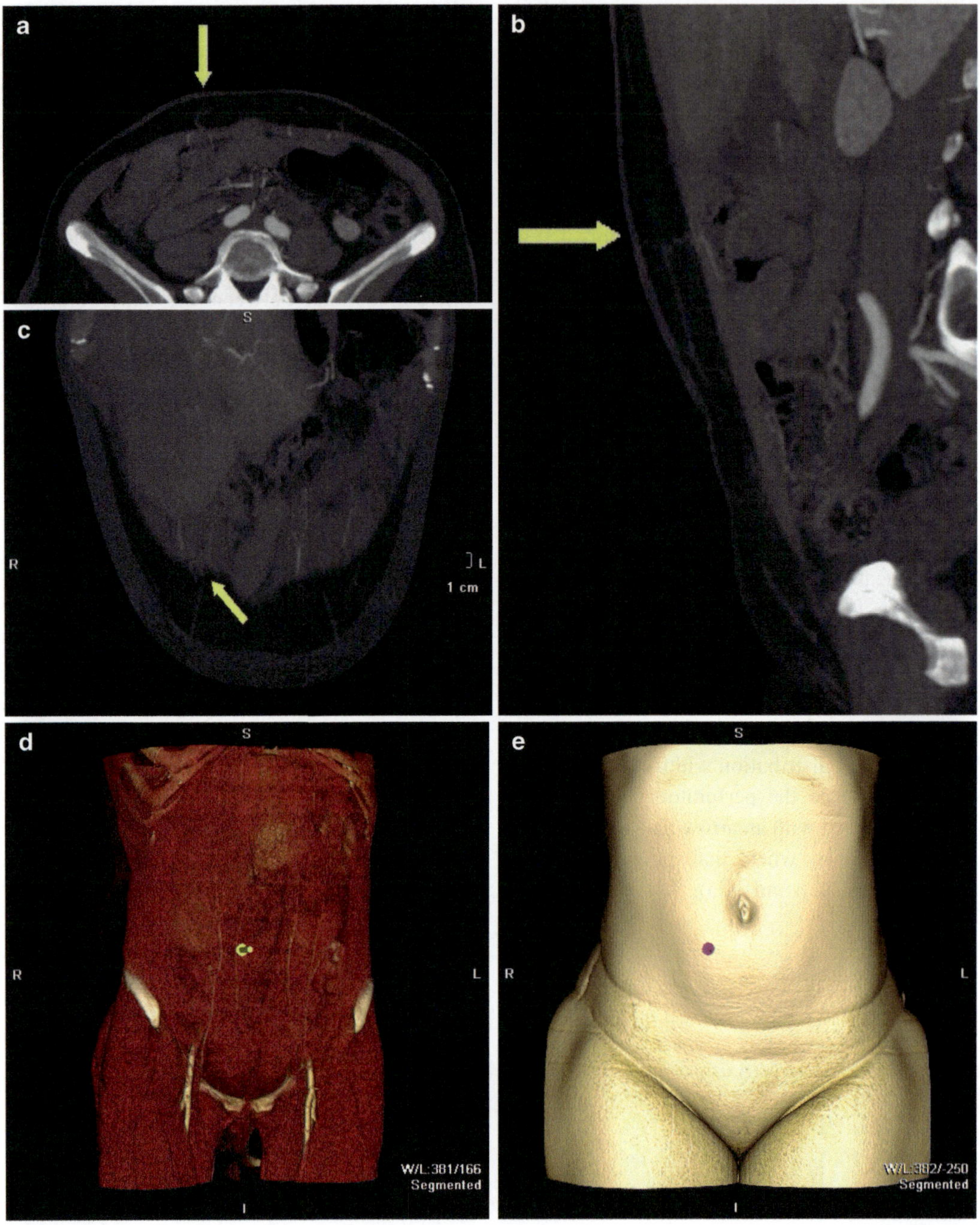

Fig. 3.1 MDCT images of a deep inferior epigastric artery perforator on the right side of the abdominal wall (the perforator is marked with a yellow arrow or a fuchsia dot). (**a**) Axial view. (**b**) Sagittal view. (**c**) Coronal view. (**d**) Three-dimensional reconstruction of deep structures of the abdominal region. (**e**) Three-dimensional reconstruction of the skin surface of the abdominal region

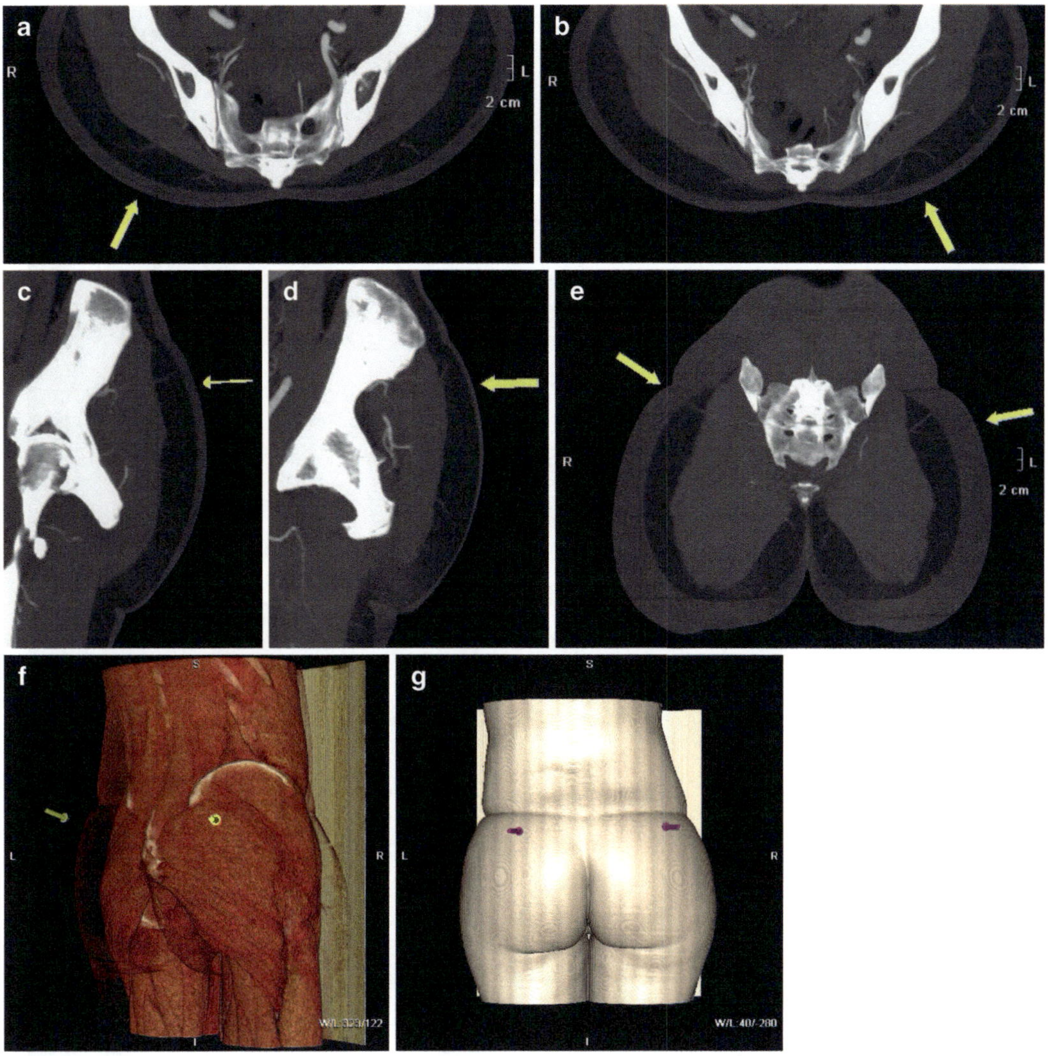

Fig. 3.2 MDCT images of two superior gluteal artery perforators (the perforators are marked with a yellow arrow or a fuchsia dot). (**a**) Axial view: a perforator on the right side. (**b**) Axial view: a perforator on the left side. (**c**) Sagittal view: the perforator on the right side. (**d**) Sagittal view: the perforator on the left side. (**e**) Coronal view: the two perforators. (**f**) Three-dimensional reconstruction of deep structures of the gluteal region: the two perforators. (**g**) Three-dimensional reconstruction of the skin surface of the gluteal region: the two perforators

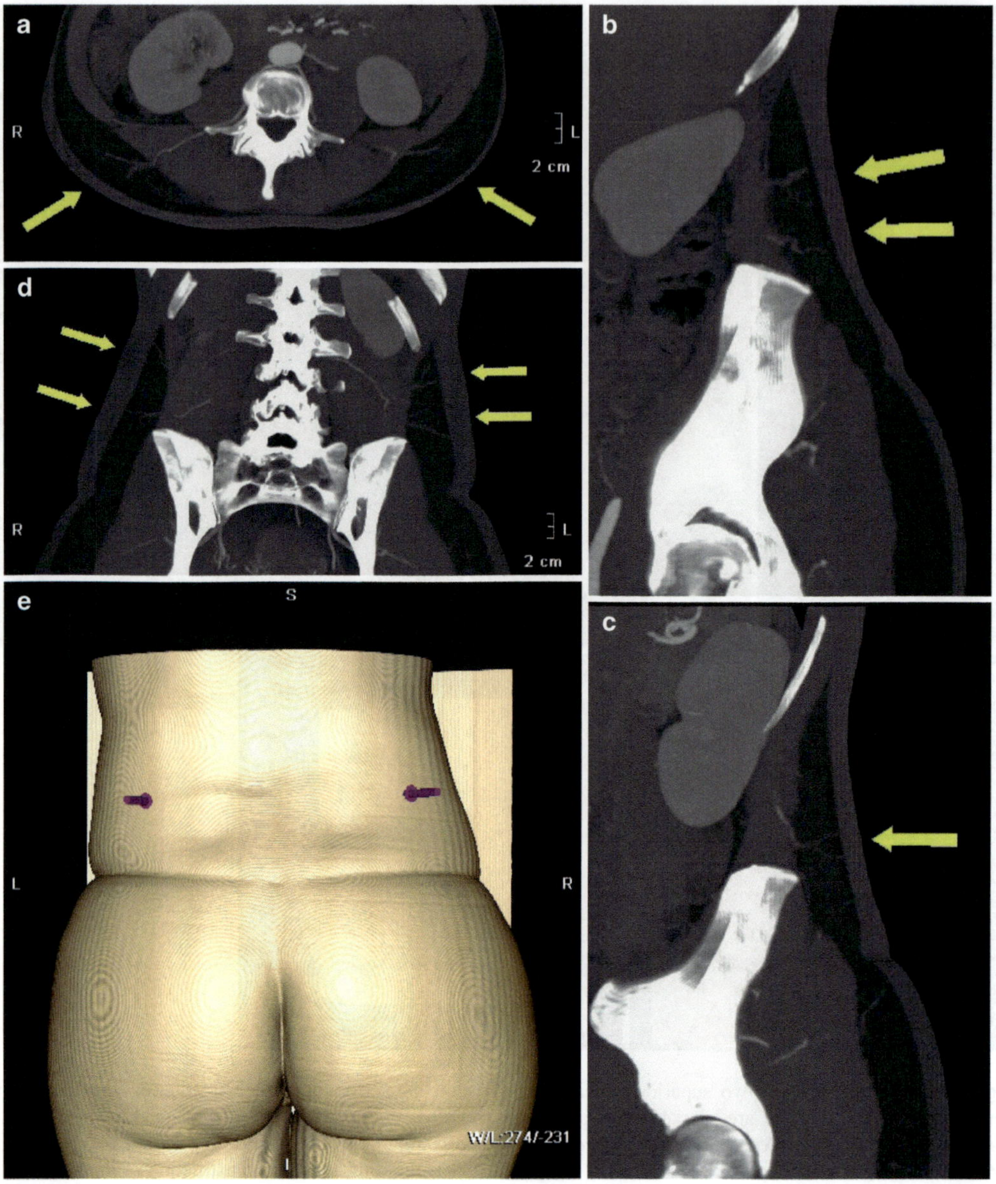

Fig. 3.3 MDCT images of lumbar artery perforators (the perforators are marked with a yellow arrow or a fuchsia dot). (**a**) Axial view: one perforator on the right side and another on the left side. (**b**) Sagittal view: two perforators on the right side. (**c**) Sagittal view: one perforator on the left side. (**d**) Coronal view: two perforators on each side. (**e**) Three-dimensional reconstruction of the skin surface of the lumbar region: the best perforator on each side

3.4 Perforator Location Coordinate System

To facilitate the precise location of each perforator, a Cartesian coordinate system is designed, where x and y axes are determined based on a reference point in the donor site region:

- On the abdomen, the zero-reference point is the umbilicus, from which two lines are drawn: a transverse line (x) extending laterally to the anterior flanks and a longitudinal line (y) extending up to the sternum and down to the pubis.
- In the anterior thoracic and thoracodorsal region, the zero-reference point is the manu-

brium of the sternum, from which two lines are drawn: a transverse line (x) extending laterally to the shoulders and a longitudinal line (y) extending downward to the xiphoid process.

- On the back, the zero-reference point is the spinous process of the C7 vertebra, from which two lines are drawn: a transverse line (x) extending laterally to the shoulders and a longitudinal line (y) extending downward to the sacrum.
- In the lumbar and gluteal region, the zero-reference point is the coccyx, from which two lines are drawn: a transverse line (x) extending laterally toward the trochanters and a longitudinal line (y) extending upward along the spinous processes of the sacral and lumbar vertebrae.
- In the upper limbs, the zero-reference point is the central part of the elbow flexure, from which two lines are drawn: a transverse line (x) that extends circumferentially to the sides and a longitudinal line (y) that extends up to the shoulder and down to the midpoint of the wrist flexure.
- In the lower limbs, the zero-reference point is the knee, from which two lines are drawn: a transverse line (x) that extends circumferentially to the sides and a longitudinal line (y) that extends up to the anterior superior iliac spine and down to the midpoint of the ankle flexure.

In this context, during the analysis of the axial view, the midpoint of the assessed region corresponds to the y axis, which intersects the regional zero-reference point. Consequently, the distance from the midline to the perforator is measured to determine the x value in the Cartesian plane (Fig. 3.4a).

Likewise, during the analysis of the sagittal view, the second measurement is recorded, that is, the distance above or below the regional zero-reference point, to determine the y value in the Cartesian plane (Fig. 3.4b).

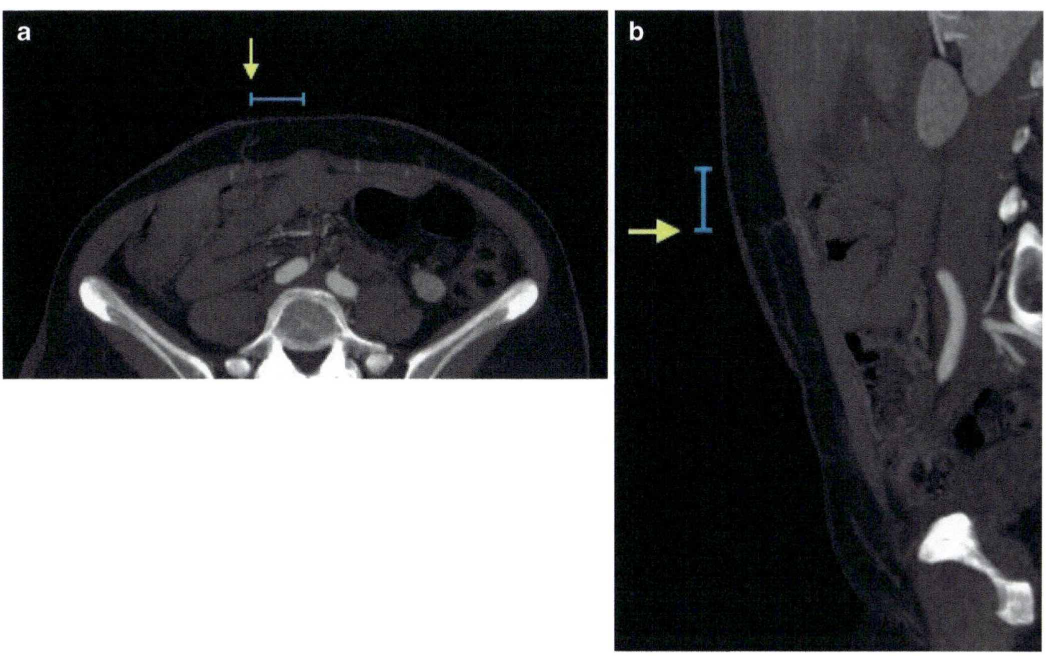

Fig. 3.4 Coordinate measurement of a deep inferior epigastric artery perforator on the right side of the abdominal wall (the perforator is marked with a yellow arrow). In the abdomen, the zero-reference point is the umbilicus. (**a**) Axial view: the distance from the midline to the perforator is measured to determine the x value. (**b**) Sagittal view: the distance from the level of the umbilicus to the perforator is measured to determine the y value

Subsequently, the information is transferred to a data sheet consisting of a 1 cm grid system, highlighting the *x* and *y* axes (Fig. 3.5). The perforators are assigned a number. Then, each perforator is specified with its coordinates and a description of its diameter, direction, and trajectory (intramuscular, septal, or direct). Below, in the same data sheet, the perforators are then marked using the grid system according to the coordinates obtained from the MDCT angiography measurements. With this coordinate format, the precise locations of the perforators can be transferred to the patient's skin before the operation.

MDCTA FOR PERFORATOR ABDOMINAL FLAPS

Patient details: Date:

RIGHT DIEPs

DEEP X Y	SUPERFICIAL X Y	CALIBER	COURSE
1			
2			
3			

LEFT DIEPs

DEEP X Y	SUPERFICIAL X Y	CALIBER	COURSE
1			
2			
3			

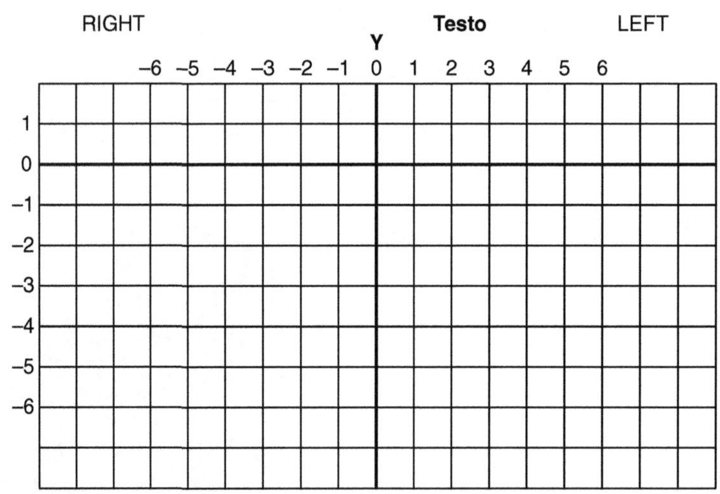

COMMENTS:

-
-

Fig. 3.5 Data form sheet where the perforator information is transferred

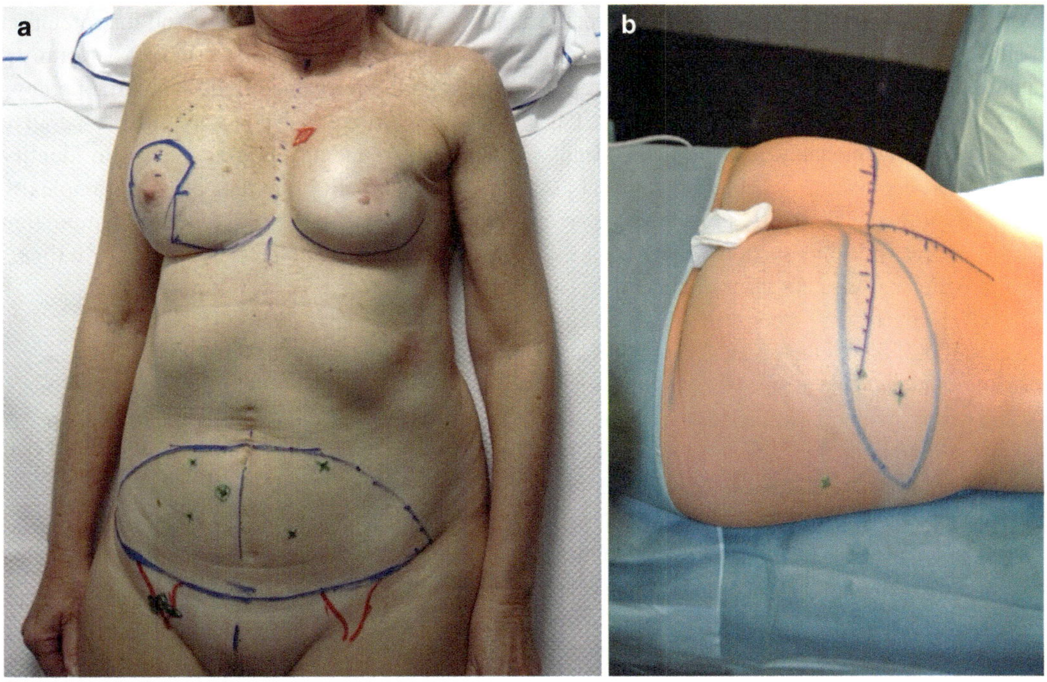

Fig. 3.6 Preoperative MDCT data transposition to the donor site skin using the coordinate system. (**a**) Abdominal region, where the umbilicus is the zero-reference point. (**b**) Gluteal region, where the coccyx is the zero-reference point

Finally, the zero-reference point and the lines corresponding to the *x* and *y* axes are drawn on the patient's skin. Using the coordinates of the data sheet, the points where the perforators emerge are marked on the patient's skin (Fig. 3.6a, b) and are then corroborated using handheld Doppler sonography. The use of the computer-to-paper-to-skin transfer method ensures that the exact point for locating the perforator is known when raising the flap.

3.5 Preoperative Perforator Selection

The role of MDCT angiography in surgical planning is to preoperatively identify the most suitable perforator on which to base the flap. The surgeon should choose the perforator based on the following criteria: caliber, location, branching pattern, and course of the perforator from the source artery to the subcutaneous tissue.

The ideal perforator is one that provides the maximum blood supply to the flap while requiring the least complex dissection. When planning a reconstruction with moderate to large dimension flaps, it is generally preferable to select the perforator with the largest caliber. The perforator should be located relatively centrally in the flap. However, if the perforator is relatively lateralized, the branching should still follow the axial direction of the flap. A perforator with a direct or septal course to the subcutaneous tissue is always desirable. If the perforators with the best characteristics have an intramuscular trajectory, it is preferable to select the one with the shortest intramuscular course. This limits muscle trauma resulting from dissection, which is particularly important in the abdominal area to prevent bulges or hernias.

3.6 Indication

MDCT angiography is mainly indicated for preoperative assessment when considering the use of large perforator-based flaps, such as the deep inferior epigastric artery perforator, superior or inferior gluteal artery perforator, or lumbar artery perforator flaps, among others. This is because identifying the anatomical features and the more suitable perforators beforehand is of utmost importance to ensure optimal perfusion of the entire flap.

This imaging modality also helps to identify anatomical anomalies, whether congenital or secondary to traumatic injury, previous surgery in the donor area (prior liposuction, scars, hernia), or certain peripheral vascular diseases that could significantly affect the reconstructive outcomes. Finally, MDCT angiography can also provide accurate information on the recipient site and vessels.

In finer or smaller flaps, such as the thoracodorsal artery perforator flap, anterolateral thigh flap, or superficial circumflex iliac artery perforator flap, among others, preoperative MDCT angiography is not essential for microsurgical planning, especially in thin patients. This is because a thin subcutaneous layer can make it challenging to reliably visualize and locate the perforators in the fascial plane. Nevertheless, MDCT angiography should be considered for preoperative assessment of these types of flaps when there are suspected anatomical anomalies at the donor site.

3.7 Drawbacks

One of the drawbacks of MDCT angiography is the potential for radiation exposure. However, low-dose protocols have allowed the dose to be decreased from 6–10 to 1.78 mSv while still providing high-resolution images. In addition, the scanning field of the study can even be reduced to include only the area of interest [19].

The other drawbacks of MDCT angiography are the possible adverse effects of iodinated contrast agents. Anaphylactoid reactions and vasospastic actions can make small-caliber vessels difficult to visualize [20]. Contraindications to the use of MDCT angiography include sensitivity to iodinated contrast medium and renal impairment.

3.8 Conclusion

MDCT angiography is presently one the most reliable imaging techniques for the preoperative planning of perforator-based flaps. This technique allows easy image acquisition and interpretation and offers precise information about perforators, with a predictive value of 100% in intraoperative anatomic findings. This maximizes operative efficiency, reducing the time needed to identify the most suitable perforator and the complexity of the total flap harvest, as well as minimizing operator stress and thus the total operative time.

References

1. Blondeel PN, Beyens G, Verhaeghe R, et al. Doppler flowmetry in the planning of perforator flaps. Br J Plast Surg. 1998;51(3):202–9. https://doi.org/10.1016/s0007-1226(98)80010-6.
2. Hallock GG. Doppler sonography and color duplex imaging for planning a perforator flap. Clin Plast Surg. 2003;30(3):347–57. https://doi.org/10.1016/s0094-1298(03)00036-1.
3. Rubin GD, Shiau MC, Schmidt AJ, et al. Computed tomographic angiography: historical perspective and new state-of-the-art using multi detector-row helical computed tomography. J Comput Assist Tomogr. 1999;23(Suppl 1):S83–90.
4. Herzog C, Dogan S, Diebold T, et al. Multi-detector row CT versus coronary angiography: preoperative evaluation before totally endoscopic coronary artery bypass grafting. Radiology. 2003;229(1):200–8. https://doi.org/10.1148/radiol.2291020630.
5. Lawler LP, Fishman EK. Multidetector row computed tomography of the aorta and peripheral arteries. Cardiol Clin. 2003;21(4):607–29. https://doi.org/10.1016/s0733-8651(03)00087-0.
6. Wintersperger BJ, Nikolaou K, Becker CR. Multidetector-row CT angiography of the aorta and visceral arteries. Semin Ultrasound CT MRI. 2004;25(1):25–40. https://doi.org/10.1053/j.sult.2003.10.004.
7. Klein MB, Karanas YL, Chow LC, Rubin GD, Chang J. Early experience with computed tomographic angiography in microsurgical reconstruction. Plast Reconstr Surg. 2003;112(2):498–503. https://doi.org/10.1097/01.PRS.0000070990.97274.FA.
8. Chow LC, Napoli A, Klein MB, Chang J, Rubin GD. Vascular mapping of the leg with multi-detector row CT angiography prior to free-flap transplantation. Radiology. 2005;237(1):353–60. https://doi.org/10.1148/radiol.2371040675.
9. Masia J, Clavero JA, Larrañaga JR, Alomar X, Pons G, Serret P. Multidetector-row computed tomography in the planning of abdominal perforator flaps. J Plast Reconstr Aesthet Surg. 2006;59(6):594–9. https://doi.org/10.1016/j.bjps.2005.10.024.
10. Vandevoort M, Vranckx JJ, Fabre G. Perforator topography of the deep inferior epigastric perforator flap in 100 cases of breast reconstruction. Plast

Reconstr Surg. 2002;109(6):1912–8. https://doi.org/10.1097/00006534-200205000-00021.
11. Saint-Cyr M, Schaverien M, Arbique G, Hatef D, Brown SA, Rohrich RJ. Three- and four-dimensional computed tomographic angiography and venography for the investigation of the vascular anatomy and perfusion of perforator flaps. Plast Reconstr Surg. 2008;121(3):772–80. https://doi.org/10.1097/01.prs.0000299338.97612.90.
12. Schaverien M, Saint-Cyr M, Arbique G, Brown SA, Rohrich RJ. Three- and four-dimensional arterial and venous anatomies of the thoracodorsal artery perforator flap. Plast Reconstr Surg. 2008;121(5):1578–87. https://doi.org/10.1097/PRS.0b013e31816b1479.
13. Schaverien M, Saint-Cyr M, Arbique G, Hatef D, Brown SA, Rohrich RJ. Three- and four-dimensional computed tomographic angiography and venography of the anterolateral thigh perforator flap. Plast Reconstr Surg. 2008;121(5):1685–96. https://doi.org/10.1097/PRS.0b013e31816b4587.
14. Ting JWC, Rozen WM, Grinsell D, Stella DL, Ashton MW. The in vivo anatomy of the deep circumflex iliac artery perforators: defining the role for the DCIA perforator flap. Microsurgery. 2009;29(4):326–9. https://doi.org/10.1002/micr.20633.
15. Wong C, Saint-Cyr M, Rasko Y, et al. Three- and four-dimensional arterial and venous perforasomes of the internal mammary artery perforator flap. Plast Reconstr Surg. 2009;124(6):1759–69. https://doi.org/10.1097/PRS.0b013e3181bf815f.
16. Allen RJ, Haddock NT, Ahn CY, Sadeghi A. Breast reconstruction with the profunda artery perforator flap. Plast Reconstr Surg. 2012;129(1):16e–23e. https://doi.org/10.1097/PRS.0b013e3182363d9f.
17. Hamdi M, Craggs B, Brussaard C, Seidenstueker K, Hendrickx B, Zeltzer A. Lumbar artery perforator flap: an anatomical study using multidetector computed tomographic scan and surgical pearls for breast reconstruction. Plast Reconstr Surg. 2016;138:343–52. https://doi.org/10.1097/PRS.0000000000002347.
18. Clavero JA, Masia J, Larrañaga J, et al. MDCT in the preoperative planning of abdominal perforator surgery for postmastectomy breast reconstruction. AJR Am J Roentgenol. 2008;191(3):670–6. https://doi.org/10.2214/AJR.07.2515.
19. Rozen W, Chubb D, Crossett M, Ashton M. The future in perforator flap imaging: a new technique to substantially reduce radiation dose with computed tomographic angiography. Plast Reconstr Surg. 2010;126:98e–100e. https://doi.org/10.1097/PRS.0b013e3181de25f9.
20. Singh J, Daftary A. Iodinated contrast media and their adverse reactions. J Nucl Med Technol. 2008;36(2):69–74; quiz 76–77. https://doi.org/10.2967/jnmt.107.047621.

MR Angiography

4

Julie V. Vasile and Joshua L. Levine

4.1 Preoperative Imaging

Preoperative anatomic imaging of vasculature markedly enhances the ability of a surgeon to devise a surgical strategy before going to the operating room. Prior to the era of preoperative perforator imaging, a surgeon had little knowledge of an individual patient's vascular anatomy until surgery was well underway. As a result, perforator selection could be a tedious and stressful decision process that occurred in the operating room at the expense of operating time and general anesthetic requirement.

4.2 Doppler

As technology has advanced, surgeons continue to explore modalities for preoperative imaging. Doppler, color Duplex sonography, thermography, and computed tomographic angiography (CTA) are other modalities that may assist in preoperative evaluation. Each of these modalities has advantages and disadvantages. A handheld Doppler ultrasound is portable and simple to use but cannot differentiate perforating vessels from superficial and deep axial vessels, nor large perforators from small ones. It cannot accurately determine the location that perforators exit the fascia or provide information on the anatomic course of a vessel [1, 2]. In comparison, color Duplex sonography provides more detailed information about the anatomy of the vessels but requires highly trained technicians with knowledge of perforator anatomy and is time-consuming [2]. The technique's most crucial drawback is an inability to produce anatomic images in a format that a surgeon can easily and independently view.

4.3 Computed Tomographic Angiography

Computed tomographic angiography (CTA) is a modality that can demonstrate vessel anatomy, assess vessel caliber, accurately locate perforators, and produce anatomic images in a format that a surgeon can easily and independently view. Although CTA can be performed quickly in as little as 15 min [1, 2], it requires that patients must be exposed to ionizing radiation. Radiation exposure precludes multiple repeated imaging

J. V. Vasile (✉)
Northern Westchester Hospital, Mt. Kisco, NY, USA

New York Eye and Ear Infirmary of Mt. Sinai,
New York, NY, USA

Stamford, CT, USA

J. L. Levine
Northern Westchester Hospital, Mt. Kisco, NY, USA

New York Eye and Ear Infirmary at Mt. Sinai,
New York, NY, USA

New York, NY, USA

J. P. Hong et al. (eds.), *Imaging for Reconstructive Microsurgery*,
https://doi.org/10.1007/978-981-97-7278-0_4

studies in one examination. CTA may expose patients to excessive and potentially unnecessary radiation [3–6]. Patients with breast cancer may have a heightened concern for any factor that can potentially increase the risk of developing a second cancer and may perceive the risks of radiation exposure even more negatively. Patients with breast cancer gene (BRCA) mutations, which confer an increased risk of developing both breast and ovarian cancers, are especially concerned about receiving radiation to the abdomen. Also, iodinated contrast to enhance vessels for CTA can be associated with small but real risks of anaphylaxis and nephrotoxicity [7, 8].

4.4 Magnetic Resonance Angiography

Magnetic resonance imaging (MRI) uses a magnetic field to uniformly align the spin of hydrogen atoms in tissue. The subsequent application of a radiofrequency pulse results in release of energy as hydrogen atoms return to their relaxed state. MRI coils detect the released energy, and computer software processes the data into anatomic images. Exposure to a magnetic field or radiofrequency pulse with MRI has not been linked to the development of cancer [9]. A paramagnetic contrast agent (gadolinium-containing) is injected to enhance vessels. Our previous papers demonstrated that MRA accurately locates perforating vessel branches and shows vessel anatomy in a format that is easily viewed by a surgeon [10–13]. However, because MRI does not use radiation, this modality has an important advantage over CTA of allowing multiple series of images to be obtained.

Disadvantages of MRA are contraindication to use with a cardiac pacemaker or an expander implant with a ferromagnetic port. An expander implant with a ferromagnetic port is placed temporarily to expand the tissue above an implant with serial injections of saline. The strong magnet in the MRI scanner can cause the expander implant to shift and flip within the pocket surrounding the expander implant. Our research demonstrated that MR imaging on a 1.5 T machine can be done safely with expander implants with ferromagnetic ports without clinical adverse outcomes. The patients in the study had breast expander implants placed to maintain or increase the breast volume after mastectomy. The expander implants were not adversely affected by the powerful magnetic field. MRI-related heating was not significant with no heating or burning of surrounding tissue observed. However, MRI artifacts that can obscure anatomy were substantial in the immediate vicinity of the tissue expander [14].

In addition, the enclosed space in the MRI machine can be problematic for claustrophobic patients. Most patients with claustrophobia can tolerate an MRI with an anxiolytic. Some patients also respond very well with a blind fold, aromatherapy, and relaxing music tracks that they bring with them to the exam. If available, scheduling of the study on an MR machine for obese patients may also be helpful. Continuing advances in MRA have decreased the procedure time for a single donor site to as little as 20 min and decreased the actual acquisition scan time to 20 s [11, 13, 15, 16]. However, the examination time could be 40 min for multiple donor site studies.

4.5 Magnetic Resonance Angiography Contrast Agents

Gadolinium-containing contrast agents used for MRA have several distinct advantages over iodinated contrast agents used for CTA. The incidence of an acute allergic reaction to iodinated contrast is 3%, which is much higher than the 0.07% incidence of allergic reaction to gadolinium contrast [7, 17]. Unlike gadolinium contrast agents, iodinated CT contrast agents can induce renal insufficiency even in patients with normal renal function [8, 18].

Gadolinium contrast agents can potentially induce nephrogenic systemic fibrosis (NSF), also called nephrogenic fibrosing dermopathy. However, reports of NSF have been limited to patients with impaired renal function [19–21]. Patients with an acute kidney injury or chronic severe renal disease (glomerular filtration rate <30 mL/min/1.73 m^2) are considered most at risk [19]. A creatinine level is drawn preoperatively in patients with a history of hypertension, diabetes, renal disease, or any other indication that renal function may be impaired. NSF is a very rare disease with about 380 cases reported worldwide [20, 21]. Since the establishment of guidelines for using gadolinium contrast agents and the increased general awareness of NSF, the occurrence of NSF has been nearly eliminated, with virtually no new NSF cases since 2008 in both patients with normal renal function and patients with renal impairment, in spite of continued use of gadolinium contrast agents, although at lower doses [22].

Gadolinium contrast agents are metabolized primarily by the kidney, and less frequently by the liver, and then excreted from the body. However, trace deposits of gadolinium have been found in the brain, liver, bone, and skin tissue of patients that received gadolinium contrast agent injections. The present consensus is that the retention of gadolinium in the brain and other tissues is not associated with adverse clinical outcomes [23–26].

A significant advance in gadolinium contrast agents was the development of blood pool contrast agents, which have a prolonged intravascular circulation time. MRI contrast agent, which effectively stays within the blood pool, allows for steady-state imaging up to 1 h postinjection of contrast [27]. This results in a decreased amount of contrast required and improved MR images and increases even further the number of donor sites that can be imaged in one study. The decreased dosage and blood pool intravascular distribution decrease the risk of nephrogenic systemic fibrosis (NSF) [28].

The blood pool contrast agents improve the vessel-to-muscle contrast ratio and vessel sharpness, mainly due to preferential enhancement of vessels compared to muscle derived from blood pool distribution [29]. This results in significantly improved images of the intramuscular course of perforating vessels, which gives valuable information for choosing the best perforating vessel and planning an intramuscular dissection of the vessel in flap reconstruction.

Because blood pool contrast agents remain intravascular for a prolonged time, there is a significantly increased amount of time to acquire images [30]. This affords the opportunity to assess many donor sites for autologous reconstruction in a single examination. A patient has time to turn their body position from prone position for imaging the posterior body (i.e., posterior thigh flaps, buttock flaps, lumbar flaps), to left and right lateral decubitus positions for imaging the lateral thorax (thoracodorsal posterior perforator flaps), and to supine position for imaging the anterior body (anterior thigh flaps, lateral thoracic intercostal perforator flaps).

In addition, flap volume estimates can be more accurately determined because the imaging is acquired with the patient in the supine, prone, or lateral decubitus positions, so that the tissue is not compressed. For example, buttock and posterior thigh flap volumes are calculated with the patient in the prone position, and abdominal DIEP flap volumes are calculated with the patient in the supine position. Knowledge of the vessel anatomy and flap volume at each donor site assists with discussion with reconstruction candidates on selecting the most suitable flap donor sites. Moreover, a patient who is found to not be a candidate for a specific perforator flap based on imaging findings, or suddenly changes his/her preference of donor site, or has a flap failure and requires another perforator flap reconstruction does not require further studies.

4.6 Magnetic Resonance Angiography Protocol

MRA is performed on a long-bore, self-shielded 3.0 T or 1.5 T scanner using a torso phased multi-array coil. The field of view is individualized to the anatomy of interest. For perforator studies, after acquiring a three-plane localizer, axial and coronal T2-weighted single-shot fast spin-echo images are acquired to screen for unexpected pathology and to help characterize any lesions detected on post-gadolinium scans. Some reconstructive patients have history of cancer, and metastatic disease is detected occasionally. This sequence is also helpful to confirm the central position of umbilicus or gluteal crease in prone position, from which perforators are measured in postprocessing. A transverse pre- and post-contrast arterial phase 3D liver accelerated volume acquisition (LAVA) sequence is acquired with imaging parameters of TR/TE/flip = 3.9/1.9/15, bandwidth = 125 kHz, slice thickness = 3 mm reconstructed at 1.5 mm intervals using twofold zero interpolation (ZIP 2), matrix = 512 × 128–256, and parallel acceleration factor = 2. Precontrast imaging is important to determine adequacy of fat suppression. Central frequency and shim field of view can be adjusted as necessary to ensure effective fat suppression over the subcutaneous tissues of interest if Dixon fat/water separation is not available. The arterial phase imaging is bolus tracked by automated triggering (Smartprep), and scanning is initiated after arrival of contrast in the suprarenal aorta. Hand injection is preferred, especially if there is a tenuous IV, because approximately one third of patients may experience some sensation at the injection site or in the pelvis related to the ionic contrast agent [24]. K-space is mapped sequentially with the absolute center of k-space collected in the middle of the scan, which is about 20 s after bolus detection for a 35-s scan duration with a 5-s pause for breath-holding instruction. This is important to provide time for the contrast to reach and fill perforating arteries. However, only the largest perforator arterial/vein bundles are adequately seen on this sequence. This is followed by equilibrium phase transverse 3D LAVA at higher resolution without parallel imaging using the following parameters: TR/TE/flip = 4/1.9/15, matrix = 512 × 512 × (172–240), bandwidth = 125 kHz, and slice thickness = 3 mm reconstructed at 1.5 mm intervals using ZIP2. Phase encoding is set to the right/left direction. This is the primary sequence utilized to generate reconstructions and create reports and also serves as a reference for the plastic surgeons. It is acquired with free breathing and typically requires 3–5-min acquisition duration with 0.9 × 0.9 × 3 mm acquired voxel dimension and 0.9 × 0.9 × 1.5 mm reconstructed voxel dimensions. Thereafter, a lower resolution coronal and sagittal plane LAVA is acquired with acquisition matrix of 512 × 256 and 512 × 224, respectively, in a single breath hold and parallel acceleration factor of 2 to evaluate internal organs.

First, the primary flap donor site is imaged, followed by a single high spatial resolution equilibrium phase imaging of other potential donor sites using free breathing 3D LAVA sequence described above. A typical complete perforator flap MR examination, including abdomen, buttocks, and upper thigh, can be 40 min.

After screening axial and coronal single-shot fast spin-echo images for unexpected pathologies, the arterial phase images are reviewed to determine the number of perforators available and to look for any enhancing lesions. High spatial resolution equilibrium phase images are used for final perforator evaluation, as perforators are best visualized on these images. The equilibrium phase series is loaded on a computer workstation for postprocessing. Coronal, sagittal, and surface-rendered reformatted images are generated. The reference point and each candidate perforator artery/vein bundle are identified. The diameter and perforator exit location at the point where the vessel pierces the superficial fascia and enters into subcutaneous fat are noted. The cephalad/caudal and right/left distances of each perforator exit site relative to the reference point are calculated to create a perforator location coordinate. The intramuscular course and length of each perforator is measured to predict vascular pedicle length. Finally, a predicted flap volume is calculated on the same workstation assuming an elliptical geometry on a slice-by-slice basis.

Coordinates identifying the location of the perforating arteries on the axial images are superimposed and displayed on volume-rendered 3D reconstructed images and coronal 3D minimum intensity projection (MIP) images. These images are especially helpful for a surgeon to locate and mark perforator vessels preoperatively in the office and also intraoperatively.

4.7 Magnetic Resonance Angiography and Perforator Selection for Flap Reconstruction

Vessel caliber in conjunction with a centralized location on the flap is the most important factor for optimal perforator selection at every donor site. Caliber measurements are uniformly performed at the point where a vessel exits the superficial fascia to perfuse the flap tissue. Location measurements are performed in reference to a landmark at each donor site. Specific considerations regarding each donor site are presented below.

4.7.1 Abdomen

First, the deep inferior epigastric vessel branching pattern is identified on each hemiabdomen. A coronal MIP image (Fig. 4.1) best illustrates the branching pattern and is included in the report. This image is helpful for confirming vessel patency and for planning when a double flap used in combination to reconstruct one breast is antici-

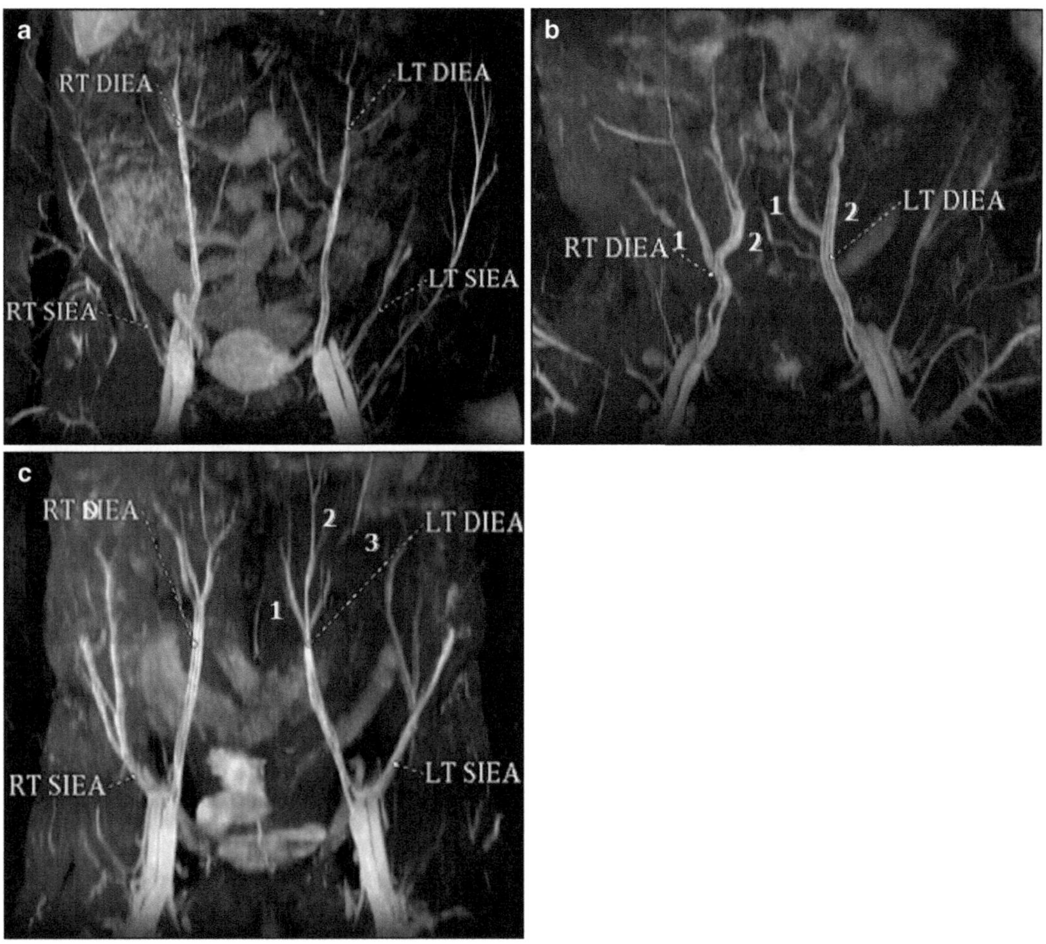

Fig. 4.1 Coronal maximum intensity projection (MIP) magnetic resonance angiography (MRA) of the abdomen. (**a**) Type 1 deep inferior epigastric branching pattern. (**b**) Type 2 deep inferior epigastric branching pattern on both sides of the abdomen with a medial and lateral branch denoted by 1 and 2. (**c**) Type 3 deep inferior epigastric branching pattern with 1, 2, and 3 denoting multiple branches from the left deep inferior epigastric vessel. *DIEA* deep inferior epigastric artery, *SIEA* superficial inferior epigastric artery, *LT* left, *RT* right. (*Used with permission* Ref. [31])

pated. Next, the location of the largest deep inferior epigastric perforators (DIEPs) is identified at the point of exit from the anterior rectus fascia and is measured in reference to the center of the base of the umbilical stalk as seen in Fig. 4.2. Vessel caliber measurements are also performed just above the anterior fascia level.

Finally, the intramuscular course or paramuscular (septocutaneous) course is examined, as seen in Fig. 4.3. The vessel course provides information for a surgeon to anticipate a tedious or straightforward dissection. The improved visualization of intramuscular perforator course on MRA allows for preoperative decision-making on harvesting more than one perforator (e.g., whether muscle transection will be required and if the pedicle has a large caliber to facilitate pedicle reanastomosis to avoid muscle transaction to harvest two perforators). It also enhances the ability of a surgeon to plan for double flaps used together to make one breast, in which one flap vessel pedicle can be connected to a second flap vessel pedicle at a branching point or at the cephalad continuation of the pedicle beyond the perforator (Fig. 4.4).

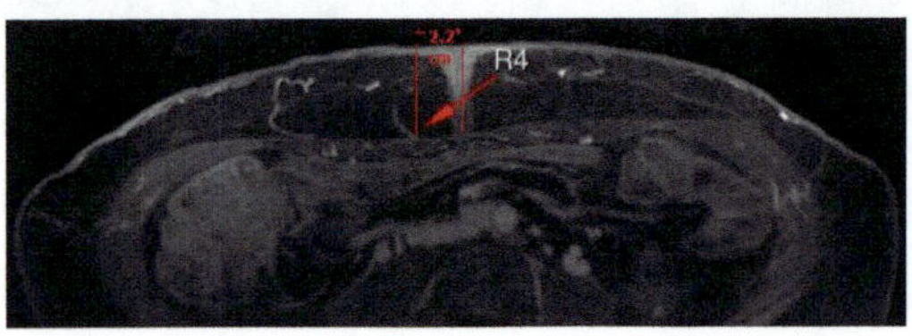

Fig. 4.2 Axial MRA of the abdomen. A DIEP location is measured at the anterior rectus fascia in relation to the center of the umbilicus at the fascia level. (*Used with permission* Ref. [31])

The location of the largest deep circumflex iliac perforators may also be identified and is measured in reference to the umbilicus (Fig. 4.5). The perforator locations and course are then superimposed onto a volume-rendered 3D reconstructed image, and this image is included in the report (Fig. 4.6).

The superficial inferior epigastric artery is evaluated and noted in the radiology report whether the superficial inferior epigastric artery shares a common origin with the superficial circumflex iliac vessels, as this will result in a larger caliber vessel for anastomosis. The superficial circumflex artery branches may also be evaluated.

A clinical example of the utility of MRA in planning bilateral breast reconstruction using an abdominal perforator flap in a patient with a midline and two right paramedian scars from several bowel surgery operations is shown in Fig. 4.7.

Spiral imaging may be employed by the radiologist to subtract venous flow to only view the SIEA (Fig. 4.8), but this is not routinely done. The largest superficial inferior epigastric vein is identified on each hemiabdomen, and the location is measured from the umbilicus at 12 cm inferior to the umbilicus.

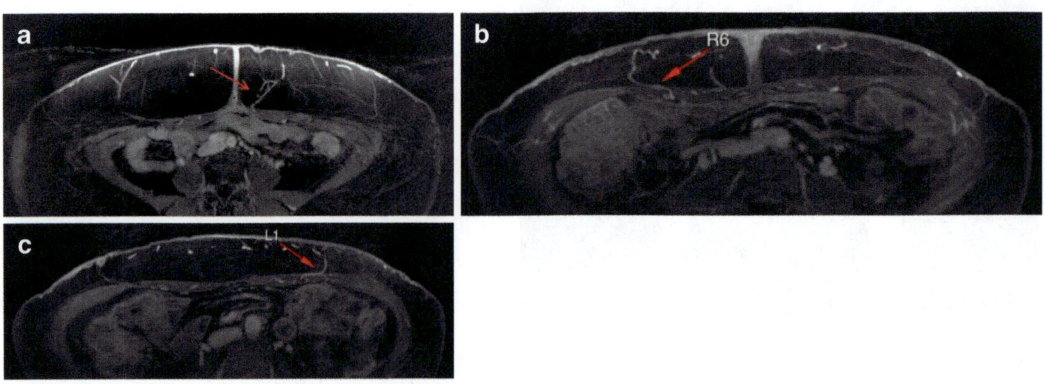

Fig. 4.3 Axial MRA of the abdomen. (**a**) Arrow pointing to a left paramuscular (septocutaneous) DIEP. (**b**) Arrow pointing to a right DIEP with short intramuscular (IM) course. (**c**) Arrow pointing to a DIEP with a longer intramuscular course, and MRA provides helpful information that this perforator has a medial course under the rectus fascia before it courses caudally. (*Used with permission* Ref. [31])

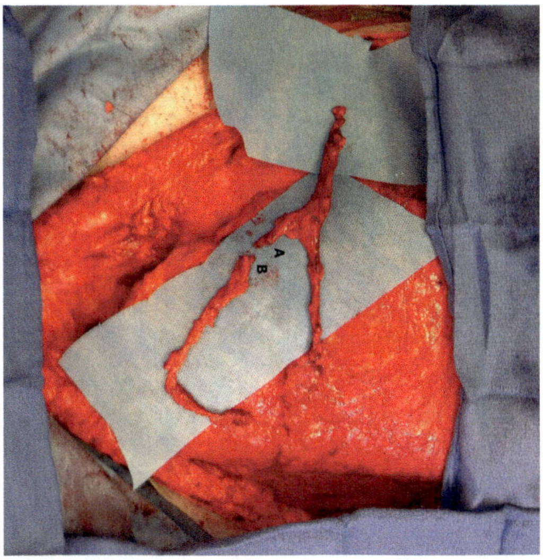

Fig. 4.4 Photograph of a DIEP pedicle lateral branch (marked as **a**) adjacent to the origin of a second DIEP pedicle (marked as **b**) in preparation for microsurgical anastomosis, in which one DIEP flap will perfuse the second DIEP flap (flow-through flap). (*Used with permission* Ref. [31])

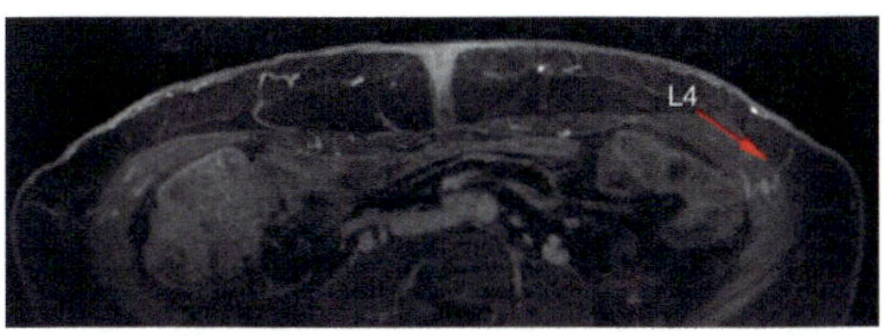

Fig. 4.5 Axial MRA of the abdomen. Arrow points to left deep circumflex iliac artery (DCIA) exiting the external oblique muscle. (*Used with permission* Ref. [31])

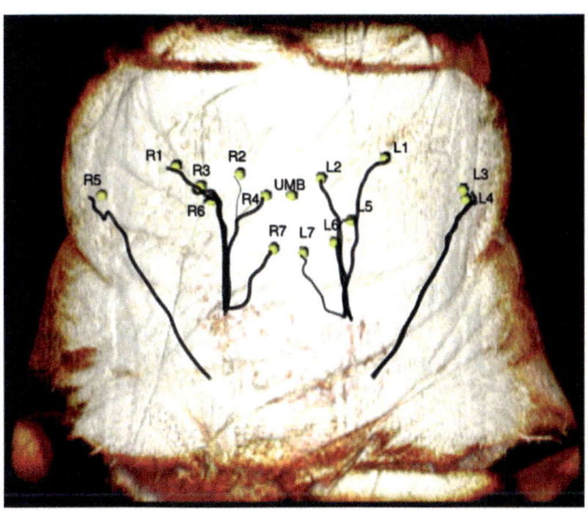

Fig. 4.6 Three-dimensional (3D) volume-rendered MRA of the abdomen with DIEP, DCIA, and umbilicus locations, and vessel courses superimposed. (*Used with permission* Ref. [31])

The branching pattern of the perforating vessels within the subcutaneous fat is also evaluated. The two-point Dixon method for fat/water signal separation at 1.5 T and LAVA Flex at 3 T are methods used by radiologists to suppress the fat signal, resulting in clearer images of DIEP arborization into the fat (Fig. 4.9). In a unilateral reconstruction, it is helpful to see a medial row DIEP with branches crossing into the subcutaneous fat on the contralateral abdomen because zone III is more likely to be well perfused, as seen in Fig. 4.10. Figure 4.11 shows a DIEP with a very lateral course into the subcutaneous fat and a corresponding photograph of a patient with inadequate venous drainage of the medial tissue. A different perforator selection and/or indocyanine green injection would have prevented this. Usually DIEP branches can be visualized in close proximity with superficial inferior epigastric venous branches, which may theoretically provide improved venous drainage through connections (Fig. 4.12).

Postprocessing software is used by the radiologist to calculate projected abdominal flap volume (Fig. 4.13). To increase accuracy of the estimated flap volume, a radiologist must first be educated in the typical markings and dimensions of an abdominal flap.

4.7.2 Buttock

A vitamin E capsule marker is placed on the skin surface at the top of the gluteal crease as a reference point from which the perforator locations are measured. The largest perforators from the superior gluteal artery (SGAP) and inferior gluteal artery (IGAP) are identified. The locations of the perforators are calculated at the point of exiting the superficial fascia, and this point is transposed onto the skin surface. Then, the distance of the perforator from the reference point is measured along the curved skin contour of the buttock (Fig. 4.14). These measurements are taken with the patient in the prone position for increased accuracy because of the compliance of the gluteal tissue. Finally, the perforator locations and reference point are superimposed onto a volume-rendered 3D reconstruc-

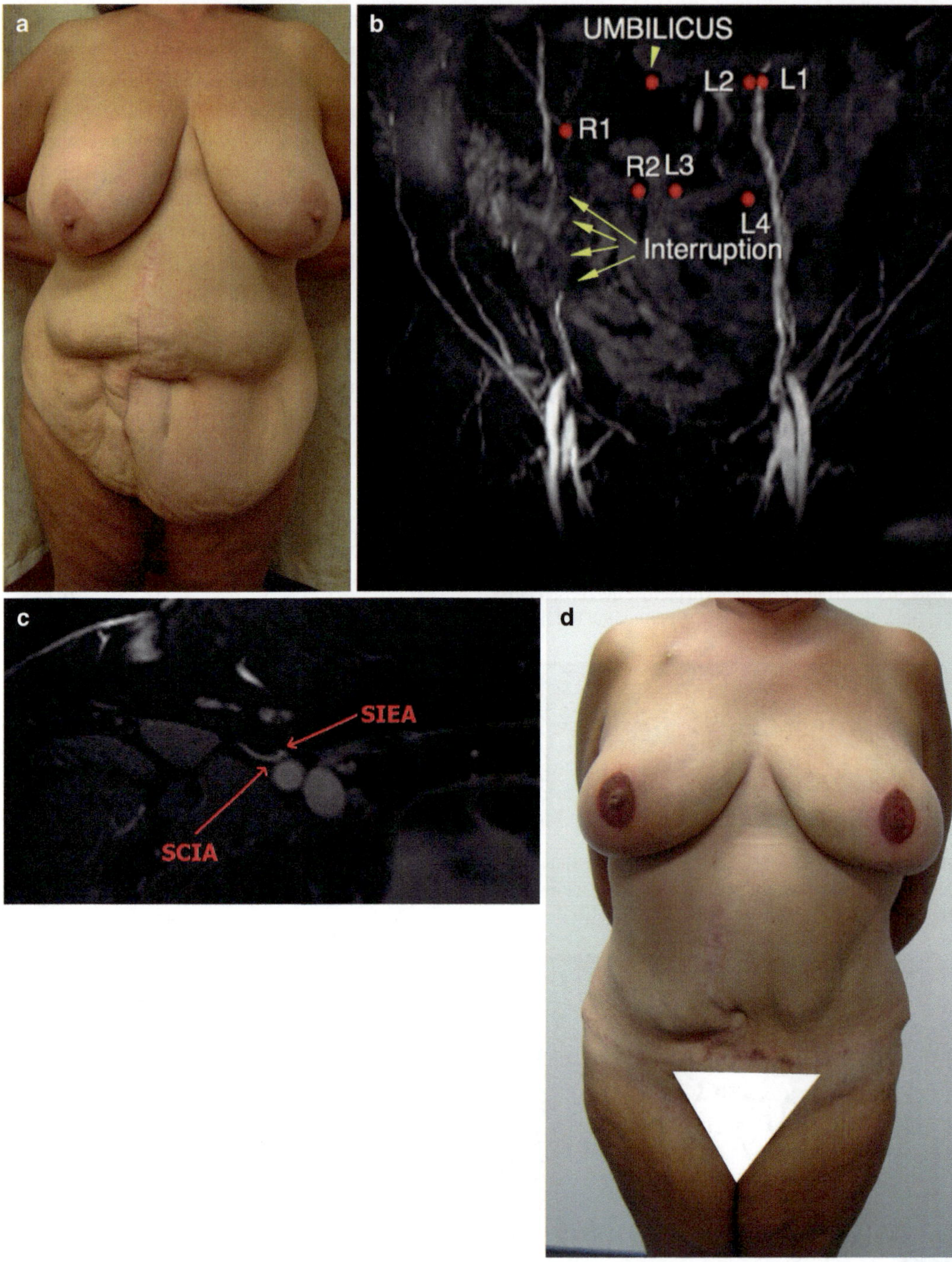

Fig. 4.7 (**a**) Photograph of a patient scheduled for a bilateral breast reconstruction with a midline and two right paramedian scars from several bowel surgery operations. She requested that the abdomen be the donor site. The estimated hemiabdominal flap volume was 1000 g, and the estimated thigh flap volume was 325 g. (**b**) Coronal MRA of the abdomen. Arrows point to an interruption in the contrast in the right DIEP pedicle secondary to previous abdominal surgery. (**c**) MRA of the abdomen. Common origin of the superficial inferior epigastric artery (SIEA) and superficial circumflex iliac artery (SCIA), measuring 2.2 mm. (**d**) Postoperative photograph of the patient with successful bilateral reconstruction with abdominal tissue (left breast SIEA flap and right breast DIEP flap). (*Used with permission* Ref. [31])

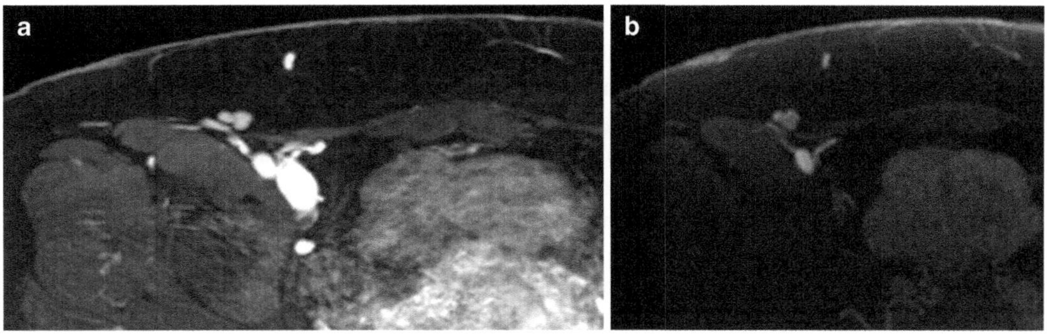

Fig. 4.8 Axial MRA of the abdomen. (**a**) Arterial and venous vessels enhanced. (**b**) Venous vessel enhancement subtracted. (*Used with permission* Ref. [31])

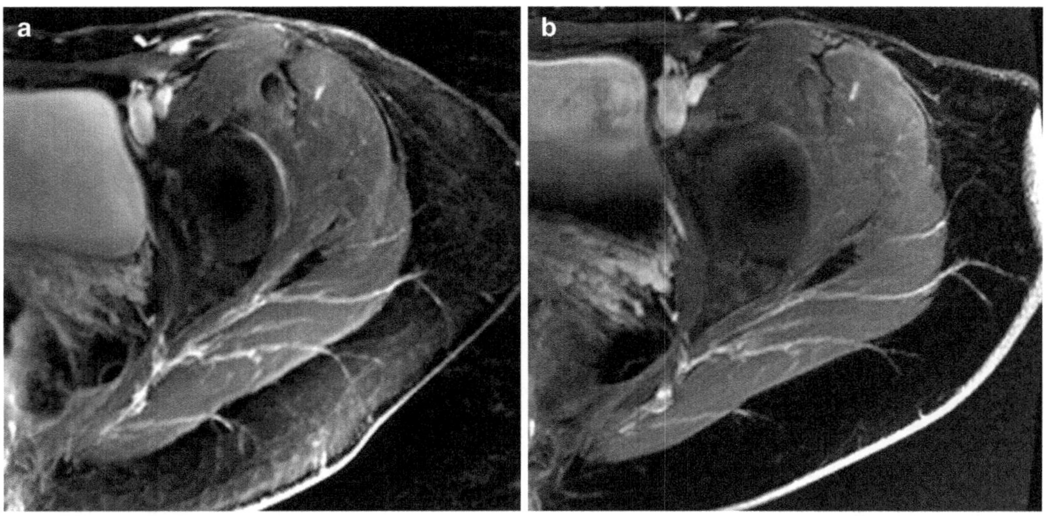

Fig. 4.9 Axial MRA of the abdomen. (**a**) Inhomogeneous fat suppression. (**b**) Liver accelerated volume acquisition (LAVA) Flex used on a 3 T image, resulting in improved visualization of DIEP arborization into the fat. (*Used with permission* Ref. [31])

tion of the buttock in the prone position so that the perforator location markings can be replicated preoperatively (Fig. 4.15).

The placement of the buttock flap skin paddle is significantly influenced by optimal perforator location. The goal is to design a flap that incorporates the optimal perforator and a backup option. Because there are usually many large caliber perforator options in the buttock, vessel location is an important determining factor in selecting the optimal vessel, taking scar location into account. Laterally positioned perforators will result in a longer pedicle, which is advantageous for flap insetting (Fig. 4.16). In addition, laterally positioned flaps may spare the central aesthetic unit in superior buttock flaps or the medial cushioning fat in lower buttock flaps. In bilateral flaps, an attempt is made to design flaps that will result in symmetrical scars by locating large perforators at a similar position bilaterally. As the familiarity of the radiologist increases with typical flap dimensions, the radiologist may calculate predicted upper and buttock flap volumes. Generally, an elliptical designed pattern measuring 6 cm in vertical dimension × 20 cm in transverse dimension is used by the radiologist.

4.7.3 Thigh

The upper thigh is imaged from the mid-gluteal region to the mid-thigh (about 12 cm caudal to the inferior gluteal crease). A transversely oriented upper thigh flap is designed from medial to predominantly posterior thigh tissue to avoid the more anteriorly located lymphatic channels. A typical elliptical flap design for calculating thigh volume is 6 cm × 20 cm. The reference point from which the perforator locations are measured is the skin surface along the midline at the bottom of the gluteal crease. The locations of profunda artery perforators (PAP flap) are calculated at the point of exiting the superficial fascia. The perforators are also located in reference to the distance to the posterior edge of the gracilis muscle, to facilitate intraoperative identification of the perforator (Fig 4.17). Similar to gluteal artery perforators, the best profunda artery perforators have an oblique course through the adductor magnus to yield a longer pedicle. Perforators that course more laterally adjacent to the femoral bone and then course cephalad into the gluteal vessels may be mistaken for profunda artery perforators. As the patients are operated in the supine position, these gluteal perforators result in a difficult dissection with difficult exposure to yield adequate caliber and length pedicles. Occasionally, there is a large medial circumflex vessel perforating through the gracilis muscle or a paramuscular (septocutaneous) medial circumflex vessel that courses around the gracilis muscle (Fig. 4.18). Perforator locations and courses and reference point are transposed onto the skin surface (Fig. 4.19).

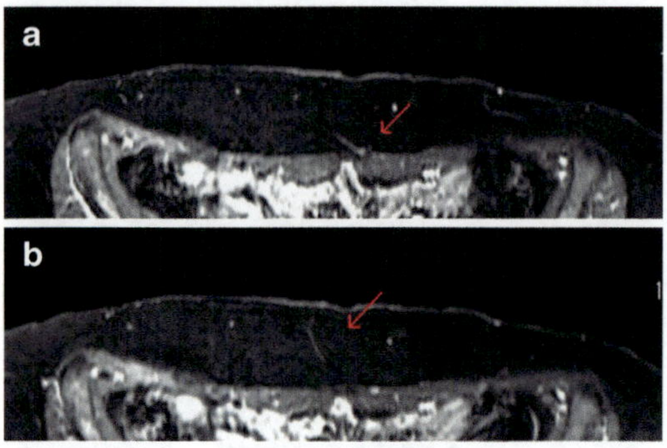

Fig. 4.10 (**a**, **b**) Sequential axial MRA cuts of the abdomen. The arrow points to a left medial DIEP with large branches crossing the midline to perfuse the contralateral abdominal tissue. (*Used with permission* Ref. [31])

Sometimes, the lateral upper thigh has a favorable fat deposition. A septocutaneous (paramuscular) lateral circumflex femoral artery perforator coursing around the tensor fasciae latae is measured in reference to the umbilicus (Fig. 4.20). Unlike posterior profunda artery perforators, the lateral circumflex femoral artery perforators are evaluated and measured in the supine position. The anterior superior iliac spine (ASIS) was initially used as a reference point, but the ASIS can be difficult to palpate on some patients with large habitus, leading to inaccuracies. It can be helpful to move the coil high enough to include the umbilicus to also use this as a reference point for perforator measurements.

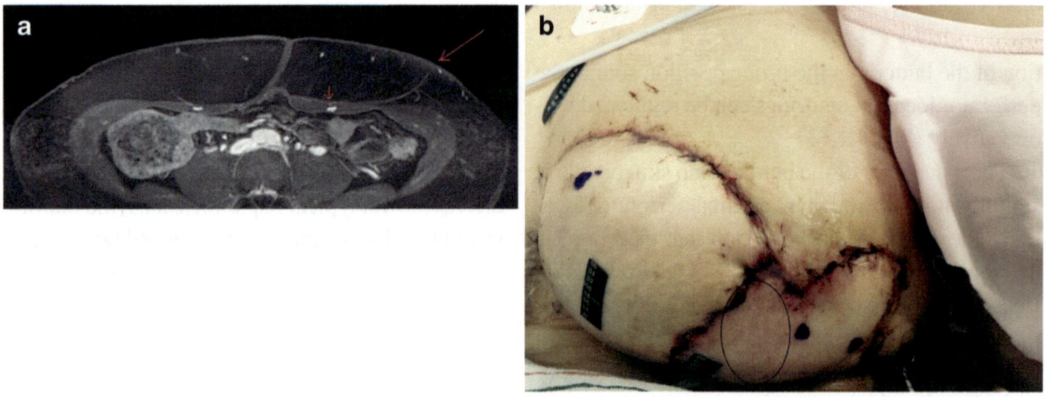

Fig. 4.11 Axial MRA of the abdomen. (**a**) Short arrow points to the location of a DIEP exiting the anterior rectus fascia. Long arrow points to the approximate location that the DIEP arborizes into the subdermal plexus. Note the very oblique course laterally. (**b**) Photograph on postoperative day 5 after double DIEP flap in a patient with a midline abdominal scar. Oval is on the medial part of the DIEP flap that has decreased venous drainage. A lateral DIEP with a very oblique lateral arborization was used in this patient. (*Used with permission* Ref. [31])

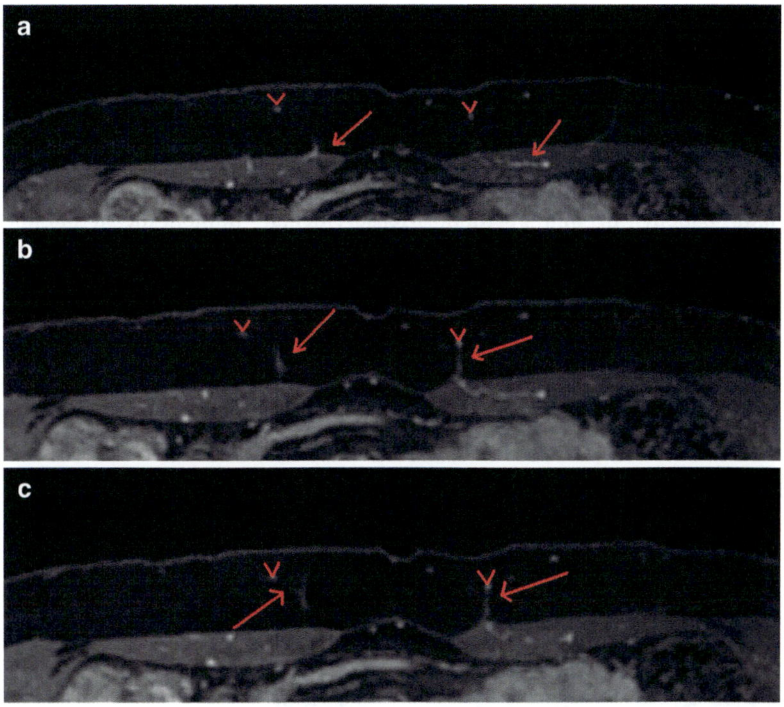

Fig. 4.12 Axial MRA of the abdomen. "V" denotes SIEV in each hemiabdomen. Arrows point to bilateral DIEPs. (**a**) Axial MRA. (**b**) Left DIEP meeting SIEV. (**c**) Right DIEP branch also meeting SIEV. (*Used with permission* Ref. [13])

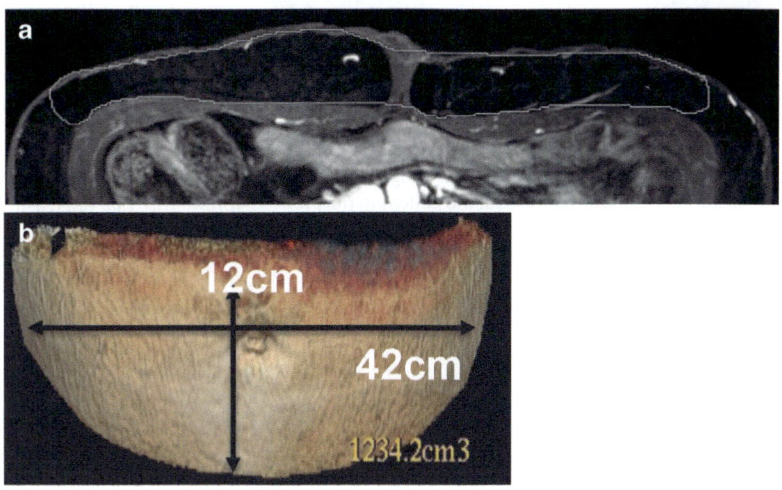

Fig. 4.13 (**a**) Axial MRA of the abdomen with the subcutaneous fat manually outlined to calculate abdominal flap volume. (**b**) 3D volume-rendered abdominal flap. (*Used with permission* Ref. [31])

4.7.4 Lower Back

Lumbar artery perforators (LAP flap) are measured in reference to the midline upper gluteal crease. The limiting factor of this flap is the short pedicle length (Fig. 4.21). Sometimes, lumbar artery perforators have an oblique course to yield a slightly longer pedicle. In general, these flaps are used as a backup option when the abdomen cannot be used, and the body habitus is not favorable for thigh or buttock flaps.

4.7.5 Upper Back

The chest is initially imaged with the patient in the supine position and the arms abducted to avoid compression of the lateral chest soft tissue. In patients with large body mass imaging for bilateral reconstruction, each side can be imaged separately so that one arm can be abducted at a time. It may be necessary for patients with a greater volume of upper arm fat to raise their arms and rest their hands on their head. Images should also be obtained of patients in the lateral decubitus position with the arm raised. Most radiology technicians are not aware that patients are positioned in the lateral decubitus position for the surgical reconstruction and part of the preoperative marking and are not accustomed to scanning patients in this position. Measurements change significantly with the patient's position and arm position. Thus, it is crucial for the radiologist to communicate the patient's position in the series that the measurements are taken from. The radiologist should be aware that preoperatively a patient may need to be turned to the lateral decubitus position to mark posteriorly located perforators, and thus this series should be used for posteriorly located perforator measurements. The reference point is the skin surface at the sternal notch and/or the nipples. The locations of thoracodorsal and internal mammary artery perforators are measured from a reference point at the sternal notch skin surface (Fig. 4.22) and transposed onto the skin surface (Fig. 4.23). Intercostal artery perforators can also be evaluated. Thoracodorsal artery perforators usually yield a longer pedicle, compared to intercostal artery perforators, which is advantageous for insetting the flap.

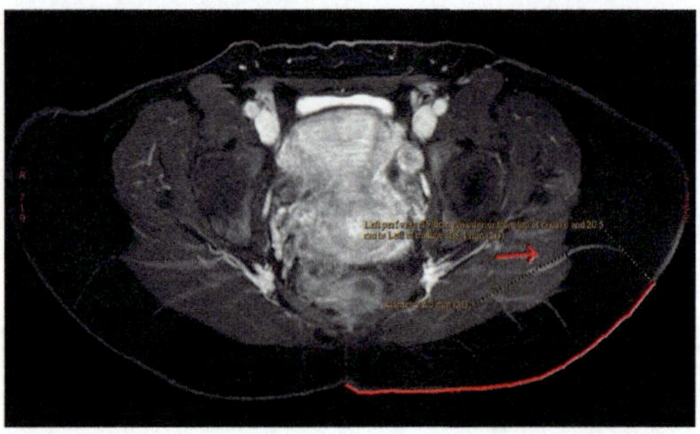

Fig. 4.14 Axial MRA of the buttock with arrows pointing to gluteal perforator. The distance from the midline reference point is calculated by measuring the distance along the curved skin surface with the patient in the prone position to increase accuracy. Vessel caliber is calculated at the superficial fascia exit point. (*Used with permission* Ref. [31])

4.7.6 Chest Recipient Site

In addition to the thoracodorsal vessels, the internal mammary (IM) vessels and internal mammary perforators can be evaluated (Fig. 4.24). The knowledge of where large IM perforators are located may assist a surgeon with avoiding the transection of these perforators, in order to maintain perfusion of the breast skin after mastectomy, or conversely may assist a surgeon with finding these perforators to preserve for anastomosis. In certain scenarios, a surgeon may want to anastomose to the IM perforator, for example, when the IM perforators have a closer diameter match to the donor vessels than the IM vessels and when additional inflow and/or outflow is

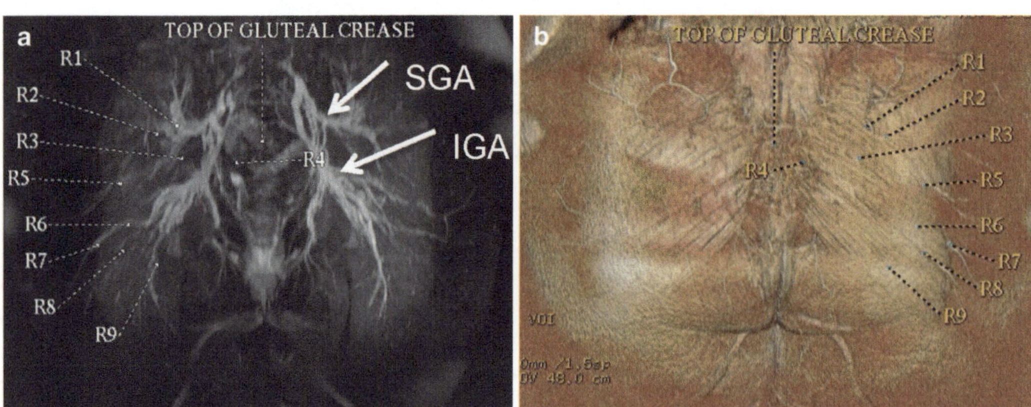

Fig. 4.15 (**a**) Coronal MRA of the buttock with the superior gluteal (SGA) and inferior gluteal (IGA) perforator locations and reference point location marked. (**b**) 3D volume-rendered MRA of the buttock with perforator locations and reference point superimposed. (*Used with permission* Ref. [31])

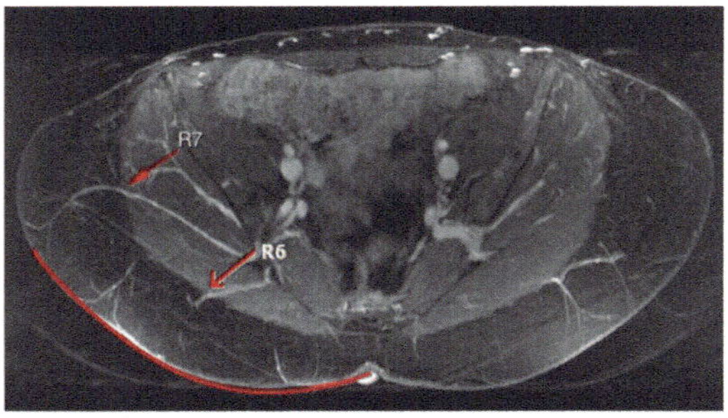

Fig. 4.16 Axial MRA of the buttock showing two superior gluteal perforators. R7 is located more lateral than R6 and has a longer intramuscular course, yielding a longer pedicle. (*Used with permission* Ref. [31])

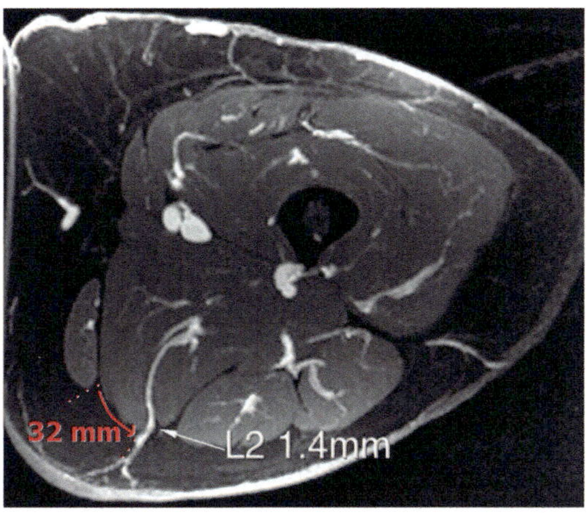

Fig. 4.17 Axial MRA of the left thigh with arrow pointing to the profunda femoral artery perforator and the distance from the posterior edge of the gracilis muscle (G) is measured. (*Used with permission* Ref. [31])

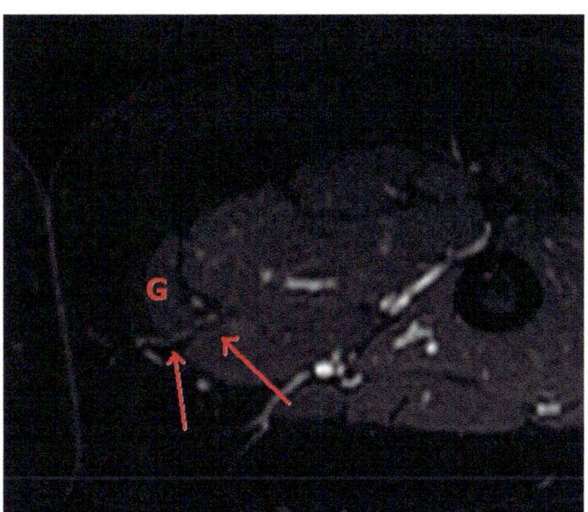

Fig. 4.18 Axial MRA of the left thigh with arrows pointing to a septocutaneous medial circumflex femoral perforator that courses around the gracilis muscle. (*Used with permission* Ref. [31])

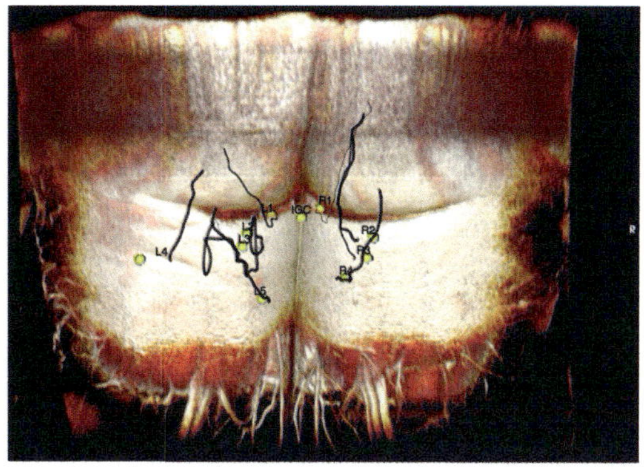

Fig. 4.19 3D volume-rendered MRA of the thigh with perforator locations and course and reference point at the inferior gluteal crease (IGC) superimposed. (*Used with permission* Ref. [31])

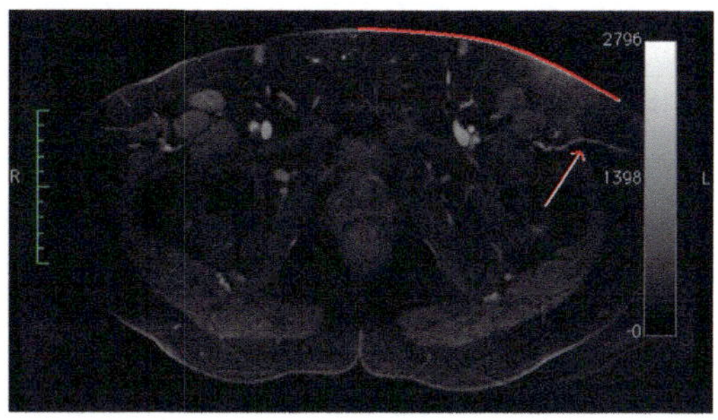

Fig. 4.20 Axial MRA of the thigh. Arrow pointing to a left septocutaneous lateral circumflex femoral perforator. (*Used with permission* Ref. [31])

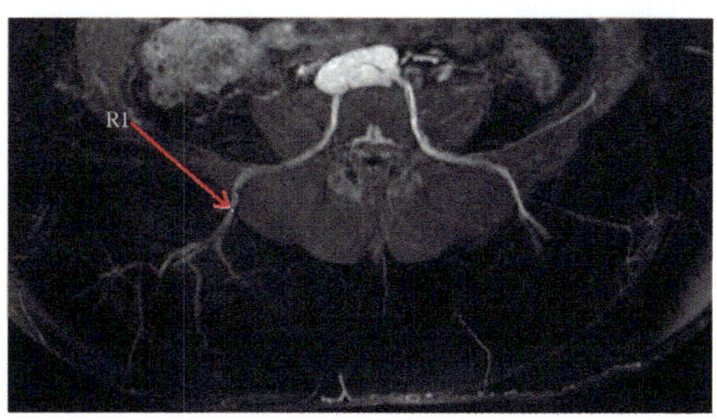

Fig. 4.21 Axial MRA of the back. Arrow pointing to a right lumbar perforator. (*Used with permission* Ref. [31])

needed. An IM perforator can be used to augment outflow by anastomosing to a second flap vein. An IM artery perforator may have a better size match with the typically smaller caliber superficial inferior epigastric artery.

The location of the intercostal space, that the internal mammary vein splits into two branches, which course medial and lateral to the internal

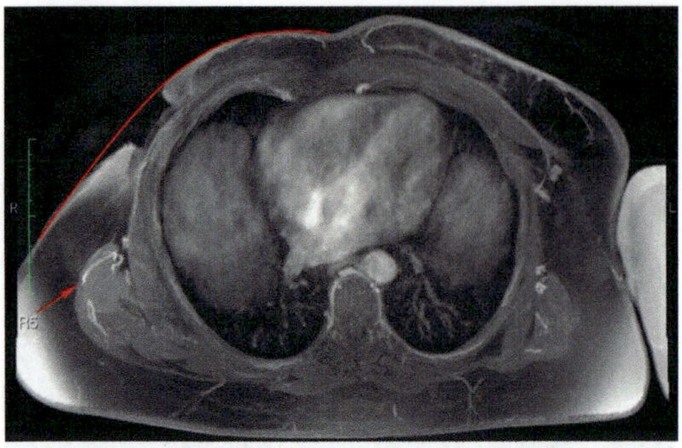

Fig. 4.22 Axial MRA of the chest in a patient with a radiated open left chest wound. Arrow points to a large thoracodorsal artery perforator, about to emerge through the anterior edge of the latissimus muscle. (*Used with permission* Ref. [31])

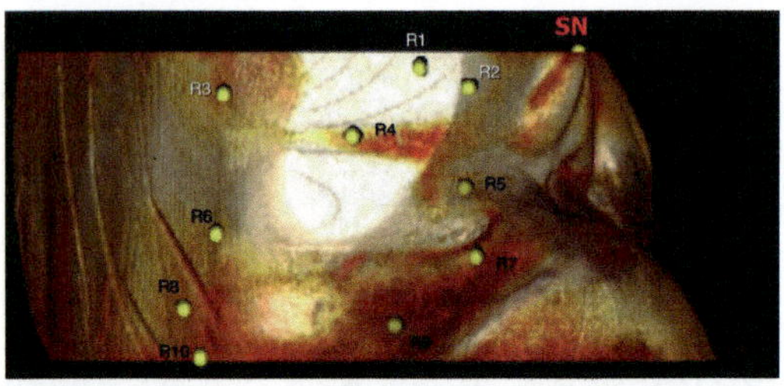

Fig. 4.23 3D volume-rendered MRA of the chest in the lateral decubitus position with perforator locations and reference point at the sternal notch (SN) marked. (*Used with permission* Ref. [31])

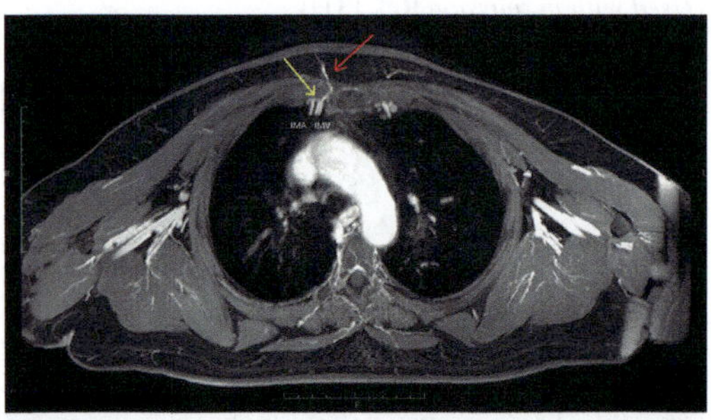

Fig. 4.24 Axial MIP MRA of the chest showing the typical anatomy of an IM vein located medial to an IM artery. Red arrow points to a large IM perforator. Yellow arrow points to the IM vein branching point

mammary artery, may assist a surgeon in choosing the optimum interspace level to dissect for anastomosis. The IM vein branching point can allow for a single larger caliber anastomosis. Alternatively, each branch can be used separately for additional outflow anastomosis options.

4.8 Conclusion

The tremendous anatomic variability in the vascular system can make perforator flap breast reconstruction challenging for surgeons at all experience levels. Accurate preoperative anatomic vascular imaging enables optimal perforator selection and improves flap design. Shifting the brunt of the perforator selection process preoperatively improves operating efficiency, which can result in reduced operating time, reduced general anesthesia requirements, and potentially increased flap success [10, 11, 13]. MRA is presently the preoperative method of choice due to the absence of radiation exposure or iodinated contrast agents and the ability for serial imaging acquisitions to visualize multiple donor sites with the patient in different positions in one examination.

References

1. Masia J, Clavero JA, Larranaga JR, et al. Multidetector-row computed tomography in the planning of abdominal perforator flaps. J Plast Reconstr Aesthet Surg. 2006;59(6):594–9.
2. Rozen WM, Phillips TJ, Ashton MW, et al. Preoperative imaging for DIEA perforator flaps: a comparative study of computed tomographic angiography and Doppler ultrasound. Plast Reconstr Surg. 2008;121(1):9–16.
3. Brenner DJ, Hall EJ. Computed tomography—an increasing source of radiation exposure. N Engl J Med. 2007;357(22):2277–84.
4. Stein R. Too much of a good thing? The growing use of CT scans fuel medical concerns regarding radiation exposure. Washington Post. 2008;F1.
5. American College Radiology Radiological Society North America, Inc. Safety in medical imaging. www.radiologyinfo.org/en/safety/index.cfm?pg=sfty_xray. Accessed 20 Oct 2015.
6. Varnholt H. Computed tomography and radiation exposure. N Engl J Med. 2008;358(8):852–3.
7. Katayama H, Yamaguchi K, Kozuka T, et al. Adverse reactions to ionic and nonionic contrast media. A report from the Japanese Committee on the Safety of Contrast Media. Radiology. 1990;175(3):621–8.
8. Parfray P. The clinical epidemiology of contrast-induced nephropathy. Cardiovasc Intervent Radiol. 2005;28(suppl 2):S3–11.
9. Shellock FG, Crues JV. MR procedures: biologic effects, safety, and patient care. Radiology. 2004;232:635–52.

10. Vasile JV, Newman T, Rusch DG, et al. Anatomic imaging of gluteal perforator flaps without ionizing radiation: seeing is believing with MRA. J Reconstr Microsurg. 2010;26(1):45–57. Epub 2009 July 10.
11. Greenspun D, Vasile J, Levine JL, et al. Anatomic imaging of abdominal perforator flaps without ionizing radiation: seeing is believing with MRA. J Reconstr Microsurg. 2010;26(1):37–44. Epub 2009 May 18.
12. Newman TM, Vasile J, Levine JL, et al. Perforator flap magnetic resonance angiography: a review of 25 deep inferior epigastric and gluteal perforator artery flap patients. J Magn Reson Imaging. 2010;31(5):1176–84.
13. Vasile JV, Newman TM, Prince MR, et al. Contrast enhanced magnetic resonance angiography. Clin Plast Surg. 2011;38(2):263–75.
14. Thimmappa ND, Prince MR, Colen KL, et al. Breast tissue expanders with magnetic ports: clinical experience at 1.5 T. Plast Reconstr Surg. 2016;138(6):1171–8.
15. Neil-Dwyer JG, Ludman CN, Schaverien M, et al. Magnetic resonance angiography in preoperative planning of deep inferior epigastric artery perforator flaps. J Plast Reconstr Aesthet Surg. 2009;62:1661–5.
16. Masia J, Kosutic D, Cervelli D, et al. In search of the ideal method in perforator mapping: noncontrast magnetic resonance imaging. J Reconstr Microsurg. 2010;26(1):29–35.
17. Dillman JR, Ellis JH, Cohan RH, et al. Frequency and severity of acute allergic-like reactions to gadolinium-containing IV contrast media in children and adults. Am J Roentgenol. 2007;189:1533–8.
18. Niendorf HP, Alhassan A, Geens VR, et al. Safety review of gadopentetate dimeglumine extended clinical experience after more than five million applications. Investig Radiol. 1994;29(suppl 2):S179–82.
19. FDA Drug Safety Communication: new warnings for using gadolinium-based contrast agents inpatients with kidney dysfunction. http://www.fda.gov/drugs/drugsafety/ucm223966.htm. Accessed 21 Sept 2010.
20. Cowper SE. Nephrogenic fibrosing dermopathy [ICNSFR Website]. 2001–2014. http://www.icnfdr.org. Accessed 24 Apr 2015.
21. Scheinfeld NS, Cowper SE. Nephrogenic fibrosing dermopathy. 2008. http://www.emedicine.com/derm/topic934.htm. Accessed 7 Aug 2008.
22. Reiter T, Ritter O, Prince MR, et al. Minimizing risk of nephrogenic systemic fibrosis in cardiovascular magnetic resonance. J Cardiovasc Magn Reson. 2012;14(1):31.
23. Gulani V, Calamante F, Shellock FG, et al. Gadolinium deposition in the brain: summary of evidence and recommendations. Lancet Neurol. 2017;16(7):564–70.
24. Mallio CA, Quattrocchi CC, Rovira A, et al. Gadolinium deposition safety: seeking the patient perspective. AJNR Am J Neuroradiol. 2020;41(6):944–6.
25. McDonald JS, McDonald RJ. MR imaging safety considerations of gadolinium-based contrast agents: gadolinium retention and nephrogenic systemic fibrosis. Magn Reason Imaging Clin. 2020;28(4):497–507.
26. Guo BJ, Yang ZL, Zhang LJ. Gadolinium deposition in brain: current scientific evidence and future perspectives. Front Mol Neurosci. 2018;11:335. https://doi.org/10.3389/fnmol.2018.00335.
27. Oliveira IS, Hedgire SS, Li W, et al. Blood pool contrast agents for venous magnetic resonance imaging. Cardiovasc Diagn Ther. 2016;6(6):508–18.
28. Ersoy H, Jacobs P, Kent CK, et al. Blood pool MR angiography of aortic stent-graft endoleak. AJR Am J Roentgenol. 2004;182(5):1181–6.
29. Zou Z, Lee HK, Cerilles M, et al. Gadofosveset trisodium enhanced abdominal perforator MRA. J Magn Reson Imaging. 2012;35(3):711–6. Epub 2011 Oct 26.
30. Agrawal MD, Thimmappa ND, Vasile JV, et al. Autologous breast reconstruction: preoperative MRA for perforator flap vessel mapping. J Reconstr Microsurg. 2015;31(1):1–11. Epub May 2014.
31. Vasile JV. Imaging for perforator flap breast reconstruction. In: Levine JL, Vasile JV, Chen CM, et al., editors. Perforator flap breast reconstruction. New York: Thieme Publishers; 2015.

5 MR Lymphangiography

Peter C. Neligan

5.1 Introduction

Patients presenting with lymphedema need a thorough multimodal assessment. There is no pathognomonic sign, no single test, and no unique characteristic that can aid the clinician in making the diagnosis. Imaging is an important facet of assessment when dealing with such a patient. There are several imaging modalities, and each has a place in patient assessment and treatment. Lymphoscintigraphy using technetium sulfur colloid (Tc99) is widely considered the gold standard for imaging the lymphatic system. Following intracutaneous injection, Tc99 is taken up by the lymphatics, and its transport within the lymphatic system can be scanned to give an objective assessment of lymphatic function. Lymphoscintigraphy gives good information on function of the lymphatic system, on the function of lymph nodes, and on the transport of Tc99 within the system [1, 2]. The transport index of Tc99 measures the time taken for the isotope to reach the draining lymph nodes and is an indication of the efficiency of the lymphatic system. Magnetic resonance is ubiquitous as an imaging modality, but its use in assessing and managing lymphedema patients is less universal. Nevertheless, it is an excellent tool for imaging the lymphatic system and can provide valuable and useful information. Using magnetic resonance to image the lymphatics was first reported in 1992 [3]. However, it has not become a widely accepted imaging modality for lymphedema until much more recently. This may be because present lymphedema treatment is dependent on detailed anatomic information. This was not as important before the introduction of the more recent physiologic procedures, lymphaticovenous bypass (LVB) and vascularized lymph node transplant (VLNT) for the treatment of lymphedema. These latter procedures rely on accurate anatomic information to help identify lymphatic channels that will be targeted surgically. There is no single imaging format that is preeminent for the evaluation of lymphedema [4]. Rather, the best information can be gleaned from multiple modalities including MR, fluorescent lymphangiography with ICG, and ultrasound [5]. When using MR lymphangiography, lymphatic channels can be visualized with [6] or without [7] contrast. Using contrast involves the injection of gadolinium in the web spaces of the fingers or toes to image the lymphatics. Like Tc99, gadolinium is taken up by the lymphatic system. It can also get into the venous system which can make interpretation of the lymphatic channels difficult. Using subtraction venography as is used in digital subtraction angiography (DSA) does not really work in MRI. For that reason, deciphering whether a structure is a lymphatic or a vein can

P. C. Neligan (✉)
Division of Plastic Surgery,
University of Washington, Seattle, WA, USA
e-mail: pneligan@uw.edu

J. P. Hong et al. (eds.), *Imaging for Reconstructive Microsurgery*,
https://doi.org/10.1007/978-981-97-7278-0_5

be very difficult. Consequently, the "dark blood" technique was introduced [8]. The lymphatics are imaged using intracutaneous gadolinium, while a second agent, ferumoxytol, is injected intravenously to suppress potentially enhancing veins, this making it easier to identify lymphatic channels with certainty and not mistake them for veins (Fig. 5.1). The mechanism by which this works is that ferumoxytol shortens the T* of arteries and veins so that by using a short and long TE (time to echo), the venous signal can be suppressed.

Fluorescent lymphangiography using ICG is probably the most widely used modality for imaging the lymphatics. It is easy to use and readily available both in clinic and in the OR. In fact, attempting lymphatic surgery without the use of ICG is difficult. Imaging penetration is a limitation of ICG as the near-infrared camera can only penetrate about 1.5 cm into the tissue. ICG therefore only images the superficial lymphatics and will not pick up a channel that is deeper than the imaging penetration. This can be a problem in patients who have significant fibro-fatty accumulation where the lymphatic channels may be deeper than anticipated. MR lymphangiography gives more detailed information about the lymphatics because of its penetration. There appears to be excellent correlation between the MRI and ICG images [9].

Ultrasound is the most recent imaging modality to achieve widespread popularity. It has been shown that ultrahigh frequency ultrasound is more efficient at identifying lymphatics than conventional ultrasound [10]. Ultrasound has the advantage of identifying veins as well as lymphatics. Finding veins which are appropriate for performing LVB is often a problem that ultrasound helps to solve.

All of the imaging modalities mentioned so far, with the exception of ICG lymphangiography, are used pre- or postoperatively, and each of these modalities has a specific advantage in assessing the lymphatic system. ICG lymphangiography can also be used intraoperatively to assess lymphatic channels in real time. Laser tomography is the most recent tool to be used for

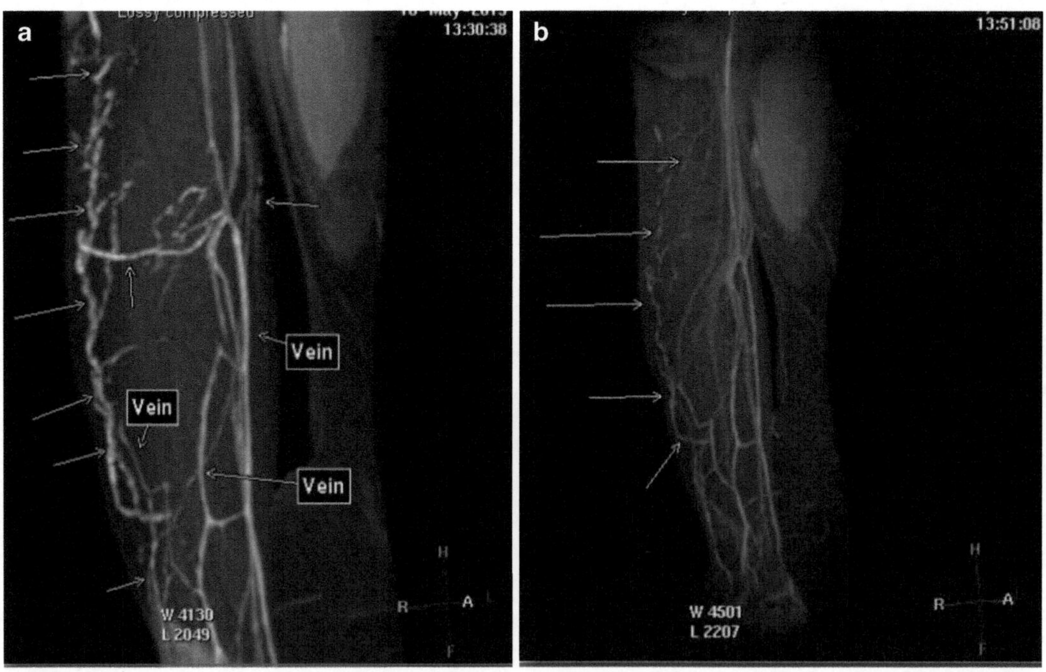

Fig. 5.1 (**a**) MR lymphangiogram of the upper extremity showing veins (labeled) and lymphatic channels (arrows). (**b**) Feraheme has allowed suppression of the enhanced venous images which makes it easier to identify the lymphatic channels

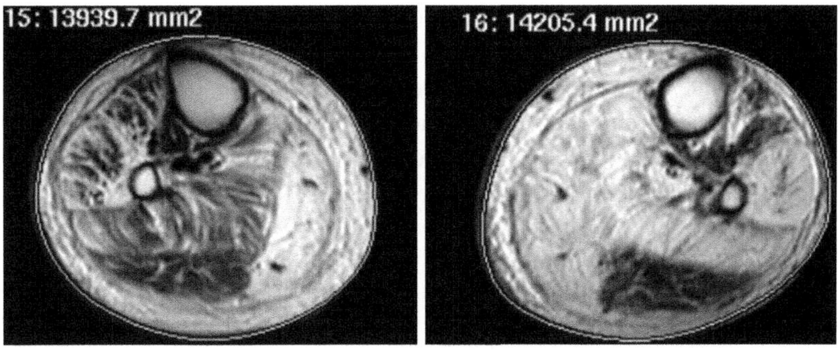

Fig. 5.2 MRI of patient presenting with bilateral lower extremity lymphedema showing fatty degeneration of the lower limb musculature

intraoperative lymphatic assessment. Laser tomography has been used in the diagnosis, management, and surveillance of ophthalmic diseases for many years [11]. It is an imaging modality that uses reflection of near-infrared light to generate images and provides high-resolution cross-sectional and optical coherence tomographic data. Hayashi et al. have reported its use in visualizing and assessing lymphatic channels intraoperatively [12].

Apart from identifying lymphatic channels, MRI can be used to identify fluid content as well as fat accumulation in the affected limb as demonstrated by Dayan [13]. This can be helpful in determining the most appropriate form of treatment. Swelling that is fluid predominant, which is generally seen in early lymphedema, is treated much differently from swelling that is mainly associated with fibro-fatty deposition as we see in more advanced stages of lymphedema. Furthermore, MR lymphangiography gives valuable information on the rest of the area being examined and not just the lymphatic system. This can change the approach to treatment or may uncover a hitherto unrecognized problem. Such is the case depicted in Fig. 5.2. This elderly patient presented with bilateral lower limb lymphedema. Imaging, however, showed fatty degeneration in his lower leg musculature. He did have lymphedema, but his lymphedema was a symptom of his muscular disease and not the primary cause of his lower extremity edema.

MR lymphangiography can be used to pinpoint a specific problem as seen in Fig. 5.3. This young male patient had a cyst removed from his thigh. He subsequently started to develop lymphedema in his left lower limb. MR lymphangiography highlighted the problem. Lymph can be seen leaking from the collecting ducts in the medial thigh. The area of damage was identified, and the leak was repaired. While direct repair was not possible, LVB could be performed on the injured lymphatic channels, thereby bypassing the area of leakage and scarring.

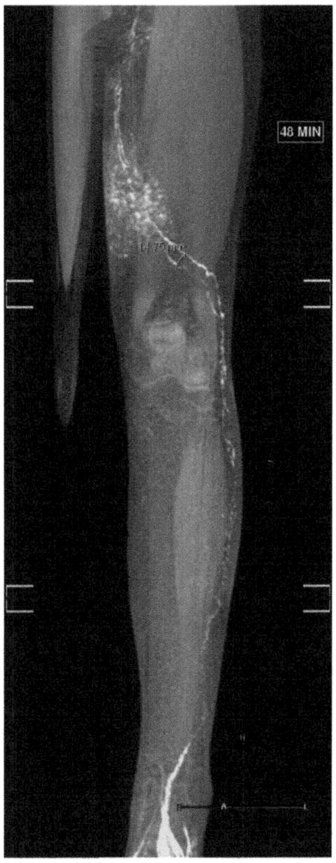

Fig. 5.3 MR lymphangiogram of left leg. Leakage from collecting ducts in the thigh is seen. This area corresponds with the site of the scar from cyst excision

A percentage of patients presenting with a swollen limb can have problems other than lymphedema; what appears to be lymphedema may turn out, on imaging, to be something else. The patient in Fig. 5.4 is such an example. A young patient presented with apparent lymphedema of his left lower extremity. MR lymphangiography revealed that he actually had a lymphangioma. The lymphangioma was excised, following which the lower extremity edema did not recur.

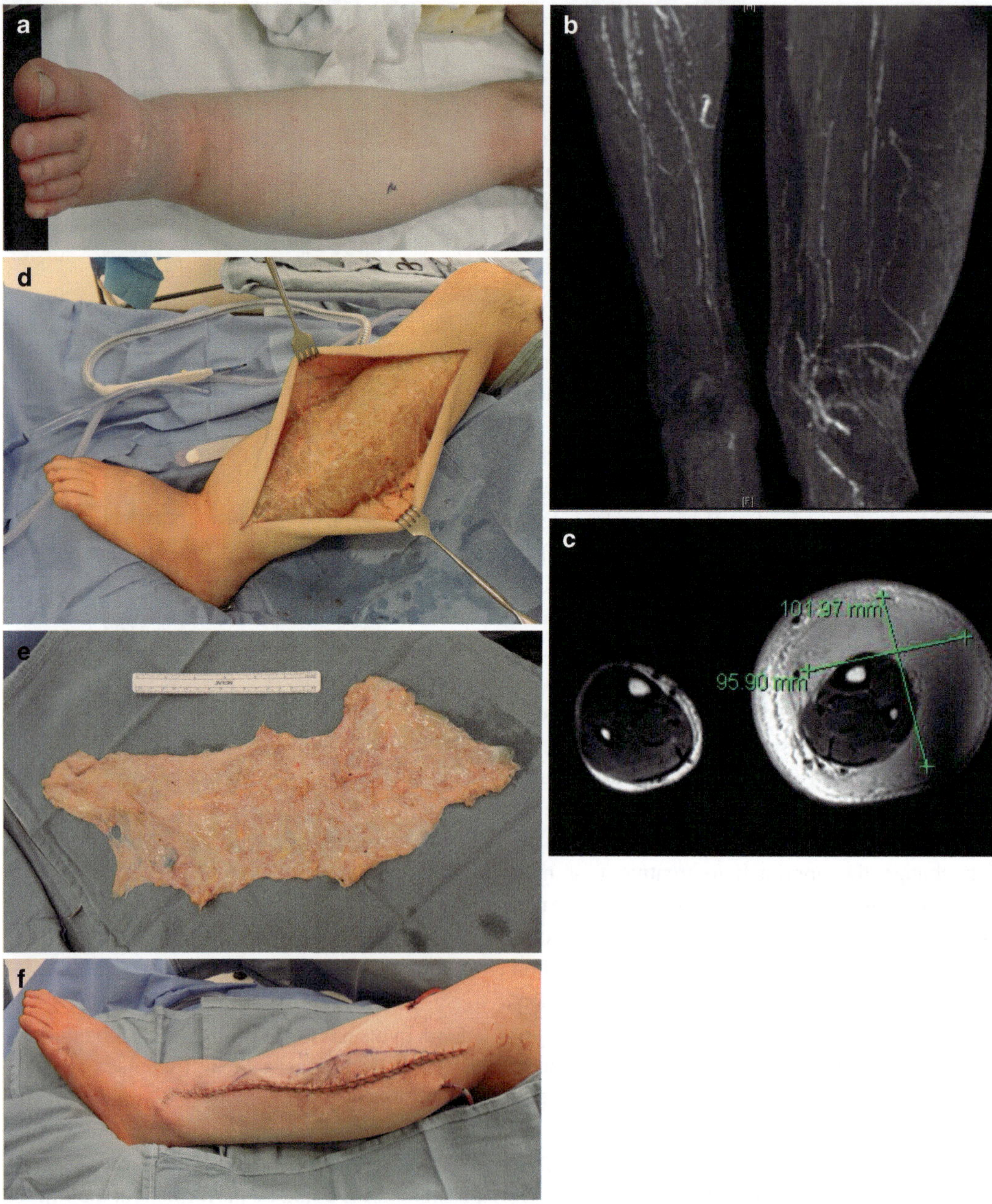

Fig. 5.4 (**a**) Patient presents with apparent lymphedema of left lower extremity. (**b**) MR lymphangiogram shows imageable lymphatic channels in both legs. (**c**) Significantly sized lymphangioma appreciated. (**d**) Lymphangioma exposed and (**e**) excised. (**f**) Limb closed following lymphangioma excision

MR lymphangiography has several advantages outlined below. However, it has also some disadvantages.

Advantages of MR lymphangiography

- Gives useful information on anatomy of lymphatic channels with high-definition images
- Documents where edema maximal
- Demonstrates areas of dermal backflow
- Documents lymphatic function
- Gives accurate limb volume measurement
- Consistent images

Disadvantages of MR lymphangiography

- Even using local anesthesia, many patients find it painful
- Time-consuming
- Expensive
- Not universally available

The fact that MR lymphangiography is time-consuming is often an issue raised by radiology departments. However, in our unit, using the protocol developed by our radiologists, the time taken to complete an examination was reduced from 4 to 1.5 h. While the advantages of MR lymphangiography outweigh the disadvantages, patients are often loathe to be subjected to repeat examinations because they find the experience uncomfortable. However, the author has found MR lymphangiography extremely valuable when assessing a patient for treatment. Follow-up examinations can easily be done with ICG lymphangiography if the patient declines further MR lymphangiograms. At that stage, information on other structures in the limb is less relevant than it is at the beginning of the patient's assessment.

References

1. Chowdhry M, Rozen WM, Griffiths M. Lymphatic mapping and preoperative imaging in the management of post-mastectomy lymphoedema. Gland Surg. 2016;5(2):187–96.
2. Chang L, et al. The role of lymphoscintigraphy in diagnosis and monitor the response of physiotherapeutic technique in congenital lymphedema. Clin Nucl Med. 2011;36(4):e11–2.
3. Case TC, et al. Magnetic resonance imaging in human lymphedema: comparison with lymphangioscintigraphy. Magn Reson Imaging. 1992;10(4):549–58.
4. Fumiere E, et al. MR imaging, proton MR spectroscopy, ultrasonographic, histologic findings in patients with chronic lymphedema. Lymphology. 2007;40(4):157–62.
5. Gentili F, et al. Comparison of indocyanine green fluorescence lymphangiography and magnetic resonance lymphangiography to investigate lymphedema of the extremities. Ann Ital Chir. 2021;92:452–9.
6. Mitsumori LM, et al. MR lymphangiography: how i do it. J Magn Reson Imaging. 2015;42:1465.
7. Arrive L, et al. Noncontrast magnetic resonance lymphography. J Reconstr Microsurg. 2016;32(1):80–6.
8. Maki JH, et al. Dark blood magnetic resonance lymphangiography using dual-agent relaxivity contrast (DARC-MRL): a novel method combining gadolinium and iron contrast agents. Curr Probl Diagn Radiol. 2015;45:174.
9. Neligan PC, Kung TA, Maki JH. MR lymphangiography in the treatment of lymphedema. J Surg Oncol. 2017;115(1):18–22.
10. Hayashi A, et al. Ultra high-frequency ultrasonographic imaging with 70 MHz scanner for visualization of the lymphatic vessels. Plast Reconstr Surg Glob Open. 2019;7(1):e2086.
11. Chen TC, et al. Spectral domain optical coherence tomography: ultra-high speed, ultra-high resolution ophthalmic imaging. Arch Ophthalmol. 2005;123(12):1715–20.
12. Hayashi A, et al. Intraoperative real-time visualization of the lymphatic vessels using microscope-integrated laser tomography. J Reconstr Microsurg. 2020;37:427.
13. Dayan JH, et al. Regional patterns of fluid and fat accumulation in patients with lower extremity lymphedema using magnetic resonance angiography. Plast Reconstr Surg. 2020;145(2):555–63.

Microvessel Visualization in Designing Perforator Flaps

6

Andreas Kehrer

Key Points

- Perforator flaps have undergone a multitude of refinements over the last decade. Finesse in preoperative design has been greatly increased and may be provided by numerous diagnostic modalities.
- Microvessel detection, imaging, and quality assessment play important roles in preoperative flap designs, especially in thin and delicate tissue transfers.
- Perforator visualization with high-resolution color-coded duplex sonography (CCDS) has the means to provide the best overall applicability of all modalities available. CCDS is a cost-effective and easy alternative that does not require radiation exposure and is not dependent on contrast media.
- CCDS has therefore become a powerful tool for microsurgeons enlarging the arsenal of techniques in reconstructive microsurgery. It may add safety and efficiency and allows to apply a "hot-zone/cold-zone" dissection concept for speedy flap elevations.
- Thin, multiple-island, chimeric, and other flap designs are simplified planning tissue transfers as the suprafascial architecture of perforators and subbranches may be assessed in real time with high-resolution imaging.
- Besides qualitative parameters as number and precise location of microvessels, quantitative parameters as vessel diameter and blood flow velocities may be measured for a better understanding of perforator flap physiology.
- The learning curve of CCDS examinations for microsurgeons is steep as they are generally open to new technology and usually used to apply micro-movements which are necessary to maneuver the ultrasound probe. Basic understanding of machine "knobology" and some practical training suffice. An in-depth physical comprehension of ultrasound is not compulsory for microvessel evaluation.
- Correct device settings for microvessel imaging is of utmost importance for a successful examination and has been described by Kehrer et al. previously [1]. Low-flow detection as present in perforators requires special ultrasound machine programming and trimming and may tremendously enhance device sensitivity for detection of microvessels.
- A highly structured approach in trimming device settings and practical methodology simplify and shorten CCDS examinations decisively.
- Reading this chapter, the reader should learn a useful sequence for a structured perforator mapping approach and be able to instantly start practicing with CCDS how to localize

A. Kehrer (✉)
Department of Plastic, Hand- and Reconstructive Surgery, University Hospital Regensburg, Regensburg, Germany

Institute for Facial Reconstruction for Facial Nerve Palsy, Ingolstadt, Germany

J. P. Hong et al. (eds.), *Imaging for Reconstructive Microsurgery*,
https://doi.org/10.1007/978-981-97-7278-0_6

and characterize microvessels for possible perforator flap designs.
- Examples of different perforator flap designs executed with CCDS have been added to this chapter and illustrate how perforators may be incorporated into modern flap transfers.

6.1 Introduction

6.1.1 Contemporary Requirements in Perforator Flap Surgery

Since Koshima and Kroll have introduced the perforator flap era more than 30 years ago, further finesse and refinements to this flap concept have continuously been added [2, 3]. In the modern era of perforator flap surgery, demands for more delicate procedures have arisen. No longer simple defect coverage constitutes the center of attention. Factors like recipient and donor site cosmesis, concealed donor sites, limited scar length, tissue replacement following the "like-with-like" principle with thin, gliding, and pliable tissue properties, and many others move into focus. As in complex reconstructions multiple reconstructive steps are often combined, consideration to a multitude of details is required. At the same time execution of flap harvest should be safe, fast, reproducible, and effective. Challenges to tackle in extremity salvage are thin flaps in obese patients, minimal donor morbidity, time constraints, and cost-effectiveness. Consequently, contemporary aims are saving time and shifting the focus away from having to find perforators through surgical dissection in favor of concentrating on other important details of reconstruction. Preoperative flap design and planning are essential for the success of microsurgical operations especially for less experienced surgeons.

6.1.2 Assessment of Color-Coded Duplex Sonography (CCDS) in the Field of Competing Diagnostic Modalities

For pre-, intra-, and postoperative perforator assessment, a multitude of modalities are presently available. Handheld Doppler (HHD), color-coded duplex sonography (CCDS), digital subtraction angiography (DSA), computed tomographic angiography (CTA), and magnetic resonance angiography (MRA) represent more widely applied techniques [4–9]. Other diagnostic modalities including MRI thermal imaging, laser-assisted ICG angiography, dynamic infrared thermography, FLIR (forward-looking infrared [FLIR] cameras), and contrast-enhanced ultrasound are less commonly utilized [10–14]. While multiple vascular diagnostics exist, no modality has gained gold standard in extremities [4–6, 8–16]. Comparing diagnostic imaging with intraoperative findings may show differing results concerning perforator size, location, anticipated course, and relation to surrounding structures [17, 18]. Furthermore, most of the named diagnostic imaging tools present disadvantages in terms of invasiveness of techniques, costs, or availability [19].

Preoperative flap planning with computed tomography angiography (CTA) is a safe option [3, 4]; however, it does imply a radiation burden and the need for the involvement of a radiology department. The disadvantage of CTA and digital subtraction angiography (DSA) is the use of a contrast medium and radiation exposure to the patient. In contrast, the higher incidence of renal dysfunction after repeated intra-arterial administration of contrast media is regarded as an indicator that various contrast agents can be responsible for kidney damage [20]. Patients with metal implants may not be candidates for some modalities.

It was reported that 1.5–2.0% of all cancers in the United States may be attributable to the radiation from CT studies [19]. FLIR may appear easy and quick in handling, but this technology has a penetration limit to superficial tissue layers and may not display the suprafascial perforator architecture in several planes to create thin perforator flaps as CCDS.

6.1.3 The Superior Role of Color-Coded Duplex Sonography (CCDS)

In the last decade, competencies of ultrasound (US)-guided microvessel visualization and blood flow imaging have improved immensely as ultrasound devices have enhanced in quality [10, 21]. However, contemporarily the handheld Doppler (HHD) is still more common for microsurgeons to use in extremities. Only qualitative nonvisual detection of perforators is possible, whereas quantitative hemodynamic information is impossible. Concordance rates between perforators found with a HHD and those found intraoperatively have been described as low as 40% [22]. Others reported ALT perforators to be more than 1 cm away from Doppler signals in 25% and 50% of cases [4].

Perforator mapping with CCDS has the means to provide the best overall applicability of all mentioned modalities [23]. CCDS is a far more cost-effective and easier alternative for perforator mapping of the perforator flaps [5–8]. It may be performed independently from a radiology department by the microsurgeon. The repeatability of the US exam without sequelae for the patient should be valued as an inherent strength.

For perforator mapping in preoperative flap planning of perforator flaps of the extremities, as the anterolateral thigh (ALT), CCDS was shown to have superior qualities compared to a HHD [12, 13]. A systematic review by Cheng et al. comparing HHD, CCDS, and CT angiography revealed that CCDS had the highest pooled sensitivity of 95.7% as well as the highest pooled positive predictive value of 94.3% to identify microvessels for perforator flaps such as the ALT flap [23–25]. Visualization of microvascular structures has been a domain of color-coded duplex sonography (CCDS) and power Doppler (PD) because of their accuracy, repeatability, and portability. Thomas et al. confirmed the superiority of CCDS to conventional Doppler US for perforator mapping and characterization prior to ALT flap harvest [26]. Kehrer et al. showed that sensitivity of PD for microvessel detection was 96.7% with a mean distance from the emergence point (true anatomy) to the projected preoperative skin marking after PD mapping (assumed anatomy) of 2.45 ± 1.90 mm (0–6 mm) [27]. These findings could be confirmed by the results of this study proving a 100% sensitivity rate for CCDS-guided perforator detection though CCDS proved to be superior compared to PD in correct assessment of microvessel diameter.

Furthermore, CCDS examinations are free of radiation exposure and are not dependent on contrast media. Overall availability, time, and cost savings are other important advantages of this fast-growing technology [26, 28–30].

High-resolution CCDS-guided vascular flow imaging has meanwhile proven as a potent instrument for microsurgeons in evaluating perforator vessels to simplify the design of perforator flaps in reconstructive surgery [10, 23]. CCDS has been shown to have great detail and precision when evaluating perforating vessels and is capable to detect vessels of 0.2 mm and greater [10, 31]. Within the last few years, it has developed impetus and may spread faster than other modalities for detection and assessment of microvessels required for preoperative microvascular flap planning [5, 10, 18, 32–35]. Anatomic and hemodynamic information may be provided in real-time imaging by CCDS of both vascular structures of the donor and recipient sites of flap reconstructions [36].

One goal is to create a safe and at the same time definite flap design before placing the first incision. Vertical vs. oblique vectors of suprafascial perforator routes have implications for different flap harvesting approaches. However, device settings for microvessel imaging are of utmost importance for a successful examination and have been described by Kehrer et al. previously [1]. Low-flow detection requires special device settings. Specific ultrasound device programming and trimming is required and may tremendously enhance device sensitivity for detection of microvessels.

CCDS perforator mapping performed by the operating surgeon has been evolved to be a key element in our practice. Having gained experience for several years now, CCDS has been found to be a convenient, inexpensive, and quickly repeatable instrument especially in small flaps such as those used for tongue reconstruction [37]. Accurate communication regarding specific flap characteristics required by the individual defect is a critical determinant for correct perforator planning and corresponding flap design.

CCDS has specific advantages compared with other cross-sectional imaging modalities including no intravenous contrast and absence of radiation exposure. Knowledge of additional parameters besides perforator course such as diameter, flow velocity, flow direction, and confluences may facilitate perforator choice. One of CCDS's drawbacks is its dependency on operator's abilities.

CCDS has the potential to change the workup for perforator flaps as well as recipient vessels for extremity reconstruction in the future from CTA/MRA to CCDS. CCDS may allow the examiner to detect, evaluate, and quantify vascular stenoses in arterial peripheral vascular disease as well as grade venous insufficiency of individual vascular systems [38, 39]. This could help estimate the success of flaps preoperatively if relevant circulatory disturbances are already known in advance.

6.1.4 Why Should the Microsurgeon Perform the CCDS Examination?

Reliably mapping perforators may seem to require scanning patients together with a specialized radiologist. However, in modern hospital settings, most disciplines face substantial time and organizational constraints. Accurate communication regarding specific flap characteristics required by the individual defect is a critical determinant for correct perforator planning and corresponding flap design. If diagnostics cannot be performed together, a substantial discrepancy between expectations of the microsurgeon and radiologist may result. These circumstances led our department to the conclusion that we should conduct perforator mapping procedures ourselves. After receiving guidance through radiologists specialized in ultrasound and a short period of supervision initially, we now perform all perforator mapping procedures ourselves, utilizing an ultrasound-based design concept. To enjoy US examination, the microsurgeon needs only little training which may be acquired through basic ultrasound courses focused on the vascular system. A structured step-by-step approach for machine settings and perforator mapping sequences has been suggested previously by Kehrer et al. [40]. We are convinced that for microsurgeons who are used to perform micromovements, scanning for diminutive vascular structures with CCDS using our system is easy to learn. Featuring high-resolution visualization properties, CCDS adds a powerful new tool to the armamentarium of microsurgeons for perforator flap design. Hereby, a safer and faster harvest of thin flaps is possible [41, 42].

6.1.5 Usage of CCDS in Planning Thin Perforator Flaps and Applying a "Hot-Zone/Cold-Zone" Dissection Concept

Due to its high resolution, CCDS can strongly simplify a thin flap design by precisely demonstrating the perforator route in the subcutaneous tissue layer. The planning of small flaps is decisively enhanced. This saves operating time and precludes unnecessary dissection of surrounding structures. The length of the donor site scar may be reduced [43].

The superficial fascial plane harvest of thin perforator flaps has been popularized by Hong et al. refining function and cosmesis of recipient and donor sites [41, 42]. Hong et al. have also popularized a superficial flap harvest using a "hot-zone/cold-zone" dissection concept [41]. As a prerequisite, the suprafascial perforator architecture must be known before incision to locate the perforator at a level within the subcutaneous tissue layer. In contrast, rare cases of unsuitable vascular constellations may be anticipated preoperatively and allow changes early in the reconstructive agenda.

Vertical vs. oblique vectors of suprafascial perforator routes have implications for different flap harvesting approaches. It requires reliable CCDS-guided preoperative diagnostics [41, 42]. Dissection of perforator flaps in superficial planes such as the suprafascial plane is simplified through preoperative perforator mapping with CCDS as the suprafascial course of perforators may be visualized [44]. The principle of a "hot-zone/cold-zone" concept of flap harvest requires knowledge of the exact perforator location.

6.1.6 Understanding Perforator Flap Physiology with CCDS

Perforator flaps are now widely performed in reconstructive surgery. Nevertheless, astonishing little knowledge exists of the altered hemodynamics within these flaps before and following transplantation. Ligating side branches of the flap's pedicle vascular system leads to an hemodynamic enhancement through an "inversion phenomenon" [45]. High perfusion pressure to the main perforator opens multiple direct and indirect vessels and connects several angiosomes, also termed perforasomes. The subsequent hyperperfusion of the skin paddle may allow the capture of the adjacent two perforasomes, explaining how a single perforator can capture larger skin territories. The amount of tissue that can be harvested based on a given skin vessel is difficult to assess. How much tissue can be carried based on a given size of perforator depends on the size and amount of pulsatility in microvessels, local vasculature anatomy, and other factors. The major cause of skin flap failure is insufficient arterial blood flow along with poor venous outflow also responsible for inadequate perfusion and subsequent flap failure.

Therefore, another novelty of integrating CCDS in flap procedures is the possibility to evaluate reproducible and comparable flow parameters of perforators. CCDS has been shown to have great detail and precision when evaluating perforating vessels [34]. Microvessel characterization by measuring quantitative parameters such as vascular diameter and blood flow velocities provides new insights in flap physiology. An ideal skin perforator as defined on CCDS is determined as having a diameter larger than 0.5 mm with an adequate waveform of pulsatile blood flow [46]. It was determined that CCDS is capable to detect vessels of 0.2 mm and greater [31]. Besides quantitative parameters, CCDS is also capable of providing static and dynamic qualitative information. Hemodynamics as flow direction of arterial and venous vascular structures, turbulences, and muscular/subcutaneous course can be assessed and visualized [47, 48].

When planning perforator-to-perforator anastomosis in flaps, recent data suggests matching flow velocity of pedicle with recipient vessels. A pulse systolic velocity (PSV) of 15 cm/s and higher was recommended as a criterion for perforator selection. Referring to the group of Suh et al. the recipient artery may be used if flow velocity is greater than 15–20 cm/s [49]. As demonstrated by Song et al. using CCDS examinations, velocity and flow of the flap are significantly different based on the rotation direction in pedicle propeller flaps. Using the preferred rotation direction with statistically higher value of velocity and flow may increase the overall outcome of the propeller flap, especially where larger flaps are used [50].

Perforators of other flaps are usually also measured at their emergence point at the level of the deep fascia. Future perspectives comprise that knowledge of flow velocities and vascular diameters in comparison with the size of the nourished angiosomes may help to gain a better estimation on how to design flap perimeters in larger flaps without vascular compromise. Experience in CCDS examinations may assist microsurgeons in a straightforward flap harvest and safer execution of perforator flaps.

6.1.7 Other CCDS Applications and Future Perspectives

Other applications of ultrasound are intraoperative vascular diagnostics and postoperative flap monitoring [51]. Multiple further applications in reconstructive surgery exist [52]. CCDS has also proven its value for postoperative perfusion monitoring in flaps lacking skin islands, e.g., free functional muscle transplants (FFMT) in facial reanimation [51]. The technology has also proved effective for the evaluation of facial musculature [53, 54]. Kehrer et al. have described how to objectively measure synkinetic dysfunction in mimetic muscles yielding a functional map that can guide therapy for facial palsy patients showing synkinesis [55].

Future perspectives suggest the idea that a well-trained microsurgeon in ultrasound techniques would perform the perforator mapping directly in the operating theater with the patient positioned on the table. Perspectives are 3D CCDS perforator imaging and contrast-enhanced US (CEUS)-guided visualization of microcirculation in flaps [10, 56]. Future perspectives are that devices will decrease in size and further enhance sensitivity and performance which will make them even more eligible for intraoperative use by the microsurgeon.

Skills then easily translate into any perforator flap design as well as chimeric flaps and perforator flaps with smaller microvasculature. In some departments, it already has therefore become routine practice that all perforator flaps (e.g., SCIP, PAP, TdAP, DIEP MSAP flaps, etc.) are planned solely with CCDS by the microsurgeon. Only recently, CCDS has reached a superb level of high resolution being able to visualize microvessels up to the level of the subdermal as well as the intradermal plexus [28, 29, 57, 58]. Therefore, CCDS applications increase in a subspecialty of microsurgery which is supermicrosurgery [29, 57, 59, 60]. With the use of US and ultrahigh-frequency (UHF) US, now smallest microvessels as arteries, veins, and lymphatics may be evaluated [29, 30].

6.2 Execution of Ultrasound Examinations

6.2.1 Technical Requirements

Any new-generation high-resolution US devices may be used. Contemporarily, suitable devices are US machines with high-performance computer chips, represented rather by the larger pushable-type device than the handheld- or notebook-type machines. Up to the year 2022, any handheld- or notebook-type devices tested by the author did not feature sufficient performance to reliably detect small microvessels and their subbranches which certainly may be subject to change in the future as computer performance and portability increase vice versa. Multifrequency linear transducers from 15 MHz and up are favorable to detect microvessels. With present technology in the 12–15 MHz range and up, any perforator detected with CCDS should be eligible for a respective perforator flap design.

6.2.2 Background Knowledge of US Technology

CCDS background knowledge may be studied from textbooks [61–64]. However, for practical purposes of US-guided microvascular imaging, in-depth physical comprehension is not compulsory. Basic understanding of machine "knobology" and practical training suffice [65].

The linear array of transducers in the probe scans a plane through the body that can be viewed as a 2D image in real time. Echogenicity is a measure of acoustic reflectance, e.g., of US waves bouncing off tissues. In B-mode (brightness mode), various acoustic impedances received from different tissue layers are displayed as a cross section of tissues. Image display is composed of bright dots representing the US echoes. The brightness of each dot is determined by the amplitude of the returned echo signal. Scanning depth is dependent on frequency: the lower the frequency the deeper, the higher the less deep is the scan. Strictly obey conventional directions of holding the probe: image screen orientation in a transverse probe position should be as in CT/MRI imaging. Axial slices are shown as looking toward the patient's head from the feet. In contrast, sagittal slices of longitudinal cuts are shown with the left of the screen displaying more proximal and the right more distal tissues in extremities. CCDS combines B-mode and color duplex imaging to noninvasively visualize and assess microvascular blood flow in real time.

CCDS provides quantitative (number, localization) as well as qualitative (static, dynamic) information about perforators [9, 20, 22]. An important quantitative static parameter is the perforator diameter at the emergence point of the perforator penetrating the deep fascia.

6.2.3 Feasible Ultrasound Modes

Modes applicable for the purposes of US-based design of perforator flaps were evaluated by the author in a busy university hospital setting. B-mode, CCDS incl. PW-mode, PD-mode, and B-flow may be used for perforator characterization.

CCDS uses the Doppler effect with the superposition of flow information displayed in a real-time image. CCDS is hereby combining modes for qualitative vessel visualization through overlaying color-flow (CF) or B-flow imaging of microvascular blood flow with grayscale US (B-mode) and pulse-wave (PW) mode. It displays the different velocities and directions of vascular blood flow. Besides qualitative parameters, CCDS is also capable of providing static and dynamic quantitative information. These modes can preoperatively identify perforators and measure hemodynamic parameters to simplify perforator vessel selection for perforator flap planning.

6.2.3.1 Qualitative Evaluation of Perforator Characteristics

Brightness (B) Mode

B-mode is a basic 2D-mode every examination is initiated with. A plane is scanned through the body by the matrix or linear arrays of transducers in the ultrasound probe. Echoes of various acoustic impedances received from different tissue layers are displayed as a cross section of tissues in a real-time grayscale picture. The brightness of each pixel is determined by the amplitude of the returned US signal. An adapted focus and depth level as well as well-selected presets can optimize B-mode images.

Color-Flow (CF) Mode

Represents the standard color-coding mode and superimposes a color box window on the B-mode image in which all Doppler information is displayed. The color visualizes blood flow direction in relation to the probe. Color intensity (or gain) reflects flow velocity. Nuances may be compared with the color bar at the display's side. Regular CF-mode was found appropriate for various tissue depth levels and vascular diameters and may differentiate venous and arterial vessels by a color-coded signal. Red color signals indicate flow toward and blue away from the transducer. Color-coding of arterial vessels in red and veins in blue simplifies a later interpretation of US images. The Invert-Button therefore has to be used for correct color-coding in some situations. In most clinical settings, the application of CF-mode is sufficient to visualize small microvessels as perforators. In high-resolution ultrasound devices, also perforator subbranches as well as the intradermal vascular plexus may be imaged by using this mode.

Power Doppler (PD) Mode

Aiming at thin suprafascial flap designs, an assessment of the perforator course in the subcutaneous adipose tissue level is of interest. Vertical vs. oblique vectors of perforator routes have implications for designing a protective cuff of adipose tissue around the superficial pedicle segments and its connection with the subdermal plexus.

Power Doppler (PD) mode and B-flow have therefore been found useful in fascial and suprafascial imaging of small microvessels. If small perforators are difficult to detect in regular color-flow (CF) mode, additional power Doppler (PD) application enhances sensitivity by a factor 3–5 [66]. PD is based on the same technique as CCDS, though its color maps only represent the intensity and velocity of blood with substantial amplification. However, PD is not capable of encoding the direction of blood flow, so that a differentiation of veins and arteries by PD only is impeded [67]. In a previous study of Kehrer et al. using the augmented power Doppler (PD) mode in CCDS, the perforator artery size was overestimated in 65.5% of the cases by 50% or more compared to the diameter observed clinically in a series of 12 PAP flaps [11].

Employing PD-mode the signal is decisively amplified. Color gain may be downregulated which may decrease background noise in terms of extravascular artifacts. PD-mode may also be employed if an acute beam angle is difficult to achieve. PD-mode offers the advantage of a more sensitive depiction of low-flow vessels displaying the blood flow intensity in colors.

B-Flow

An US technique enabling a highly sensitive visualization of perforator vessels is B-flow. This digital subtraction technique does not rely on the Doppler effect but visualizes the echogenicity signal of erythrocytes, whereas background noises are lowered. Blood flow signals are displayed in the entire field of view without being angle dependent. The flow intensity and direction are thus not affected by the interrogation angle as it is with color Doppler (CF-mode). B-flow is capable of imaging true flow hemodynamics with a spatial resolution comparable to that of the grayscale image of B-mode. Therefore, an angiography-like, simultaneous imaging of slow- and high-flow vessels is enabled. While quantification of flow velocities is not possible, color-coding of B-flow may be selected. Blooming artifacts or wall overwriting as in color Doppler or PD-mode may not be expected. Another advantage is the suppression of extravascular reflexes as moving corpuscular elements are detected. B-flow may allow studying the microvascular network at the subfascial level with precision.

6.2.3.2 Quantitative Evaluation: Blood Flow Velocity Measurements in Pulse-Wave (PW) Mode

As CCDS combines the advantages of PW-mode and CF imaging, measurements of hemodynamic parameters are possible. An acoustic, optical, and nominal differentiation between arterial and venous as well as lymphatic characters of a vessel is possible. Perforator blood flow may be displayed in a frequency spectrum with characteristic spectral curves representing the hemodynamics depending on cardiac cycle in relation to time. Peak velocities of 5–30 cm/s are expected inside perforator vessels. Usually, a monophasic pattern is displayed. Peak systolic velocity (PSV) and end diastolic velocity (EDV) may be measured to evaluate blood flow by placing the adaptable sample volume inside the vascular lumen. The sample volume axis should be parallel to the vessel; otherwise, an angle correction should be performed (30°–60°), though velocity measurements are more precise with an angle <50°. PSV, EDV, and RI are representative parameters of hemodynamics. Along with measurement of microvessel diameter using the measurement tool, they can be used for comparison of different microvessels.

Table 6.1 provides a brief summarization of different feasible ultrasound modes for perforator evaluation and characterization.

Table 6.1 Brief description of different US modes and specific qualification for perforator assessment

Brief description of different US modes and specific qualification for perforator assessment	
B-mode	In B-mode (brightness mode), various acoustic impedances received from different tissue layers are displayed as a cross section of tissues. Each tissue layer interface has a particular echogenicity. Image display is composed of bright dots representing the US echoes. The brightness of each dot is determined by the amplitude of the returned echo signal. Basic US mode for tissue layer identification (e.g., deep fascia level)
Color-flow (CF)-mode	Color duplex = velocity information is presented as a color-coded overlay on top of a B-mode image in a color box. Technique estimates the average relative velocity of vascular flow by color-coding the information; the blood flow direction is expressed through color red or blue, indicating flow toward or away from the transducer. Different flow velocities may be compared with the color scale bar at the side of the screen; variable top velocities are defined by the examiner through the PRF (pulse-repetition frequency)/scale
Power Doppler (PD)-mode	Technique that utilizes the amplitude of Doppler signal to detect motion of particles. Independent of direction (no aliasing artifacts), single color not showing direction of flow. Independent of angle, allowing detection of smaller velocities than color Doppler, sensitivity is increased by factor 3–5x

(continued)

Table 6.1 (continued)

Brief description of different US modes and specific qualification for perforator assessment	
Pulse-wave (PW)-mode	Usually combined with B-mode image together with color Doppler. Measurements of hemodynamic parameters are displayed in a frequency spectrum with characteristic curves depending on the examined vessel. Doppler information is sampled from only a small sample volume placed inside the targeted vessel (defined in 2D image) and presented on a timeline in curves; different blood flow velocity parameters may be measured
B-flow	Digital subtraction mode which highlights weak flow reflectors (mainly red blood cells) and suppresses signals from the surrounding stationary tissues by subtraction of two serial pulse-echo cycles. Blood flow echoes are visualized, different gray intensities reflect speed and dynamics, and color enhancement with overlaying B-mode is possible. Advantages: High spatial resolution and relative independence from beam angle. Disadvantages: Imaging of flow direction and quantification of velocity are limited. Angiography-like, simultaneous imaging of slow- and high-flow vessels. B-flow is an alternative to Doppler ultrasound

6.3 Practical Methodology

6.3.1 Knobology of Ultrasound Machines

Before scanning patients, microsurgeons should become familiar with the specific knobology of the ultrasound device used. Although there is no real standard, different ultrasound devices usually feature quite similar ultrasound panels. Knobs, switches, and buttons to adjust parameters may be categorized into functional groups as well as fairly arranged in a rational chronological order:

1. **Pre-exam buttons**: patient data button, probe selection button (usually different linear and convex probes), and on-screen buttons for different program presets.
2. **Knobs to classify ultrasound findings for saved pictures**: body pattern ellipse and text editing button.
3. **Adjusting contrast, frequency, and focus**: time-gain-control (TGC) switches, gain of B-mode picture, automated contrast, focus, and frequency.
4. **Basic knobs, switches, and buttons used in every mode**: trackball, enter button, keyboard, depth, freeze, and save button (fixed images and cine loops).
5. **Mode-selection knobs and control dials**: B-mode, CF-mode, and PW-mode.
6. **Special sub-mode buttons**: PD-mode and B-flow.
7. **Knobs to adjust CF-mode image**: CF-mode frequency, color box size button, angular correction/steer for color box adjustment, invert, pulse-repetition frequency/scale, and CF-mode gain.
8. **Knobs to adjust PW-mode image**: sample volume adjustment, angular correction, pulse-repetition frequency/scale, baseline correction, invert, and freeze.
9. **Buttons for measurements**: measure, trackball, and enter.

Figure 6.1 illustrates the knobology of a typical ultrasound panel highlighting important features for microvessel assessment.

6.3.2 Selection of Transducer, Preset Programs, and Device Properties

The higher frequency and multifrequency linear probes, e.g., 6–15 MHz and up, show superior imaging qualities than the linear transducer with lower US frequencies. Selection of the "breast" or "thyroid" preset program provides the best overall contrast of the B-mode picture and optimized color-flow presettings for microvessel interpretation. Relevant settings to optimize the CF-mode image are adjustment of CF-mode frequency, pulse-repetition frequency (PRF)/scale, color gain, color box size, angular correction/steer for color box orientation, and usage of the invert button. Key steps to fine-tune PW-mode

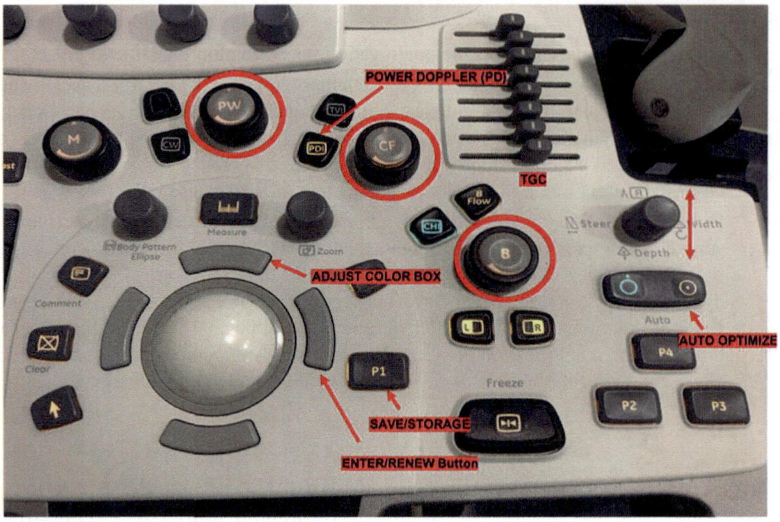

Fig. 6.1 Knobology of a standard ultrasound device panel. Many ultrasound devices share strong similarities of steering panels. Knobology of a standard ultrasound device panel is outlined for the microsurgeon. Less obvious but important buttons are illustrated for simplified usage. Different modes are indicated by red circles; power Doppler (PD) mode is initiated in color-flow (CF) mode. Time gain controls (TCG) may be all set in a middle position. Depth is varied by upper and lower lever actions (far right, up). The "Auto Optimize" button harmonizes image quality. The "Adjust Color Box" button changes the size of the color box in combination with the "Trackball." In pulse-wave (PW) mode, the "Enter/Renew" button starts/restarts flow velocity measurements. P1 may be programmed to save/store images (in freeze) or cine loops (in nonfrozen visualization)

image are sample volume adjustment, angular correction, pulse-repetition frequency/scale, and baseline correction. The renew calculation button, invert button, and switching on the automatic value calculation of the frozen image greatly help to speed up blood flow diagnostics, and the "Measure" button may be used to determine microvessel diameter. Inserting patient data before saving images/cine loops and adjusting body pattern pictograms and possibly text edit findings on the screen allow a subsequent interpretation of images later. Measurements in B-flow mode minimize the error of blooming artifacts with vessel wall overlap seen in CF-mode and overamplified vascular diameter in PD-mode.

6.3.3 General Considerations Before the CCDS Exam

A motivated perforator flap surgeon and basic knowledge about ultrasound device handling are needed. Start with thin patients and sufficient time. With an increasing level of experience, the examination may be performed in the OR immediately before patient preparation. Enough gel which may be pre-warmed, skin markers (different colors), and a 50–60-cm ruler are needed. Mapping procedures either confirm previously found vessels "on the table" or identify perforators from scratch. Device calibration with adequate settings through the following guiding principles and just little practice should also enable beginners of CCDS and less experienced microsurgeons to successfully achieve a level of expertise where "what you see is what you get intraoperatively."

If skin markings must be saved for the subsequent day or later they may be protected by transparent sticky foil. Prepping the patient using a non-alcohol, iodine-based scrub simplifies maintenance of markings before refreshing them on the table.

6.3.4 Improving Ergonomics for the Microsurgeon

Position yourself and ultrasound device on the same side next to the patient and dim room lighting. Imaging should be conducted on the patient side where the flap is planned. The examiner needs to learn to perform exams with either hand for a relaxed work posture. Always insert patient data and ID into system, save important images and videos (cine loops). Perform a pinch test to the patient's subcutaneous tissue layer to assess approximate thickness in cm. Strictly obey conventional directions of holding the probe: image screen orientation in a transverse probe position should be as in CT/MRI imaging. Axial slices of the patient are shown as looking toward the patient's head from the feet. Gently touching the edge of the probe after applying gel helps with orientation. In contrast, sagittal slices of longitudinal cuts are shown with the left of the screen displaying more proximal and the right more distal tissues in extremities. Use enough gel and place probe in full contact with the skin. Hold transducer between thumb and middle finger close to its end, and fixate against index and ring finger. Avoid compression disturbing blood flow. Resting the examiner's wrist on the patient's thigh helps to maneuvering with micro-movements. Use enough gel and place probe in full contact with the skin; have skin marker and cloth ready. Always slightly tilt probe. The ultrasound beam angle in relation to the focused level should be less than 90° for qualitative and less than 60° for quantitative evaluation for improved visualization and precise measurements (PW-mode). Before saving images, adjust body pattern ellipse pictogram and possibly text edit findings on the screen.

6.3.5 Importance of Practical Sequence and Structured Approach

A highly structured approach simplifies and shortens examination times decisively. Perforator evaluation should be performed the day before surgery and be repeated for verification on the operating table before preparation.

Each ultrasound mode should be adjusted and optimized individually with an identical sequence for efficiency. A systematic approach can be applied to all perforator flaps. Dermis and subcutaneous tissue may be assessed in various parts of the body to plan flaps providing different properties and tissue qualities regarding pliability, elasticity, and mechanical strength (Fig. 6.2). Examinations should be performed in double-imaging mode using overlaid B-mode and CCDS as a standard. Downregulation of pulse-repetition frequency (PRF)/scale to adapt device sensitivity to low blood flow velocities is mandatory to visualize microvessels. Switching to PW-mode should become a standard tool for vascular characterization. Acoustic Doppler signals and characteristic waveforms may clearly differentiate the vessel type. The endoluminal blood flow is displayed as spectral curves.

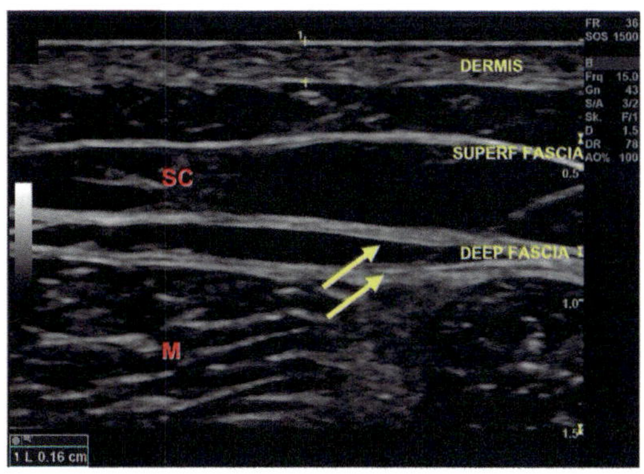

Fig. 6.2 Superficial brightness (B) mode scan of thigh tissues. Assessment of thigh tissues with a superficial high-resolution scan in B-mode. Morphology of skin, fascia, subcutaneous, and muscle tissues is depicted. The centimeter bar located at the right side of the screen helps in identification and distinction of tissue layers. Dermis and deep fascia are hyperechoic (bright). In between, fatty components of subcutaneous tissue appear less echoic (darker in comparison to dermis). Here in this skinny patient the deep fascia was found in a depth of less than 1 cm. The thickness of the dermis was determined with 1.6 mm using the measuring tool, setting two cursors (yellow crosses). Adipose lobules of the subcutaneous tissue (SC) are encompassed in ellipsoid frames of fibrous tissue representing the superficial fascia (SF). The SF may often be visualized as a bright band separating a more superficial from the deep adipose layer. It often shows various depth levels and separate layers. The deep fascia is identified as a thick hyperechoic (bright) stratum separating the subcutaneous layer from deeper muscle bellies. Here two separate laminae of the deep fascia may be distinguished (yellow arrows). Deep to the DF hypoechoic skeletal muscle appears dark, whereas intra- and intermuscular septa appear bright

6.3.6 Specific CCDS Device Settings for Perforator Mapping and Characterization

Examinations should start in B-mode and, following image improvement, should then be performed in double-imaging mode using overlaid B-mode and CCDS. Breast/vascular/thyroid preset programs will provide enhanced contrast of the B-mode picture and optimize color-flow presettings.

In B-mode, the morphology of skin, fascia, subcutaneous, and muscle tissues is depicted. Just deep to skin level, adipose components of subcutaneous tissue will appear iso- or slightly hyperechoic with skeletal muscle (both dark). In contrast, subcutaneous lobules of fatty tissue are encompassed in larger and thicker ellipsoid frames of fibrous tissue representing the superficial fascia. If identification of the deep fascia and muscle bellies is troublesome, the patient may be asked to activate his muscles causing muscle bellies appear more round than ellipsoid and gliding individually against each other. This will usually help for easier muscle belly distinction and identification of intermuscular septa. For instance, in planning ALT flaps, it appears useful to differentiate septal from intramuscular perforators. Flexing of the quadriceps muscle complex by the patient will cause the septum between rectus femoris and vastus lateralis change from an oblique to more vertical direction and simplifies its identification. Perforators may then be characterized to one of the two before mentioned categories accordingly.

Duplex mode is started by adding the color-flow (CF) mode. Optimization of device settings decisively increases image quality. Each mode has to be enhanced individually, e.g., upregulation of frequency.

Placing the field of view (FoV) over the targeted area shows the direction of flow. The FoV is a square color box in which all color Doppler information is displayed [64]. Size and location are adjustable, affecting image resolution and quality. It should be chosen rather small to maximize frame rate and usually tilted to a rhomboid using the "steer" button at an acute angle in relation to the vascular axis [68]. Thus, an angular correction (angle <60°) is granted for detection of low-flow vessels. The color visualizes blood flow direction in relation to the probe. Color intensity (or gain) reflects flow velocity [69]. Nuances may be compared with the color bar at the display's side. Pulse-repetition frequency (PRF/scale) or velocity range must be adjusted to present flow velocities. To detect microvessels featuring low velocities, 0.5–20 Hz is recommended [70]. Respectively, the adjusted flow velocity in the color bar at the side of the image should indicate values from 3 to 10 cm/s. If the velocity scale setting is lower than the arterial flow velocity, aliasing artifacts will be present. Multicolor aliasing artifacts are artificial flow reversals in a physiological vessel. Synchronous pulsatile flow with a corresponding vessel is typical for perforator architecture.

Color gain should then be set as high as possible without displaying too much background color noise or massive artifacts outside vessels [68]. It should be balanced avoiding an over- or underestimation of the diameter of perforators. Color-coding is red if flow is directed toward the transducer and blue away from it. If colors are shown reversed, an inverse/reverse button in the on-screen menu may be used for correction.

The wall filter (WF) eliminates low frequency noise that may arise from vessel wall motion below an operator-defined frequency threshold. WF settings are usually preset by manufacturer [68]. It may be linked to the focus function adjusting itself automatically with setting the focus depth. If flow is very low, a manual reduction of wall filter frequency (<20 Hz) or turning it off is recommended. The frame rate can be slightly lowered leading to a minored acquisition of images per time (<25 frames/s ideally) to increase sensitivity.

If small perforators are still difficult to detect, additional power Doppler (PD) application enhances sensitivity by a factor 3–5 [66]. Also, B-flow may be applied providing an angiography-like, simultaneous imaging of slow- and high-flow vessels. Color-coding B-flow is possible and features more graphic imaging. The advantage of B-flow is fully exploited when small superficial low-flow vessels and larger profound high-flow vessels should be visualized at the same time.

Figure 6.3 provides an image of a suprafascial perforator with correct color-coding extending from its emergence point up to the subdermal and intradermal plexus. An ultrahigh-resolution image of a is superficial perforating vessel is shown in Fig. 6.4.

Quantitative measurements of hemodynamic parameters, e.g., peak systolic and end diastolic velocity (PSV, EDV), are possible by application of PW-mode and positioning of the adaptable sample volume inside the target vessel. The endoluminal blood flow is displayed as spectral curves representing the hemodynamics depending on cardiac cycle in relation to time. Besides lowering the PRF/scale in order to measure low flow velocities, the baseline has to be set from a medium to slightly lowered level to depict the corresponding flow pattern. After placing the sample volume inside the vessel, it must be adapted to two thirds of the vascular diameter to obtain representable velocity values. A separate angle correction should always be adjusted by automation (pressing the automated button) first and then fine-tuning. Fine-tuning is possible through altering the adjustable line within the sample volume by turning the knob clock or

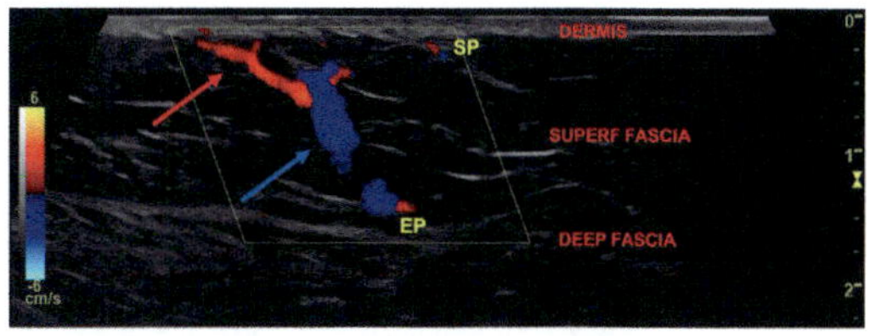

Fig. 6.3 Color-flow (CF) scan of a suprafascial perforator. CF image of a suprafascial perforator after consequent device trimming with a penetration depth of the scan of roughly 2 cm (note centimeter bar at right side of image). A high-quality visualization of the targeted microvessel allows for precise evaluation of the vascular architecture. Increasing frequency and lowering PRF/scale is mandatory to image low-flow microvessels as perforators. The adjusted blood flow velocity at the side of the image in the color bar in this example shows a range from—6 to 6 cm/s. Consecutively, the superficial low-flow perforator vessel could be imaged from its emergence point (EP) at the deep fascia level up to the subdermal plexus (SP) with CCDS at the same time. Color-flow artifacts outside an artery should be removed by decreasing the gain. The perforator artery (red) may be differentiated from the vein (blue arrow). Even arterial subbranches (red arrow) to the subdermal plexus are visualizable. Duplex sonography; *CF* color flow, *PRF* pulse-repetition frequency

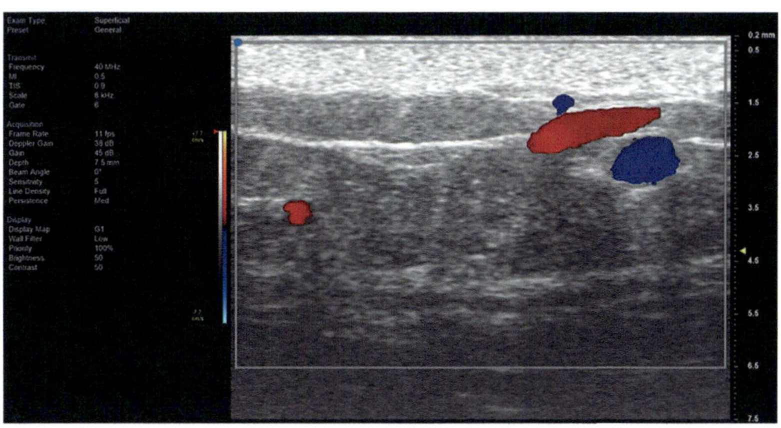

Fig. 6.4 Ultrahigh-resolution image of superficial perforating vessel (CF-mode). Ultrasound devices with high-resolution transducers are capable of visualizing smallest microvessels at very superficial tissue levels. Using a 48-MHz transducer, the penetration depth of this scan was set at 7.5 mm. Superficial arterial and venous branches of a perforator are visualized in the upper right aspect of the image in a depth of about 2 mm. Thickness of the epidermis and dermis may be assessed with about 1.5 mm. Flap design of capillary and pure dermal flaps may be executed with an ultrahigh-resolution approach. (Image courtesy of Prof. Akitatsu Hayashi, Director of Kameda Lymphedema Center, Kameda-honchō, Japan)

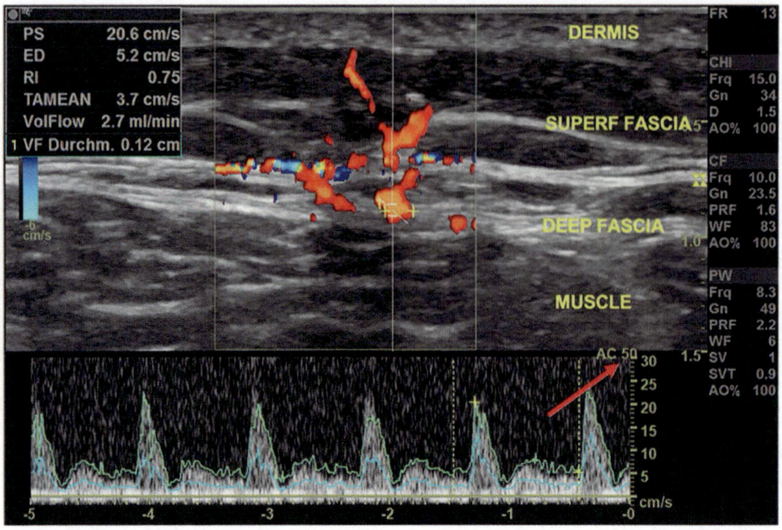

Fig. 6.5 Pulse-wave (PW) mode for quantitative evaluation of perforator blood flow. Measuring quantitative parameters in perforators helps to gain a better understanding of the physiology of perforator flaps. In this image, a perforator microvessel with several subbranches is visualized taking its course from the deep fascia to the subdermal plexus. PW-mode was used to determine flow characteristics. The characteristic monophasic waveform (lower part of image) of an arterial perforator may be perceived. After adjustment of the sample volume to about two thirds of the vascular diameter, a fine-trim of the angular correction was manually performed to 50° (red arrow). A pulse systolic velocity (PS) of 20.6 cm/s was measured. Additionally, the perforator's diameter was measured at the level of the deep fascia with 1.2 mm, deeming it suitable to base a perforator flap on it. If raised at the deep fascia level, the flap's thickness will be just about 1 cm in this patient, as to be noted from the cm bar at the right side of the image (deep fascia at 1 cm depth)

counterclockwise. The sample volume's line should roughly follow the vessel's direction by adaptation of the angle for correct parameter measurements to <60°. For precise velocity measurements, the selected angle displayed should be <50°. The number of the angle usually turns from red to green when realistic angles are fine-tuned. Figure 6.5 shows how PW-mode is employed to scrutinize a perforator vessel regarding hemodynamic values and diameter (Fig. 6.5).

6.3.7 CCDS Settings for Vascular Diameter Measurements

Sizable perforators were defined as ≥0.5 mm in diameter. With present technology in the 6–15 MHz range, any perforator detected with CCDS should be eligible for a respective perforator flap design. Using the measurement tool lets the examiner position two cursors at the vascular boundaries of the targeted microvessel. Placing the measuring points, the "leading-to-leading edge" method should be used [71]. Adjusting depth and magnification may help to increase precision. Measurements in B-flow mode minimize the error of blooming artifacts with vessel wall overlap seen in CF-mode and overamplified vascular diameter in PD-mode.

6.4 Step-by-Step Approach: A Useful Sequence for a Structured Perforator Mapping and Characterization

Color-coded duplex sonography (CCDS) has proven to be a powerful tool for preoperative perforator characterization when using a structured approach and mapping algorithm [9, 11].

Any operation starts with a mapping procedure either confirming previously found vessels "on the table" or identifying perforators from scratch. Perform a pinch test to assess thickness of skin and subcutaneous tissue layer. Tissue morphology of skin, fascia, subcutaneous, and muscle tissues is always assessed first. Apply moderate pressure on probe not to compromise perforator flow for better identification.

1. Start in B-mode, appreciation of different tissue layers, and identification of deep fascia.
2. Add CF-mode, and locate perforator(s) at deep fascia level. Change to PD-mode if small vessels are to be traced in very superficial levels. Assess infra- and suprafascial vascular course. Store cine loops.
3. Start PW-mode to verify an arterial signal. Measure PSV and ED at the deep fascia level or close to it. Angular correction <50° for realistic measurements. Store frozen images containing nominal values.
4. Return to CF-mode. Then switch to B-Flow. Freeze. Measure diameter of perforators at EP. Store pictures.
5. Take note of qualitative and quantitative perforator characteristics. Skin mark EP(s). May additionally label skin markings with quantitative values (e.g., PSV and diameter).

Figure 6.6 provides a useful strategy on how to perform a fluent ultrasound examination employing different modes in a logical sequence.

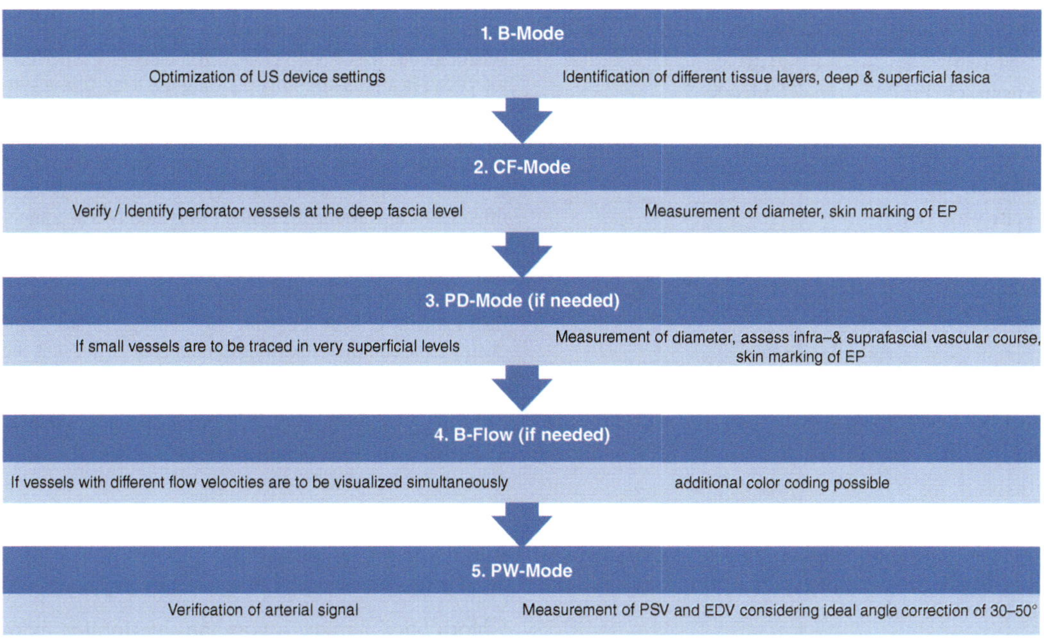

Fig. 6.6 Structured approach using different ultrasound (US) modes for perforator evaluation. Algorithm of a sequential structured usage of different ultrasound (US) modes for perforator mapping. To enjoy US examination, the microsurgeon needs only little training, which may be acquired through basic ultrasound courses focused on the vascular system. A highly structured approach simplifies and shortens the US examination decisively. Each US mode should be adjusted and optimized individually with an identical sequence for efficiency, e.g., setting of frequency and gain in B- and CF-modes. A useful sequence is as follows: (1) Start in B-mode, appreciation of different tissue layers, identification of deep fascia. *B* brightness. (2) Add CF-mode, and locate perforator(s) at the deep fascia level. Measure the diameter of perforators at EP. Change to PD-mode if small vessels are to be traced in very superficial levels. Assess infra- and suprafascial vascular course. Store cine loops. *CF* color flow, *EP* emergence point, *PD* power Doppler. (3) Start PW-mode to verify an arterial signal. Measure PSV and ED at the deep fascia level or close to it. Angular correction <50° for realistic measurements. Store frozen images containing nominal values. *ED* end diastolic, *PSV* peak systolic velocity, *PW* pulse wave. (4) Return to CF-mode. If desired, switch to B-flow or color-coded B-flow. Freeze. Store pictures. *CF* color flow. (5) Take note of qualitative and quantitative perforator characteristics. Skin mark EP(s). May additionally label skin markings with quantitative values (e.g., PSV and diameter). *EP* emergence point, *PSV* peak systolic velocity

Table 6.2 provides data of suitable CCDS settings for microvessel detection and assessment. With most of the devices and transducers, the ideal settings should be in the range or close to the range of values presented (Table 6.2). Fig. 6.7 shows a deep color-flow (CF) scan of thigh tissues.

Table 6.2 CCDS settings for microvessel detection and assessment

Quantitative characterization	
B-mode (B)	
Probe selection	Linear (optimal 15 MHz)
Frequency (Frq)	15 MHz
Gain (Gn)	25–35 dB
Depth (D)	2–3 cm
Focus	1–2 cm
Color flow (CF)	
Wall filter (WF)	Minimum
Gain (Gn)	10–20 dB
Frequency (Frq)	5–7.5 MHz
PRS/scale	5–9 cm/s

Qualitative characterization	
Pulse wave (PW)	
Frequency (Frq)	6.3 MHz
Gain (Gn)	30–35 dB
Wall filter (WF)	100–200 Hz
PRS/scale	6–12 cm/s

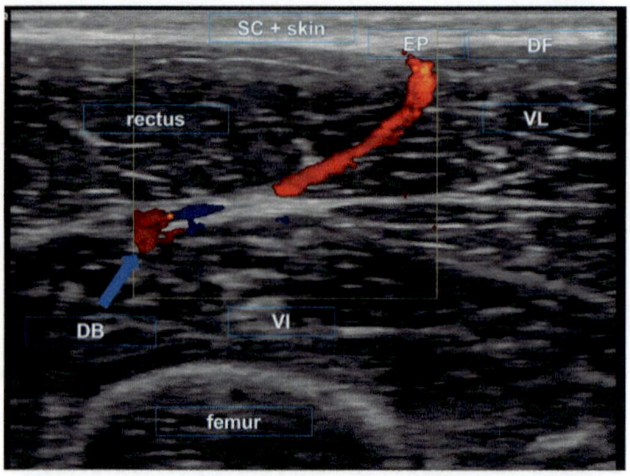

Fig. 6.7 Deep color-flow (CF) scan of thigh tissues. Deep scan with a 15-MHz probe in CF-mode: hemodynamic and morphological information gained by a transverse scan of the thigh depicting the perforator topography of an ALT flap. The B-mode picture displays femur with cortical hyperechogenicity, vastus intermedius (VI), rectus femoris, vastus lateralis (VL) with a separation of both by the intramuscular septum, deep fascia (DF), skin, and subcutaneous tissue (SC) clearly. Indicative for a perforator vessel is a pulsatile flow piercing the deep fascia synchronous with the DB (descending branch) as shown in the figure. In the left aspect of the duplex window frame, the arterial and venous anatomy of the DB of the lateral circumflex femoral artery (LCFA) is visualized. It is identified featuring a pulsatile center artery and two accompanying veins. The DB is sending off a septal perforator, which runs exactly in between muscle bellies of rectus femoris (recuts) and vastus lateralis (VL) toward the deep fascia and the emergence point (EP). This perforator demonstrated a complete extra-muscular course through the intermuscular septum which was confirmed upon microsurgical dissection. Note the short segment of the perforator lateral of the DB missing in this visualization, because it is located in a different plane than this transverse cut

6.5 Conclusion

Color-coded duplex sonography perforator mapping and evaluation enhances the microsurgeon's ability to design and elevate flaps by capturing dominant vessels and maximizing flap survival. It is a reliable and easy tool which can be used to make the planning of perforator flaps safer. Specific ultrasound device trimming for low-flow detection is required and decisively enhances sensitivity for microvessel imaging. Conducted by microsurgeons trained in CCDS, more sophisticated thin perforator flaps and multiple skin island chimeric perforator flaps are simplified and open to a greater number of microsurgeons [72–76].

6.6 Design of Perforator Flaps

6.6.1 Case Examples

The following examples of patients receiving different free tissue transfers illustrate the design of perforator flap reconstructions using a CCDS approach.

1. Head and neck ALT flap reconstruction: a 55-year-old female suffered from a temporal and galeal defect of 13 × 8 cm involving the skull after resection of an orbital fibroma with subsequent radiation therapy. In another hospital, several reconstructive operations also had failed with a titanium mesh implantation, tissue expansion, and necessary explanation of foreign material due to infection. Several attempts at placement of titanium mesh plates resulted in recurrent infection requiring subsequent removal of hardware. Failed tissue expansion resulted from infected expanders and device removal. A duplex ultrasound-guided ALT flap reconstruction was planned. The patient did not wish another alloplastic implant. Figure 6.8 shows the reconstructive planning for defect reconstruction before flap transfer to the superficial temporal vessels. Perforator mapping on CCDS examination detected three suitable ALT perforators. Figure 6.8 also demonstrates the exact intra-

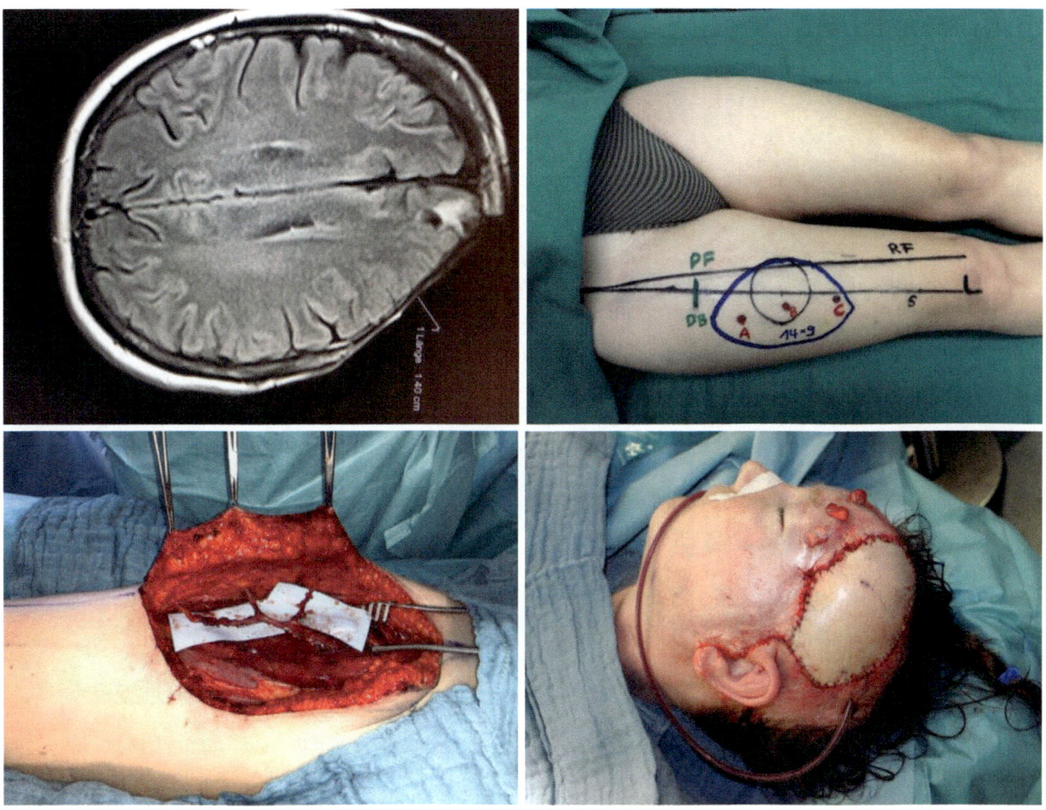

Fig. 6.8 Preoperative ultrasound-guided ALT flap planning. Upper left: CT scan of the defect demonstrates a bony gap of several centimeters as well as the depth of the defect. Upper right: ultrasound-guided ALT flap planning involves marking the RF and septum line as well as marking suitable perforators at their emergence point on the thigh. In this case, A, B, and C perforators were detected, and the template was marked in reference. DB marks the exit point of the descending branch (DB) of the LCFA stemming from the profunda femoral (PF) artery making an estimation of the anticipated length of flap pedicle possible. Lower left: intraoperative view of the respective three perforators in correspondence with skin markings. Lower right: ALT flap after inset at the end of the operation

operative correspondence with preoperative markings.

2. Upper extremity ALT flap reconstruction: a 25-year-old male was involved in a rollover vehicle accident as a passenger with composite soft tissue loss of his lower arm including fracture of distal radius, ulnar, and multiple carpal fractures. Through components of friction burn, avulsion, and crush injury, the patient demonstrated substantial loss of flexor carpi radialis (FCR), abductor pollicis longus (APL), and extensor pollicis brevis (EPB) tendon substance, palmar fascicles of median nerve, complete rupture of the radial artery, and a 30 cm × 9 cm defect of the soft tissue envelope. Following two debridements, reconstruction was planned with ultrasound-guided perforator mapping involving a thin two-perforator ALT flap. Further reconstructive steps included two tendon grafts solidified by doubling of contralateral plantaris and palmaris tendons, arterial vessel graft of the distal LCFA, and a total of six cable grafts of contralateral sural nerve in a single operation (Fig. 6.9).
3. Lower extremity ALT flap reconstruction—ALT flap design for Achilles tendon repair + fascia legend: a 72-year-old lady with multi-

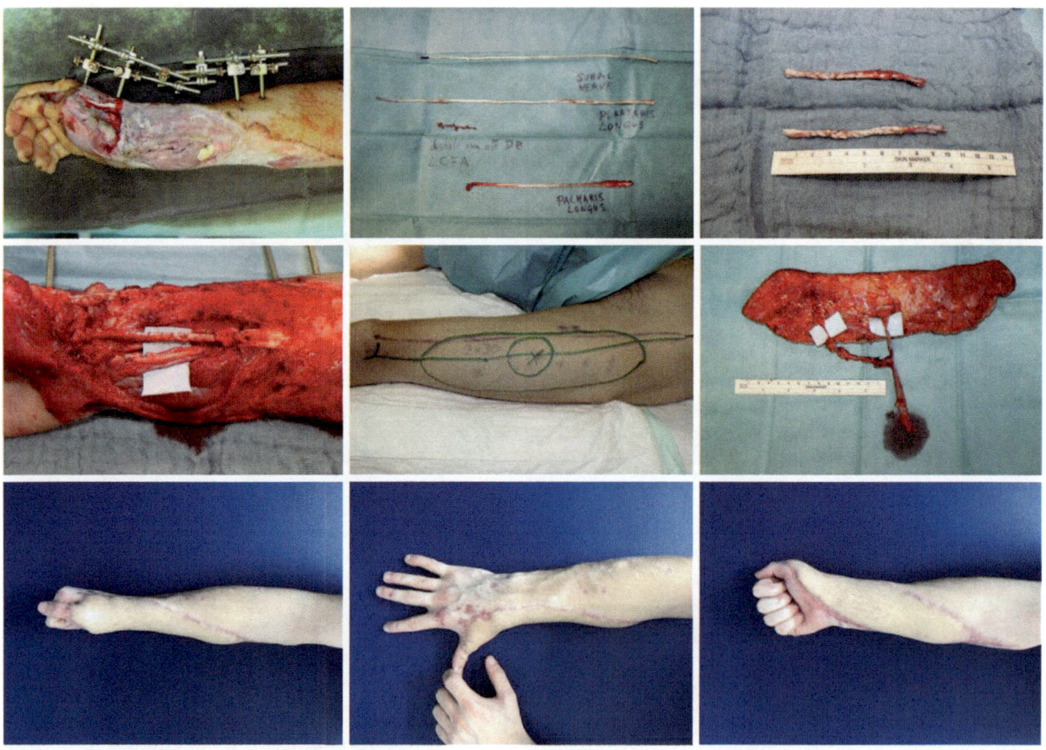

Fig. 6.9 Complex upper extremity reconstruction using preoperative ultrasound-guided ALT flap planning. **Upper left**: the image demonstrates the composite full-thickness soft tissue loss. Defect size measured 30 × 9 cm. The complex character of the injury involved a substantial loss of FCR and APL/EPB tendon substance, palmar fascicles of median nerve, and a complete rupture of the radial artery accompanied by a 30 × 9 cm defect of the soft tissue envelope. **Upper middle**: different components for defect reconstruction were harvested—sural nerve for median nerve reconstruction, palmaris and plantaris longus tendon for EPB and FCR tendon grafting, and distal LCFA for bridging the gap of the radial artery. **Upper right**: contralateral plantaris and palmaris tendon grafts were solidified by doubling. **Middle left**: a total of six cable grafts were used to reconstruct the median nerve defect. **Middle middle**: an ultrasound-guided ALT flap planning was chosen for coverage of the wrist and carpal joint spanning defect. **Middle right**: a two-perforator ALT flap was chosen for coverage of the wrist and carpal joint spanning defect. **Low left, middle, and right**: the thin ALT flap provided good coverage and elastic properties for the joint spanning defect. An extensor indicis transfer still has to be planned

ple comorbidities, including peripheral vascular disease, liver cirrhosis, and kidney failure, was suffering from a complete loss of about 8-cm Achilles tendon combined with 14 × 7 cm skin defect secondary to degenerative rupture, initial repair, re-rupture, and soft tissue infection. The defect reconstruction was planned with a modified Silfverskiöld repair [72] of the tendon combined with a chimeric musculocutaneous ALT flap design for dead space obliteration. The chimeric design was simplified by easy ALT-perforator selection and inclusion of a muscle component of vastus lateralis. Four months post-op, the lady could demonstrate standing on her toes with intact tendon function (Fig. 6.10).

4. A 55-year-old gentleman suffered from a melanoma formation of the plantar area (Fig. 6.11).
5. Soft tissue loss by a motorbike accident of a 17-year-old female ballet dancer (Fig. 6.12).
6. Obese patient with an extensive soft tissue defect of the dorsum of the foot. It resulted after a consequent debridement following a soft tissue infection with necrotizing fasciitis (Fig. 6.13).

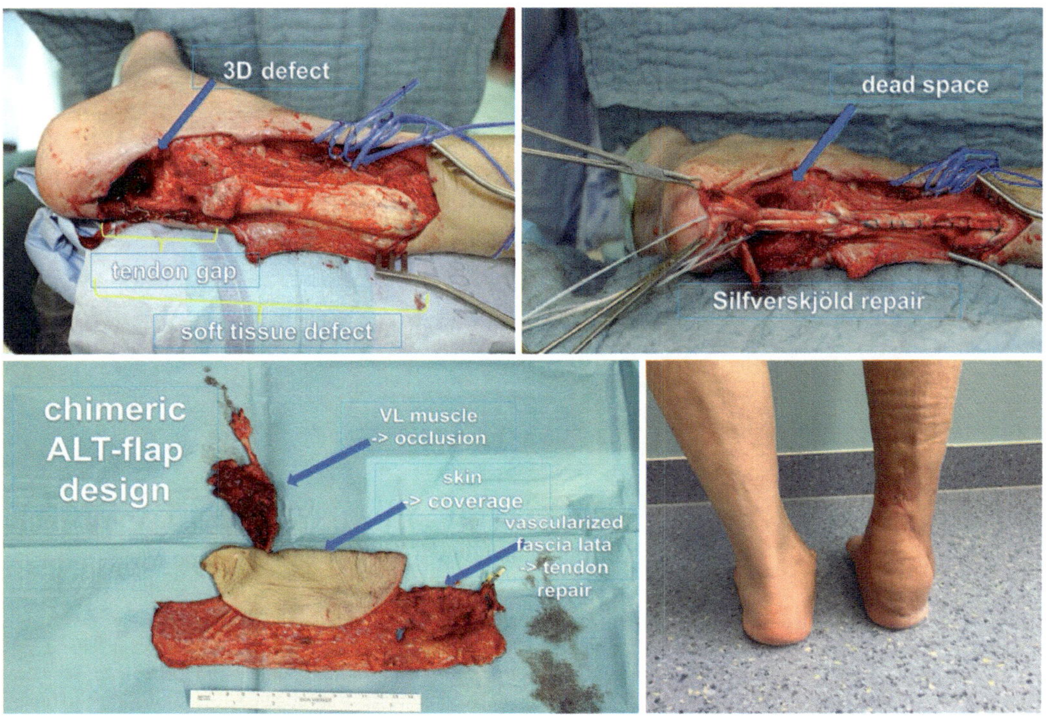

Fig. 6.10 Ultrasound-guided chimeric ALT flap design for Achilles tendon reconstruction. This patient demonstrated a complete loss of 8-cm Achilles tendon combined with 14 cm × 7 cm skin defect and severe comorbidities (upper left). Upper right: the tendon gap was reconstructed with a modified Silfverskiöld repair [72] and subsequently solidified with ALT fascia/vascularized fascia lata. Lower left: a chimeric ALT flap design was chosen with an inclusion of vascularized fascia, a VL muscle component for dead space occlusion, and a fasciocutaneous flap element for final coverage. Anterior tibial vessels were used as recipient vessels. Lower right: adequate flap cosmesis is seen 4 months post-op. The patient could demonstrate standing on her toes with intact tendon function

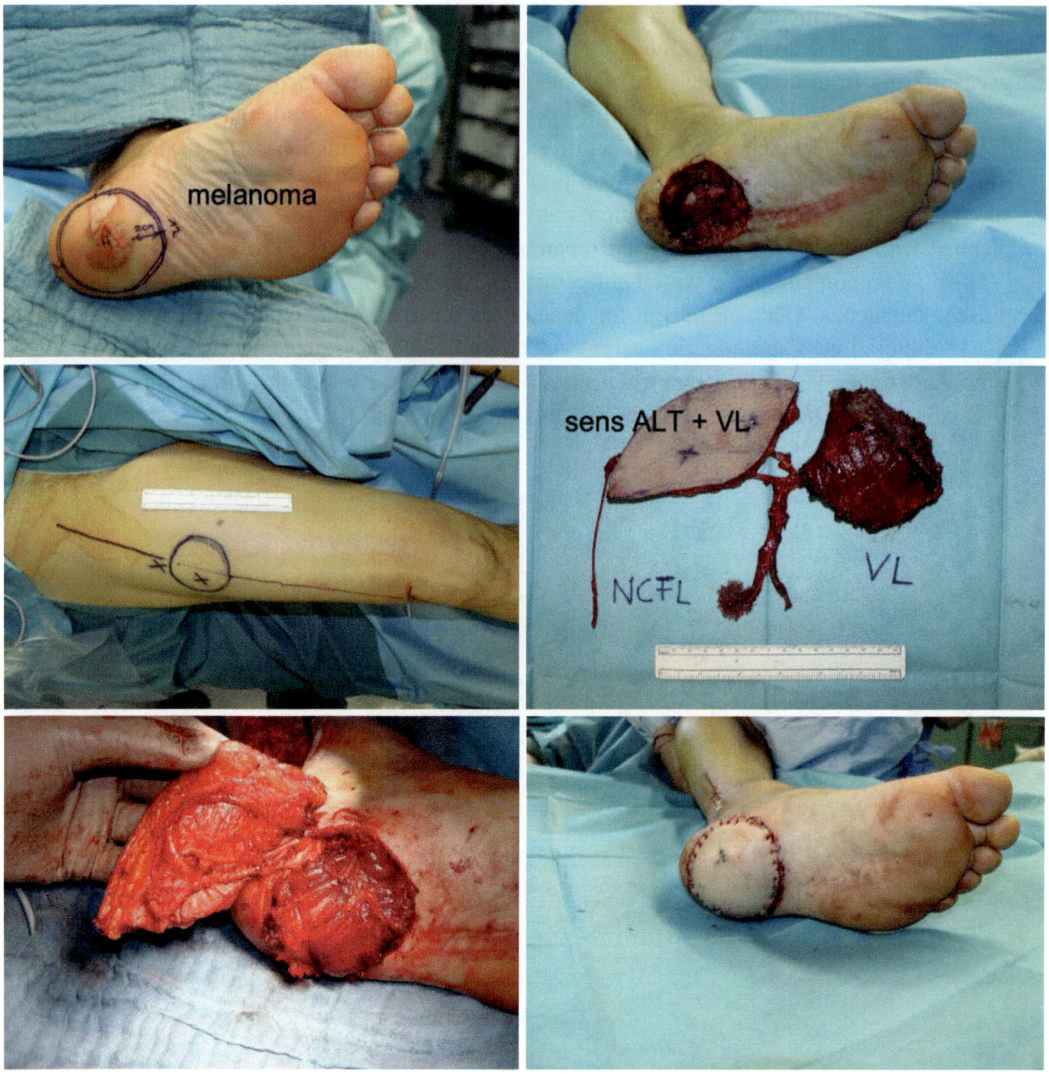

Fig. 6.11 Sensate ALT flap design with ultrasound planning for reconstruction of sole of the foot. Upper left: melanoma of the weight-bearing area of the left heal. Upper right: wide excision resulted in a 7.5 × 7.5 × 3 cm three-dimensional soft tissue defect. Middle left: a sensate chimeric ALT flap featuring a VL muscle component was planned with CCDS. Lower left: VL muscle was used to obliterate the defect. The sensate ALT skin island was used for skin coverage. The branch of the lateral femoral cutaneous nerve was coapted to a skin branch. Lower right: final result of the flap coverage

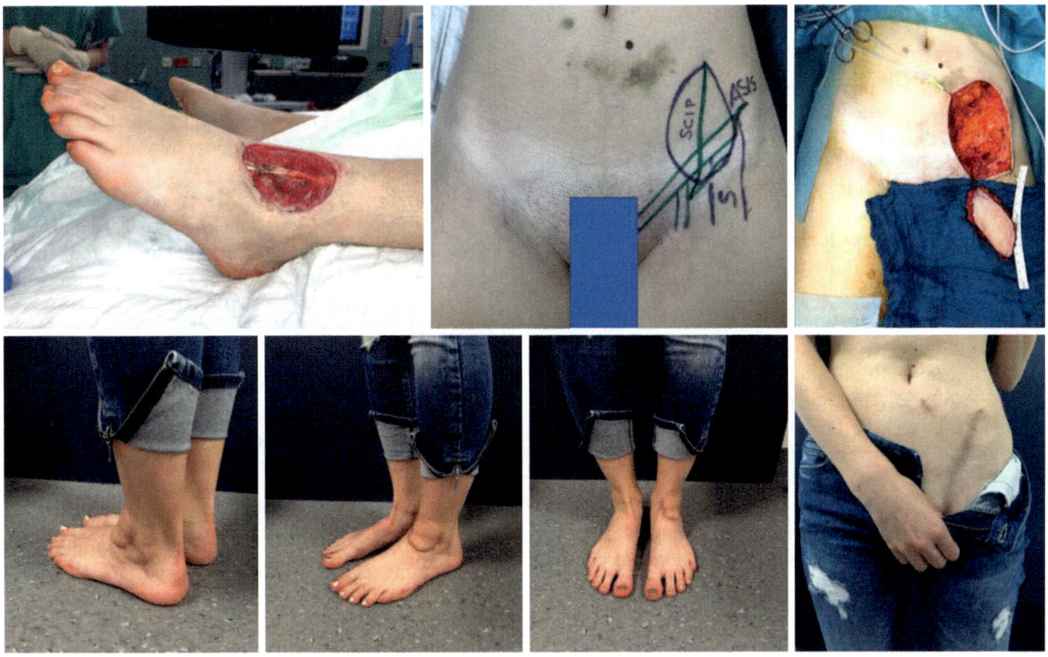

Fig. 6.12 Simplified design of superficial circumflex iliac artery (SCIP) perforator flap with US. Upper left: soft tissue defect anteriorly of left ankle joint with exposed tendons. Upper middle: planning of a superficial circumflex iliac artery (SCIP) perforator flap in the groin region. Upper right: situation after harvest of the tissue transfer at the level of the superficial fascia. Lower three left images: the thin tissue properties of the SCIP flap achieved a pleasing function and cosmesis reconstructing well the contour of the thin tissue envelope of distal lower limb. Lower far right: the harvesting site is inconspicuously positioned and covered well by regular clothing

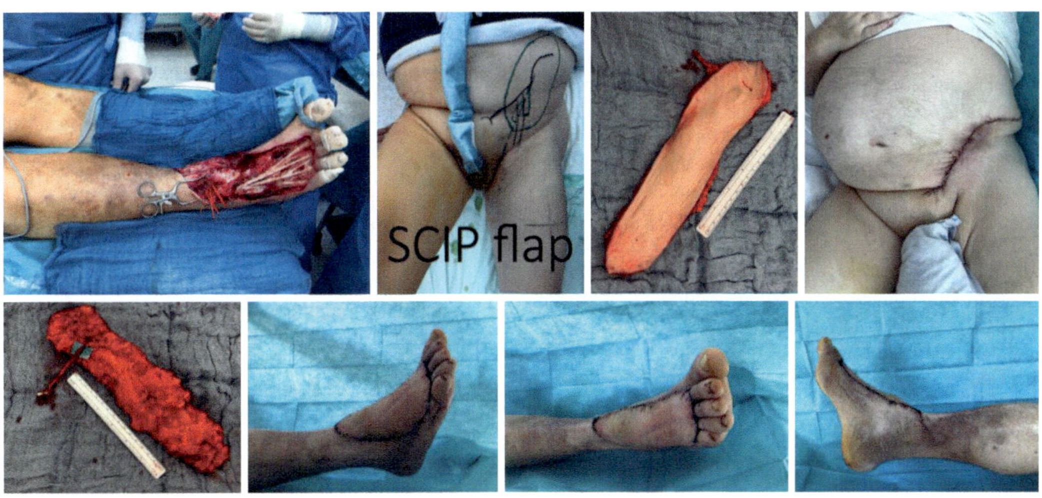

Fig. 6.13 Thin SCIP flap planned with color-coded duplex sonography (CCDS) in an obese patient. Upper left: soft tissue defect with exposed extensor tendons. Upper middle two images: a thin SCIP flap from the left groin and lower abdominal area was designed with CCDS. Upper right: primary closure of the harvesting site was possible. Lower left: SCIP flap before transfer. Lower three right images: the SCIP flap featured thin tissue properties and adequate contour restoration

References

1. Kehrer ASN, Platz Batista da Silva N, Jung EM, Prantl L, Hong JP. Step by step guide to ultrasound based design of ALT flaps by the microsurgeon—device settings and application. In: American Society of Reconstructive Microsurgery (ASRM); Palm Desert, CA, USA. 2019.
2. Kroll SS, Rosenfield L. Perforator-based flaps for low posterior midline defects. Plast Reconstr Surg. 1988;81(4):561–6.
3. Koshima I, Soeda S. Inferior epigastric artery skin flaps without rectus abdominis muscle. Br J Plast Surg. 1989;42(6):645–8.
4. Yu P, Youssef A. Efficacy of the handheld Doppler in preoperative identification of the cutaneous perforators in the anterolateral thigh flap. Plast Reconstr Surg. 2006;118(4):928–33. discussion 34–5.
5. Ensat F, Babl M, Conz C, Rueth MJ, Greindl M, Fichtl B, et al. The efficacy of color duplex sonography in preoperative assessment of anterolateral thigh flap. Microsurgery. 2012;32(8):605–10.
6. Rozen WM, Anavekar NS, Ashton MW. Magnetic resonance angiography in preoperative planning of deep inferior epigastric artery perforator flaps. J Plast Reconstr Aesthet Surg. 2010;63(1):e120–1.
7. Wong C, Nagarkar P, Teotia S, Haddock NT. The Profunda artery perforator flap: investigating the perforasome using three-dimensional computed tomographic angiography. Plast Reconstr Surg. 2015;136(5):915–9.
8. Newman TM, Vasile J, Levine JL, Greenspun DT, Allen RJ, Chao MT, et al. Perforator flap magnetic resonance angiography for reconstructive breast surgery: a review of 25 deep inferior epigastric and gluteal perforator artery flap patients. J Magn Reson Imaging. 2010;31(5):1176–84.
9. Cina A, Salgarello M, Barone-Adesi L, Rinaldi P, Bonomo L. Planning breast reconstruction with deep inferior epigastric artery perforating vessels: multidetector CT angiography versus color Doppler US. Radiology. 2010;255(3):979–87.
10. Su W, Lu L, Lazzeri D, Zhang YX, Wang D, Innocenti M, et al. Contrast-enhanced ultrasound combined with three-dimensional reconstruction in preoperative perforator flap planning. Plast Reconstr Surg. 2013;131(1):80–93.
11. Onoda S, Azumi S, Hasegawa K, Kimata Y. Preoperative identification of perforator vessels by combining MDCT, Doppler flowmetry, and ICG fluorescent angiography. Microsurgery. 2013;33(4):265–9.
12. Sheena Y, Jennison T, Hardwicke JT, Titley OG. Detection of perforators using thermal imaging. Plast Reconstr Surg. 2013;132(6):1603–10.
13. Phillips BT, Munabi NC, Roeder RA, Ascherman JA, Guo L, Zenn MR. The role of intraoperative perfusion assessment: what is the current state and how can I use it in my practice? Plast Reconstr Surg. 2016;137(2):731–41.
14. de Weerd L, Mercer JB, Setsa LB. Intraoperative dynamic infrared thermography and free-flap surgery. Ann Plast Surg. 2006;57(3):279–84.
15. Wong C, Nagarkar P, Teotia S, Haddock N. The Profunda artery perforator flap: investigating the perforasome using 3D CT angiography. Plast Reconstr Surg. 2015;136:915.
16. Pappalardo M, Jeng SF, Sadigh PL, Shih HS. Versatility of the free anterolateral thigh flap in the reconstruction of large defects of the weight-bearing foot: a single-center experience with 20 consecutive cases. J Reconstr Microsurg. 2016;32(7):562–70.
17. Hallock GG. Attributes and shortcomings of acoustic Doppler sonography in identifying perforators for flaps from the lower extremity. J Reconstr Microsurg. 2009;25(6):377–81.
18. Saito A, Furukawa H, Hayashi T, Oyama A, Funayama E, Yamamoto Y. Intraoperative color Doppler sonography in the elevation of anterolateral thigh flap. Microsurgery. 2011;31(7):582–3.
19. Brenner DJ, Hall EJ. Computed tomography—an increasing source of radiation exposure. N Engl J Med. 2007;357(22):2277–84.
20. Kooiman J, Le Haen PA, Gezgin G, de Vries JP, Boersma D, Brulez HF, et al. Contrast-induced acute kidney injury and clinical outcomes after intra-arterial and intravenous contrast administration: risk comparison adjusted for patient characteristics by design. Am Heart J. 2013;165(5):793–9. 9 e1
21. Tashiro K, Yamashita S, Araki J, Narushima M, Iida T, Koshima I. Preoperative color Doppler ultrasonographic examination in the planning of thoracodorsal artery perforator flap with capillary perforators. J Plast Reconstr Aesthet Surg. 2016;69(3):346–50.
22. Tsukino A, Kurachi K, Inamiya T, Tanigaki T. Preoperative color Doppler assessment in planning of anterolateral thigh flaps. Plast Reconstr Surg. 2004;113(1):241–6.
23. Cheng HT, Lin FY, Chang SC. Diagnostic efficacy of color Doppler ultrasonography in preoperative assessment of anterolateral thigh flap cutaneous perforators: an evidence-based review. Plast Reconstr Surg. 2013;131(3):471e–3e.
24. Cheng HT, Lin FY, Chang SC. Diagnostic efficacy of preoperative 64-section multidetector computed tomographic angiography in identifying the cutaneous perforators in the anterolateral thigh flap: an evidence-based review. Plast Reconstr Surg. 2012;130(5):771e–2e.
25. Cheng HT, Lin FY, Chang SC. Evaluation of diagnostic accuracy using preoperative handheld Doppler in identifying the cutaneous perforators in the anterolateral thigh flap: a systematic review. Plast Reconstr Surg. 2012;129(4):769e–70e.
26. Thomas B, Warszawski J, Falkner F, Nagel SS, Schmidt VJ, Kneser U, et al. A comparative study of preoperative color-coded Duplex ultrasonography versus handheld audible Dopplers in ALT flap planning. Microsurgery. 2020;40(5):561–7.
27. Kehrer A, Hsu MY, Chen YT, Sachanandani NS, Tsao CK. Simplified profunda artery perforator (PAP) flap

design using power Doppler ultrasonography (PDU): a prospective study. Microsurgery. 2018;38(5):512–23.
28. Visconti G, Hayashi A, Bianchi A, Salgarello M. Technological advances in lymphatic surgery: the emerging role of ultrasound. Plast Reconstr Surg. 2019;144:940e.
29. Visconti G, Bianchi A, Hayashi A, Salgarello M. Pure skin perforator flap direct elevation above the subdermal plane using preoperative ultra-high frequency ultrasound planning: a proof of concept. J Plast Reconstr Aesthet Surg. 2019;72:1700.
30. Hayashi A, Giacalone G, Yamamoto T, Belva F, Visconti G, Hayashi N, et al. Ultra high-frequency ultrasonographic imaging with 70 MHz scanner for visualization of the lymphatic vessels. Plast Reconstr Surg Glob Open. 2019;7(1):e2086.
31. Schwabegger AH, Bodner G, Rieger M, Jaschke WR, Ninkovic MM. Internal mammary vessels as a model for power Doppler imaging of recipient vessels in microsurgery. Plast Reconstr Surg. 1999;104(6):1656–65.
32. Feng S, Min P, Grassetti L, Lazzeri D, Sadigh P, Nicoli F, et al. A prospective head-to-head comparison of color Doppler ultrasound and computed tomographic angiography in the preoperative planning of lower extremity perforator flaps. Plast Reconstr Surg. 2016;137(1):335–47.
33. Gravvanis A, Karakitsos D, Dimitriou V, Zogogiannis I, Katsikeris N, Karabinis A, et al. Portable duplex ultrasonography: a diagnostic and decision-making tool in reconstructive microsurgery. Microsurgery. 2010;30(5):348–53.
34. Dorfman D, Pu LL. The value of color duplex imaging for planning and performing a free anterolateral thigh perforator flap. Ann Plast Surg. 2014;72(Suppl 1):S6–8.
35. Debelmas A, Camuzard O, Aguilar P, Qassemyar Q. Reliability of color Doppler ultrasound imaging for the assessment of anterolateral thigh flap perforators: a prospective study of 30 perforators. Plast Reconstr Surg. 2018;141(3):762–6.
36. Gravvanis A, Petrocheilou G, Tsoutsos D, Delikonstantinou I, Karakitsos D. Integrating imaging techniques in lower limb microsurgical reconstruction: focusing on ultrasonography versus computed tomography angiography. In Vivo. 2013;27(3):371–5.
37. Fernandez-Riera R, Hung SY, Wu JC, Tsao CK. Free profunda femoris artery perforator flap as a first-line choice of reconstruction for partial glossectomy defects. Head Neck. 2017;39(4):737–43.
38. Rafailidis V, Sidhu PS. Vascular ultrasound, the potential of integration of multiparametric ultrasound into routine clinical practice. Ultrasound. 2018;26(3):136–44.
39. Rubenthaler J, Reiser M, Clevert DA. Diagnostic vascular ultrasonography with the help of color Doppler and contrast-enhanced ultrasonography. Ultrasonography. 2016;35(4):289–301.
40. Kehrer A, Sachanadani NS, da Silva NPB, Lonic D, Heidekrueger P, Taeger CD, et al. Step-by-step guide to ultrasound-based design of alt flaps by the microsurgeon—basic and advanced applications and device settings. J Plast Reconstr Aesthet Surg. 2020;73(6):1081–90.
41. Hong JP, Choi DH, Suh H, Mukarramah DA, Tashti T, Lee K, et al. A new plane of elevation: the superficial fascial plane for perforator flap elevation. J Reconstr Microsurg. 2014;30(7):491–6.
42. Hong JP, Chung IW. The superficial fascia as a new plane of elevation for anterolateral thigh flaps. Ann Plast Surg. 2013;70(2):192–5.
43. Kehrer A, Hsu MY, Chen YT, Sachanandani NS, Tsao CK. Simplified profunda artery perforator (PAP) flap design using power Doppler ultrasonography (PDU): a prospective study. Microsurgery. 2017;38:512.
44. Kehrer A, Heidekrueger PI, Lonic D, Taeger CD, Klein S, Lamby P, et al. High-resolution ultrasound-guided perforator mapping and characterization by the microsurgeon in lower limb reconstruction. J Reconstr Microsurg. 2020;37:75.
45. Rubino C, Coscia V, Cavazzuti AM, Canu V. Haemodynamic enhancement in perforator flaps: the inversion phenomenon and its clinical significance. A study of the relation of blood velocity and flow between pedicle and perforator vessels in perforator flaps. J Plast Reconstr Aesthet Surg. 2006;59(6):636–43.
46. Lin CT, Huang JS, Hsu KC, Yang KC, Chen JS, Chen LW. Different types of suprafascial courses in thoracodorsal artery skin perforators. Plast Reconstr Surg. 2008;121(3):840–8.
47. Alzaraa A, Gravante G, Chung WY, Al-Leswas D, Morgan B, Dennison A, et al. Contrast-enhanced ultrasound in the preoperative, intraoperative and postoperative assessment of liver lesions. Hepatol Res. 2013;43(8):809–19.
48. Hallock GG. Doppler sonography and color duplex imaging for planning a perforator flap. Clin Plast Surg. 2003;30(3):347–57.
49. Suh HS, Oh TS, Lee HS, Lee SH, Cho YP, Park JR, et al. A new approach for reconstruction of diabetic foot wounds using the angiosome and supermicrosurgery concept. Plast Reconstr Surg. 2016;138(4):702e–9e.
50. Song S, Jeong HH, Lee Y, Powers H, Suh YC, Christoffi P, et al. Direction of flap rotation in propeller flaps: does it really matter? J Reconstr Microsurg. 2019;35(8):549–56.
51. Kehrer A, Mandlik V, Taeger C, Geis S, Prantl L, Jung EM. Postoperative control of functional muscle flaps for facial palsy reconstruction: ultrasound guided tissue monitoring using contrast enhanced ultrasound (CEUS) and ultrasound elastography. Clin Hemorheol Microcirc. 2017;67(3–4):435–44.
52. Oni G, Chow W, Ramakrishnan V, Griffiths M. Plastic surgeon-led ultrasound. Plast Reconstr Surg. 2018;141(2):300e–9e.
53. Volk GF, Sauer M, Pohlmann M, Guntinas-Lichius O. Reference values for dynamic facial muscle ultrasonography in adults. Muscle Nerve. 2014;50(3):348–57.

54. Sauer M. Instructions for sonography of the facial muscles/Anleitung zur Sonographie der mimischen Muskulatur. 2015.
55. Kehrer ARM, Klebuc M, Platz Batista da Silva N, Lonic D, Heidkrueger P, Jung EM, Prantl L, Knoedler L. Objectifying the role of the depressor anguli oris muscle in synkinetic smile formation with high-resolution ultrasound—a prospective study. Plast Reconstr Surg. 2023;152:866–70.
56. Sidhu PS, Cantisani V, Dietrich CF, Gilja OH, Saftoiu A, Bartels E, et al. The EFSUMB guidelines and recommendations for the clinical practice of contrast-enhanced ultrasound (CEUS) in non-hepatic applications: update 2017 (short version). Ultraschall Med. 2018;39(2):154–80.
57. Hayashi A, Visconti G, Yamamoto T, Giacalone G, Hayashi N, Handa M, et al. Intraoperative imaging of lymphatic vessel using ultra high-frequency ultrasound. J Plast Reconstr Aesthet Surg. 2018;71(5):778–80.
58. Visconti G, Hayashi A, Yoshimatsu H, Bianchi A, Salgarello M. Ultra-high frequency ultrasound in planning capillary perforator flaps: preliminary experience. J Plast Reconstr Aesthet Surg. 2018;71(8):1146–52.
59. Visconti G, Bianchi A, Hayashi A, Cina A, Maccauro G, Almadori G, et al. Thin and superthin perforator flap elevation based on preoperative planning with ultrahigh-frequency ultrasound. Arch Plast Surg. 2020;47(4):365–70.
60. Czedik-Eysenberg M, Steinbacher J, Obermayer B, Yoshimatsu H, Hara H, Mihara M, et al. Exclusive use of ultrasound for locating optimal LVA sites—a descriptive data analysis. J Surg Oncol. 2020;121(1):51–6.
61. Hofer M, Antoch G. Teaching manual of color duplex sonography: a workbook on color duplex ultrasound and echocardiography; 2004
62. Schäberle W, Herwig B. Ultrasonography in vascular diagnosis: a therapy-oriented textbook and atlas. Springer International Publishing; 2018.
63. Smith J. Ultrasound teaching manual: the basics of performing and interpreting ultrasound scans. Ultrasound. 2013;21(4):234.
64. Dietrich CF. EFSUMB course book on ultrasound. EFSUMB; 2012.
65. Ihnatsenka B, Boezaart AP. Ultrasound: basic understanding and learning the language. Int J Shoulder Surg. 2010;4(3):55–62.
66. Naqvi TZ, Perese S. Noninvasive vascular appropriateness criteria—review and comments on the American College of Cardiology (ACC) Guidelines. J Am Soc Echocardiogr. 2013;26(5):A34.
67. Zwiebel WJ, Pellerito JS, Zwiebel WJ. Introduction to vascular ultrasonography. 5th ed. Philadelphia: Elsevier Saunders; 2005. p. 723.
68. Hwang JY. Doppler ultrasonography of the lower extremity arteries: anatomy and scanning guidelines. Ultrasonography. 2017;36(2):111–9.
69. Kruskal JB, Newman PA, Sammons LG, Kane RA. Optimizing Doppler and color flow US: application to hepatic sonography. Radiographics. 2004;24(3):657–75.
70. Saba L, Atzeni M, Rozen WM, Alonso-Burgos A, Bura R, Piga M, et al. Non-invasive vascular imaging in perforator flap surgery. Acta Radiol. 2013;54(1):89–98.
71. Borgbjerg J, Bogsted M, Lindholt JS, Behr-Rasmussen C, Horlyck A, Frokjaer JB. Superior reproducibility of the leading to leading edge and inner to inner edge methods in the ultrasound assessment of maximum abdominal aortic diameter. Eur J Vasc Endovasc Surg. 2018;55(2):206–13.
72. Pajala A, Kangas J, Siira P, Ohtonen P, Leppilahti J. Augmented compared with nonaugmented surgical repair of a fresh total Achilles tendon rupture. A prospective randomized study. J Bone Jt Surg Am. 2009;91(5):1092–100.
73. Yamamoto T, Yamamoto N, Fuse Y, Kageyama T, Sakai H, Tsukuura R. Subdermal dissection for elevation of pure skin perforator flaps and superthin flaps: the dermis as a landmark for the most superficial dissection plane. Plast Reconstr Surg. 2021;147(3):470–8.
74. Vaienti L, Cottone G, De Francesco F, Borelli F, Zaccaria G, Amendola F. The suprafascial course of lower leg perforators: an anatomical study. Arch Plast Surg. 2020;47(2):165–70.
75. Kehrer A, Lonic D, Heidekrueger P, Bosselmann T, Taeger CD, Lamby P, et al. Feasibility study of preoperative microvessel evaluation and characterization in perforator flaps using various modes of color-coded duplex sonography (CCDS). Microsurgery. 2020;40(7):750–9.
76. Cho MJ, Kwon JG, Pak CJ, Suh HP, Hong JP. The role of duplex ultrasound in microsurgical reconstruction: review and technical considerations. J Reconstr Microsurg. 2020;36(7):514–21.

Ultra High Frequency Ultrasound

7

Akitatsu Hayashi

7.1 Introduction

Ultrahigh-frequency ultrasound (UHFUS) is a recently introduced preoperative and intraoperative imaging technique in reconstructive microsurgery and supermicrosurgery, characterized by the use of ultrasound (US) frequencies in the range between 30 and 70 MHz. The use of higher frequency US affords improved spatial resolution at the expense of a shallower depth of penetration, compared to conventional high-frequency ultrasound (CHFUS).

In recent years, research on small animals promoted advances in diagnostic imaging technologies, such as UHFUS, which were first introduced at the beginning of the 2000s in the preclinical setting and have recently been approved. This novel device has recently been approved for use in humans. In particular, initial applications of UHFUS predominantly involved dermatology and angiology, where conventional US techniques were already available and widely employed. Subsequently, the development of more performing UHFUS appliances for clinical use led to the dissemination of the technique in other medical fields as it made it possible to obtain submillimeter resolution of small structures. At present, UHFUS is employed for vascular, musculoskeletal, dermatological, and small parts applications.

This chapter introduces the potential role of ultrahigh-frequency ultrasonography in the imaging workup of reconstructive microsurgery and supermicrosurgery in the light of the present applications of the technique.

7.2 Ultrasound in Reconstructive Microsurgery

US is a widely used, noninvasive, real-time imaging technique that finds application in clinical practices. The operating principle of US is based on the reflection of sound waves when encountering different tissues. Especially, the degree of reflection of the US waves depends on the acoustic impedance of the tissue, which is the result of tissue density and beam's angle of incidence [1]. When at the interface between two different tissues a large difference in impedance is present, the acoustic energy can be either reflected or scattered depending on the beam's angle, while a reduced difference in impedance allows the majority of the sound waves to be transmitted deeper in the tissue [2]. The acoustic impedance also determines the characteristic echo pattern of

Supplementary Information The online version contains supplementary material available at https://doi.org/10.1007/978-981-97-7278-0_7.

A. Hayashi (✉)
Lymphedema Center, Kameda General Hospital, Kamogawa, Japan

J. P. Hong et al. (eds.), *Imaging for Reconstructive Microsurgery*,
https://doi.org/10.1007/978-981-97-7278-0_7

a tissue, which is of great importance when performing diagnosis on US images. A tissue can be defined as anechoic, hypoechoic, or hyperechoic depending on the type of signal produced, based on the echo pattern [1, 2].

The choice of the frequency depends on the clinical situation. There is an inverse proportionality between the US frequency and wavelength, which results in a different degree of penetration in the tissues. Lower US frequencies are characterized by a higher depth of penetration of the US wave, at the expense of image resolution. In contrast, higher US frequencies provide better image resolution but limited depth of penetration.

Presently, we are in the era of reconstructive microsurgery and supermicrosurgery, in which microsurgeons preserve major vessels, decreased operative time, initial debulking of the flap, and increased flexibility for the reconstructive surgeons [3]. As these reconstructions frequently utilize vessels that are smaller than a single millimeter, understanding of location of lymphatic vessels and perforator anatomy preoperatively is essential. While ultrasound has advantages of low cost and no radiation, computed tomography angiography (CTA) has become the primary imaging of choice, and ultrasound is typically used as a means to confirm the CTA imaging, because disadvantages of ultrasound include steep-learning curve and operator dependency.

To change with the times, the role of US has changed from an adjunct to primary imaging of the choice in reconstructive surgery such as supermicrosurgery and lymphedema surgery [4]. CHFUS and color Doppler ultrasonography (CDU) became a valuable tool, because these procedures require a detailed preoperative planning with mapping the perforators and lymphatic vessels, intraoperative assessment, and postoperative monitoring. The need for high-resolution imaging of superficial anatomical structures of reduced dimensions has favored the application of CHFUS frequencies >15 MHz. High-frequency CDU allows us to minimize guessing, perform faster dissection, anticipate anatomical variations, and determine information on flap physiology in real time. The use of CDU can help one obtain information that is needed to make enhanced decision in reconstructive surgery [5].

Recently, the introduction of ultrahigh US frequencies (>30 MHz) for the imaging of lymphatic vessels, capillary perforators, and intradermal plexus has responded to the previously unmet need for a submillimeter resolution imaging of small anatomy and superficial tissue layers.

7.3 Ultrahigh-Frequency Ultrasound: New Modality for Supervision

UHFUS is defined as an ultrasonographic technique involving the use of ultrasound frequencies higher than 30 MHz, which allow to obtain submillimeter resolution of superficial anatomical structures [6]. UHFUS was developed in the mid-1990s in the preclinical setting, where it found application for the study of pharmacokinetics of drugs, tumor biology, and several pathologic conditions in small animals. Especially, UHFUS allowed to monitor tumor growth in animal models and their changes after antineoplastic therapy, to visualize the microvascularization of neoplastic masses, and to study the progression of atherosclerotic lesions and the medium-intimate thickness of the arterial wall in murine models [7–10].

In the early 2000s, UHFUS was introduced in the clinical setting. As axial resolution proportionally increases with ultrasound frequency, the use of ultrahigh frequencies provides submillimeter image resolution, although the shorter wavelength limits the depth of penetration of the ultrasound beam. From this viewpoint, UHFUS appears suitable for the investigation of small structures located within the first centimeters from the surface of application of the probe.

Recent developments in UHFUS systems provide frequencies as high as 70 MHz and capability resolution as fine as 30 μm within 10.0 mm from the surface and frequencies as high as 48 MHz and capability resolution as fine as 50 μm within 23.5 mm from the surface which

Table 7.1 UHFUS features

UHFUS frequency	70 MHz	48 MHz
Bandwidth	29–71 MHz	20–46 MHz
Image width (maximum)	9.7 mm	15.4 mm
Image depth (maximum)	10.0 mm	23.5 mm
Focal depth	5.0 mm	9.0 mm
Axial resolution	30.0 μm	50.0 μm
Lateral resolution	65.0 μm	110.0 μm

UHFUS ultrahigh frequency ultrasound

could allow more precise imaging of small anatomical structures (Table 7.1). Therefore, the improved degree of visualization of superficial anatomical structures has favored the diffusion of UHFUS in all the fields where the detailed investigation of small anatomy is required.

7.4 UHFUS for Perforator Flaps

Perforator flaps represent nowadays a gold standard in reconstructive surgery. However, when the aim of the reconstruction is resurfacing rather than creating volume or filling spaces, traditional perforator flaps may result in suboptimal results due to their bulkiness.

The latest evolution of perforator flap was represented by the introduction of thin and superthin skin flaps. They became increasingly popular for resurfacing purposes, which are based on very peripheral vascular structures. Moreover, a growing evidence is coming out on the reliability of smaller perforators also called "capillary" perforator in sustaining those dermis flap metabolic demands, which may further expand reconstructive freedom and reduce morbidity. However, for resurfacing of very thin area of the body such as face, foot, hand, ankle, and knee, thin and superthin flaps may result still bulky, and a pure skin perforator (PSP) would be optimal to achieve primary reconstruction.

The first study describing the planning of perforator flap surgery and visualizing capillary perforators using UHFUS was the one by Visconti et al. [11]. The study reported that the authors were able to precisely visualize the capillary perforators piercing the superficial fascia and to follow their course in the hypodermis layer up to and within the dermis layer, thus allowing to precisely mark the superficial fascia perforator location and to precisely trace vascular axiality to optimize flap design orientation. This information goes over the ability of CTA, frequently used in preoperative planning of traditional perforator flaps.

Visconti et al. described the feasibility of PSP direct harvesting above the subdermal plane using preoperative planning with UHFUS [12]. In this study, the authors were able to locate the main perforator vessels and then trace them till the dermis entry point in all PSP flaps. UHFUS is able to provide unprecedented clear images of perforator branches directly piercing the dermis, nearby subdermal venules coming from the dermis and connecting to the comitantes perforator venules as well as intradermal arterioles and venules. By using these preoperative findings, PSP are directly harvested above the subdermal plane using the "hot and cold zone" technique reported by Hong [13] Visconti et al. also reported preoperative planning with UHFUS for thin and superthin perforator flap based on this knowledge [14].

In a study of Yoshimatsu et al. they demonstrated visualization of the intradermal plexus using UHFUS for elevating dermis flap [15]. UHFUS permit observation of small arteries entering the dermis layer (Video 7.1). The artery is observed to give off branches after entering the dermis, in effect constituting an "intradermal plexus." Knowledge of the existence of the intradermal plexus makes it possible to discard nearly all subdermal adipose tissue quickly and safely in their study.

Superficial circumflex iliac artery (SCIA) perforator (SCIP) flap is one of representatives of thin flap. During the elevation of the SCIP flap, conversion of the flap pedicle from the superficial branch to the deep branch of the SCIA often occurs, complicating and prolonging the procedure. In a study of Yoshimatsu et al. they demonstrated the feasibility of UHFUS to decrease the conversion rate by making a comparison with CHFUS and CDU [16]. The use of a preoperative UHFUS significantly decreases the intraoperative conversion rate, thus notably facilitating the

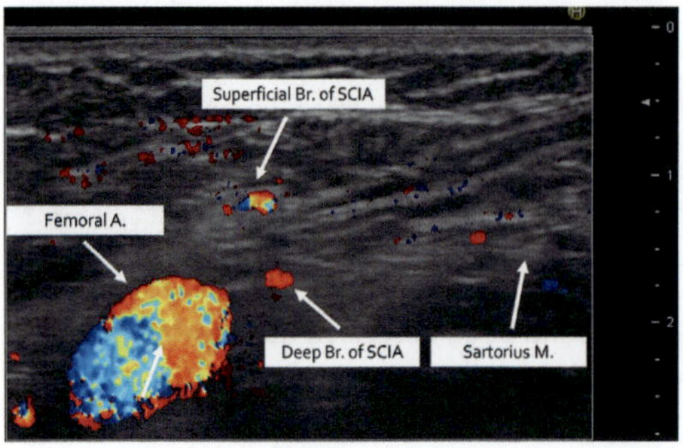

Fig. 7.1 UHFUS can detect superficial and deep branch of SCIA easily and clearly

procedure (Fig. 7.1). A large skin paddle based on the superficial branch of the SCIA is safely procured after accurate preoperative examinations are made using UHFUS, requiring only one venous anastomosis in most cases and resulting in shorter operative time.

7.5 UHFUS for Lymphatic Supermicrosurgery

Among the surgical procedures for lymphedema, lymphaticovenular anastomosis (LVA) is an effective and minimally invasive surgical treatment for refractory lymphedema. Preoperative and intraoperative identification of functional lymphatic vessels is essential for success of the surgery.

Indocyanine green (ICG) lymphography has been reported to be a minimally invasive imaging modality that can evaluate the severity of lymphedema but also allows a live visualization of superficial lymphatic vessels as linear patterns [17–19]. However, ICG lymphography cannot visualize lymphatic flow that is masked beneath dermal backflow patterns, particularly in stardust and diffuse patterns, in the extremities affected with severe lymphedema. For detection of lymphatic vessels in a region masked by dermal backflow pattern or in patients with allergic reactions to ICG, CHFUS has been reported to be useful as a substitute for ICG lymphography even in the limbs severely affected by lymphedema [20, 21]. In CHFUS, lymphatic channels show as intermittent, homogeneous, hypoechoic, and specular misshapen images. Ultrasound-guided detection of lymphatic vessels for lymphedema results in more effective LVA surgery.

Disadvantages of CHFUS system are that it is highly operator dependent and that it is difficult to distinguish the lymphatic vessels with the subcutaneous veins or the nerves when the lymphatic vessels are smaller than 0.3 mm, even if the operator uses CDU [21]. Precise imaging of small anatomical structures is often difficult with conventional ultrasound.

The first study describing detection of lymphatic vessels using UHFUS was the one by Hayashi et al. [22]. This study revealed high sensitivity and specificity of UHFUS for detection of the lymphatic vessels when compared with those of CHFUS. This study also showed UHFUS could detect the lymphatic vessels with smaller diameter and larger number of lymphatic vessels in the upper and lower extremities. In addition, from the results of this study, this advanced ultrasound showed not only unprecedented clear image of the lymphatic vessels, even ones with diameters smaller than 0.3 mm, but also new characteristics and imaging findings that could not be observed using CHFUS. The lymphatic vessels are less likely to collapse when pressure is applied to the skin with the transducer (Fig. 7.2), and mosaic pattern cannot be seen in the lymphatic vessel because of its slow flow speed (Video 7.2). Thus, the lymphatic vessels can be distinguished from other structures by not only shape and echogenic texture but also adopting this pressure application technique. Lymphatic fluids moving inside the lumen and functioning valves were visualized in some lymphatic vessels with UHFUS (Video 7.3). Moreover, for the lymphatic vessels, low echoic area can be detected while narrows and spreads and these areas merge from distal to proximal in UHFUS (Video 7.4). UHFUS may have the big advantage of identification of functional lymphatic vessels.

In a study of Bianchi et al. they evaluated the accuracy of UHFUS in detecting the lymphatic vessels and in evaluating their degeneration status, including wall and lumen characteristics,

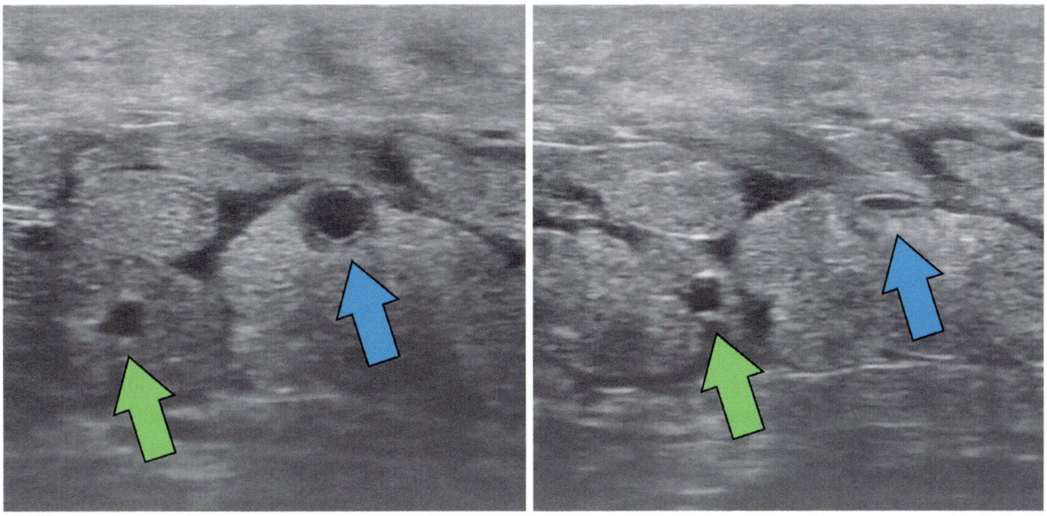

Fig. 7.2 (Left) Cutaneous vein (blue arrow) and lymphatic vessel (green arrow) were detected using ultrahigh-frequency ultrasound. (Right) The lymphatic vessels were less likely to collapse when pressure was applied to the skin with the transducer

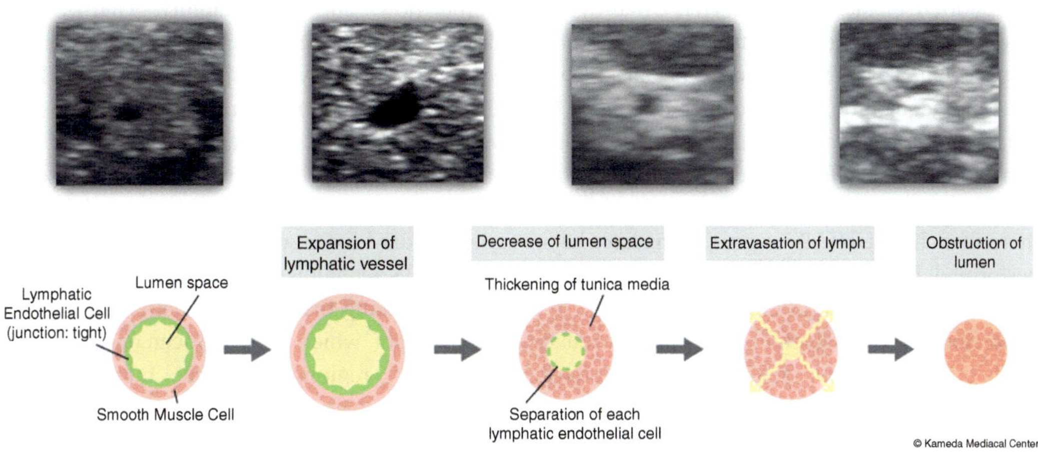

Fig. 7.3 From the image of lymphatic vessel in ultrahigh-frequency ultrasound, high echoic region around the low echoic region shows degenerative status of smooth muscle cells and hyperplasia of collagenous fibers in the lymphatic vessels

compared with direct histology observation through the procedure of LVA [23]. UHFUS preoperative and intraoperative analysis of lymphatic channels strongly correlates with their histology. This represented a step forward in lymphatic surgery. Preoperatively, UHFUS can be used as an effective and reliable method for the detection of functional and overloaded lymphatic vessels, which should be targeted for LVA to obtain the maximum therapeutic effect, aiding surgeons in locating the best incisions for LVA, beyond the ICG lymphography (Fig. 7.3). Intraoperatively, UHFUS aids the surgeon in selecting the lymphatic channels suitable for anastomosis when multiple channels are found in the same incision.

The surgeon may be in the frustrating condition of finding a valuable lymphatic channel to bypass but lacking a recipient venule through LVA. This situation may bring to lengthen the incision still without the certainty of finding a good recipient venule, leading to failure in performing LVA. Visconti et al. reported usefulness of UHFUS for helping the surgeon to know all those information before the surgery [24]. They found the venule rerouting a simple and effective method to overcome the unfavorable situation of incision devoid of vein in LVA surgery. This method also allows optimizing the surgical scars, which are kept to minimum, this being advantageous under both a functional and a cosmetic point of view.

7.6 Insights into a Role for UHFUS in Reconstructive Supermicrosurgery

As reported in the literature, UHFUS provides several advantages in reconstructive supermicrosurgery. Our UHFUS experience began in 2018 with the acquisition in our center of Vevo MD ultrasound device (FUJIFILM VisualSonics, Amsterdam, the Netherlands) equipped with 48 MHz and 70 MHz transducers. Since then, more than 1200 UHFUS examinations have been performed in reconstructive supermicrosurgery. UHFUS has benefited us enormously.

Recently, CDU, which the surgeon previously used for preoperative marking of perforator, addresses the issues of CTA and thus is commonly used to identify and evaluate the vessels. The resolution of US images decreases, however, when the CDU is used. Another setback of conventional US devices is the relatively high rate of false-positive identification of flap pedicles. A peculiar characteristic of the UHFUS is that arteries and veins can be distinguished, thanks to the images' high resolution: the arteries can be seen to pulsate, and the venous flow is observed as fluctuating mosaic patterns inside the lumen. Moreover, with the use of preoperative UHFUS, the pedicle can be traced further distally, allowing a flap design that ensures the inclusion of the vessels in the distal regions of the skin paddle. This contributed to the absence of partial necrosis of the flaps.

Free flaps have evolved from musculocutaneous flaps to perforator-based cutaneous flaps. The subdermal plexus is now thought to play a significant role in skin paddle perfusion. The feasibility of superthin flap, dermis flap, and PSP direct harvesting above the subdermal plane using preoperative planning with UHFUS may further expand freedom in reconstructive surgery and may increase safety, predictability, and time efficiency in flap harvesting.

US-guided detection of lymphatic vessels leads the surgeon to efficient and effective LVA. US is an effective and reliable method to detect functional yet overloaded lymphatic vessels, which has the greatest importance to obtain the maximum therapeutic effect in LVA surgery. UHFUS makes possible the selection of lymphatic channels suitable for anastomosis, both preoperatively and intraoperatively, by evaluation of wall composition related to the lumen, lymph flow, and expandability. UHFUS has already been shown to be the best tool for the venule preoperative mapping, and UHFUS allows a precise flow evaluation and valve visualization even in the smallest branches. UHFUS-based preoperative planning is the quintessence of LVA surgery and should be considered the new gold standard for preoperative planning of LVA.

UHFUS technique has some limitations, the main one being the limited penetration depth of the US beam, which allows to scan only the more superficial regions of the human body. Additionally, a training period for the operators is usually required to achieve the manual skills to properly manage the probe during the scan and the confidence for an accurate interpretation of the images (Table 7.2).

Our experience supports the extreme versatility and applicability of UHFUS to surgical planning due to its noninvasiveness and repeatability. Its features give insight into the potential role of UHFUS in the diagnosis, surgical planning, and follow-up of various pathologic conditions in other reconstructive microsurgeries. The literature on UHFUS is still evolving, but ultra-high frequencies seem the answer to surgical planning related to the high-resolution investigation of both normal perforator anatomy and tissue degenerating status of lymphatic vessels. The

Table 7.2 Summary of ultrasound for reconstructive microsurgeons

UHFUS frequency (MHz)	Low (5–12)	High (12–20)	Ultrahigh (>20)
Resolution	★	★★	★★★
Depth of penetration	★★★	★★	★
Lymphatic imaging		★	★★★
Perforator imaging	★	★★★	★★
Learning curve	★★★	★★	★
Cost	★	★★	★★★

★ indicates the relative value
UHFUS ultrahigh frequency ultrasound

advantages of ultrasonographic techniques in terms of noninvasiveness, repeatability, and relatively low cost make UHFUS the avant-garde in ultrasonography, which has still to be fully explored in all its possibilities.

7.7 Conclusion

UHFUS application involves an increasing number of reconstructive supermicrosurgery field. The high spatial resolution and the superb image quality achievable allow to foresee a wider use of this novel technique, which has the potential to bring innovation in supermicrosurgical imaging. UHFUS is a valuable and powerful tool for any reconstructive surgeons who are interested in performing supermicrosurgery. As the demand for customized flaps using superthin flaps, PSP, perforator-to-perforator anastomosis, and lymphedema supermicrosurgery increases, understanding and becoming versatile in UHFUS will be essential.

References

1. Wortsman X. Ultrasound in dermatology: why, how, and when? Semin Ultrasound CT MR. 2013;34:177–95.
2. Schmid-Wendtner MH, Dill-Müller D. Ultrasound technology in dermatology. Semin Cutan Med Surg. 2008;27:44–51.
3. Badash I, Gould DJ, Patel KM. Supermicrosurgery: history, applications, training and the future. Front Surg. 2018;5:23.
4. Oni G, Chow W, Ramakrishnan V, Griffiths M. Plastic surgeon-led ultrasound. Plast Reconstr Surg. 2018;141(02):300e–9e.
5. Cho MJ, Kwon JG, Pak CJ, et al. The role of duplex ultrasound in microsurgical reconstruction: review and technical considerations. J Reconstr Microsurg. 2020;36(7):514–21.
6. Izzetti R, Vitali S, Aringhieri G, et al. Ultra-high frequency ultrasound, a promising diagnostic technique: review of the literature and single-center experience. Can Assoc Radiol J. 2020;72:418.
7. Gan LM, Grönros J, Hägg U, et al. Non-invasive real-time imaging of atherosclerosis in mice using ultrasound biomicroscopy. Atherosclerosis. 2007;190:313–20.
8. Lavaud J, Henry M, Coll JL, Josserand V. Exploration of melanoma metastases in mice brains using endogenous contrast photoacoustic imaging. Int J Pharm. 2017;532:704–9.
9. Carotenuto AR, Cutolo A, Petrillo A, et al. Growth and in vivo stresses traced through tumor mechanics enriched with predator-prey cells dynamics. J Mech Behav Biomed Mater. 2018;86:55–70.
10. Fernandes DA, Kolios MC. Intrinsically absorbing photoacoustic and ultrasound contrast agents for cancer therapy and imaging. Nanotechnology. 2018;29:505103.
11. Visconti G, Hayashi A, Yoshimatsu H, et al. Ultrahigh frequency ultrasound in planning capillary perforator flaps: preliminary experience. J Plast Reconstr Aesthet Surg. 2018;71(8):1146–52.
12. Visconti G, Bianchi A, Hayashi A, et al. Pure skin perforator flap direct elevation above the subdermal plane using preoperative ultra-high frequency ultrasound planning: a proof of concept. J Plast Reconstr Aesthet Surg. 2019;72(10):1700–38.
13. Hong JP, Choi DH, Suh H, et al. A new plane of elevation: the superficial fascial plane for perforator flap elevation. J Reconstr Microsurg. 2014;30(7):491–6.
14. Visconti G, Bianchi A, Hayashi A, et al. Thin and superthin perforator flap elevation based on preoperative planning with ultrahigh-frequency ultrasound. Arch Plast Surg. 2020;47(4):365–70.
15. Yoshimatsu H, Hayashi A, Yamamoto T, et al. Visualization of the "intradermal plexus" using ultrasonography in the dermis flap: a step beyond perforator flaps. Plast Reconstr Surg Glob Open. 2019;7(11):e2411.
16. Yoshimatsu H, Karakawa R, Fuse Y, et al. Use of preoperative high-resolution ultrasound system to facilitate elevation of the superficial circumflex iliac artery perforator flap. J Reconstr Microsurg. 2021;37:735. https://doi.org/10.1055/s-0041-1726395.
17. Yamamoto T, Narushima M, Doi K, et al. Characteristic indocyanine green lymphography findings in lower extremity lymphedema: the generation of a novel lymphedema severity staging system using dermal backflow patterns. Plast Reconstr Surg. 2011;127:1979–86.
18. Yamamoto T, Matsuda N, Doi K, et al. The earliest finding of indocyanine green lymphography in asymp-

tomatic limbs of lower extremity lymphedema patients secondary to cancer treatment: the modified dermal backflow stage and concept of subclinical lymphedema. Plast Reconstr Surg. 2011;128:314e–21e.
19. Yamamoto T, Yamamoto N, Doi K, et al. Indocyanine green-enhanced lymphography for upper extremity lymphedema: a novel severity staging system using dermal backflow patterns. Plast Reconstr Surg. 2011;128:941–7.
20. Hayashi A, Yamamoto T, Yoshimatsu H, et al. Ultrasound visualization of the lymphatic vessels in the lower leg. Microsurgery. 2016;36:397–401.
21. Hayashi A, Hayashi N, Yoshimatsu H, et al. Effective and efficient lymphaticovenular anastomosis using preoperative ultrasound detection technique of lymphatic vessels in lower extremity lymphedema. J Surg Oncol. 2018;117:290–8.
22. Hayashi A, Giacalone G, Yamamoto T, et al. Ultra high-frequency ultrasonographic imaging with 70 MHz scanner for visualization of the lymphatic vessels. Plast Reconstr Surg Glob Open. 2019;7(1):e2086.
23. Bianchi A, Visconti G, Hayashi A, et al. Ultra-high frequency ultrasound imaging of lymphatic channels correlates with their histological features: a step forward in lymphatic surgery. J Plast Reconstr Aesthet Surg. 2020;73(9):1622–9.
24. Visconti G, Bianchi A, Hayashi A, et al. Ultra-high frequency ultrasound preoperative planning of the rerouting method for lymphaticovenular anastomosis in incisions devoid of vein. Microsurgery. 2020;40(6):717–8.

Thermographic Imaging as Applied for Reconstructive Microsurgery

8

Geoffrey G. Hallock

8.1 Introduction

A thermogram is a visible portrayal of radiative heat loss from the skin to its surroundings [1]. The latter is the basic physics for maintenance of body temperature equilibrium [1]. Core heat transfer primarily is via the vascular system, thereby ensuring a good correlation between skin temperature and the quality of skin perfusion [1, 2]. What then is perceived as heat loss by the body is in the form of infrared radiation, whose wavelength falls within the nonvisible range (700 nm–1 mm) of the electromagnetic spectrum [3]. Increments in the quantity of infrared radiation that is emitted will cause demonstrable alterations of the skin temperature, which directly correlates to variations in the cutaneous blood flow that in turn relies on cutaneous perforators [3, 4].

Thermal imaging cameras necessary for capturing a thermogram actually have been available for over three decades [5]. Observed static "hot spots" as differentiated by the chosen thermal palette will correspond to regions where greater heat had been emitted, as via a "dominant" perforator (Fig. 8.1a), and dynamic studies over time often can demonstrate the extent of the surrounding vascular network and interconnections so served by that perforator which today might correspond to a functional perforasome [1–4, 6–8]. Such thermogram images have proven to complement quite accurately other means for preoperative studies used for preoperative perforator identification, such as computed tomography (CT) angiography [4], auditory Doppler [8], and flow Doppler ultrasound [7].

Over time, thermal imaging cameras have become not only more sensitive but less expensive. Today, incredibly inexpensive miniature thermal imaging cameras (FLIR ONE Pro [FLIR Systems, Inc., Wilsonville, OR], FLIR.com/FLIRONE/Start) are available for anyone. These may be attached to any type of the ubiquitous smartphone so that rapid real-time thermogram still or video images can be digitally merged with the visible light camera photograph on the smartphone using an app provided by the manufacturer [9], thereby enabling acquisition of this technology with virtually no learning curve.

Perhaps, unfortunately, the smartphone applied thermal imaging camera provides a lower resolution image, and the temperature detection range is narrower than the hundred times more expensive professional camera [8, 9]. Professional cameras are also superior as temperature differences as little as 0.04 °C can be differentiated [3,

Supplementary Information The online version contains supplementary material available at https://doi.org/10.1007/978-981-97-7278-0_8.

G. G. Hallock (✉)
Division of Plastic Surgery, St. Luke's Hospital, Sacred Heart Division, Allentown, PA, USA

J. P. Hong et al. (eds.), *Imaging for Reconstructive Microsurgery*,
https://doi.org/10.1007/978-981-97-7278-0_8

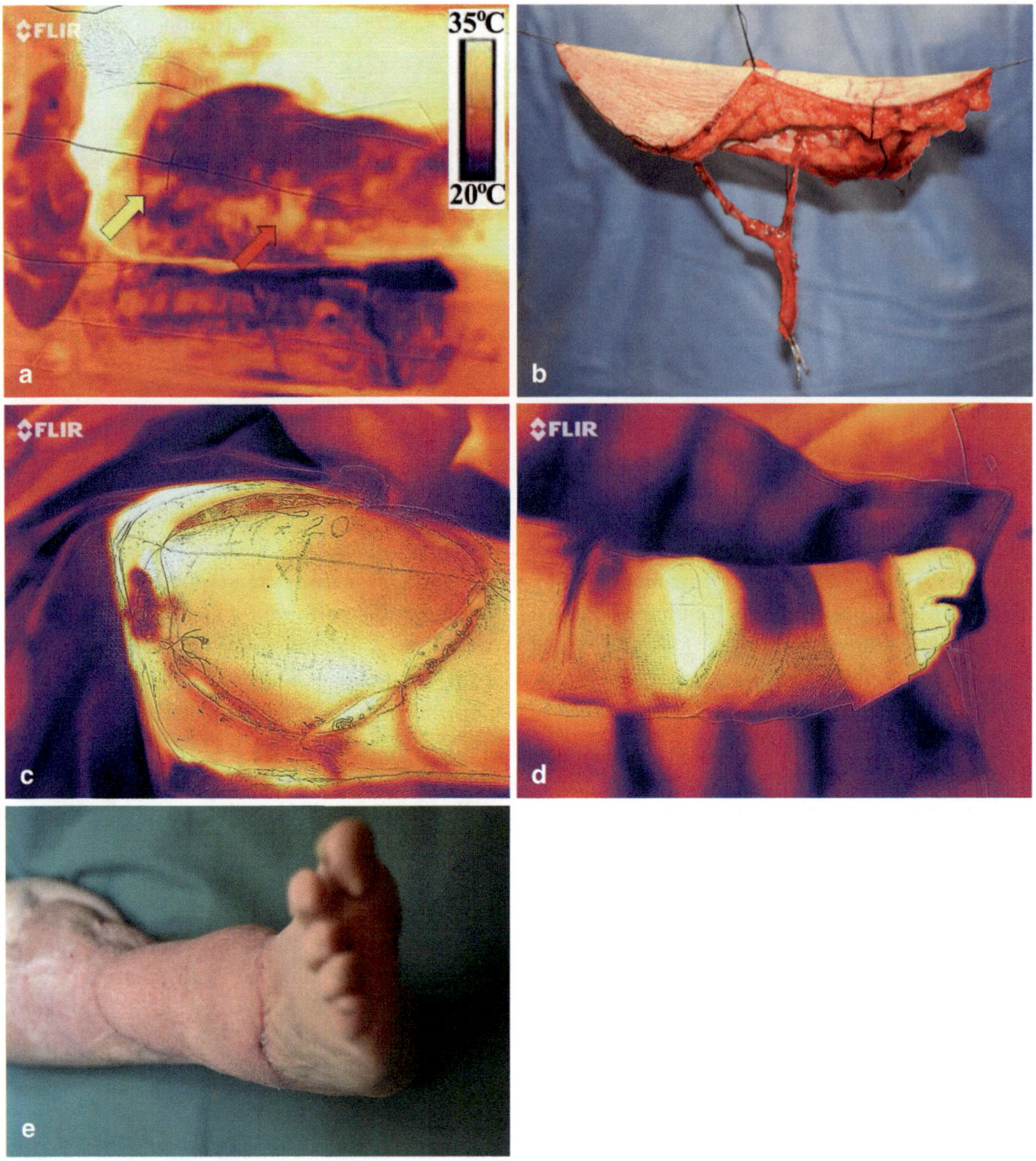

Fig. 8.1 Thermograms of anterolateral thigh donor site: (**a**) during this "cold challenge," the hottest "hot spot" (red arrow) was just posterior to the midpoint of the line drawn between the anterior superior iliac spine and the superior lateral border of the patella. A separate "hot spot" was suggested more proximally (yellow arrow). Be wary of the offset of the thermal image from the visible camera image (thermal palette inset). (**b**) Perforators seen emanating from this anterolateral thigh free flap were found exactly as marked and predicted by the thermogram. (**c**) Still pedicled anterolateral thigh flap in situ. Homogeneous warmth seen throughout flap except diminished at distal border where exposed to ambient air. Note "hot spots" at the "x" points previously noted where perforators found on thermal image were marked. (**d**) Monitoring on postoperative day 1 shows acceptable warmth of flap compared to surrounding dressings, implying viability, (**e**) as indeed was the case at follow-up 3 months later of this ALT flap used to cover unstable burn injury of the anterior ankle

10], in contrast to smartphone accuracy that is only within a 3.0 °C or 5% range [11]. Yet the latter is enough for smartphone perforator detection IF preceded by a thermal stress or "cold challenge" that will initiate an adequate modulation of the infrared emission [7]. Termed dynamic infrared thermography (DIRT), this will primarily be a preferable adjunct when using the less sensitive smartphone thermal imaging camera [1–3, 12, 13].

8.2 Technique

8.2.1 Preoperative

To detect perforator location, whatever is the chosen donor site must first be cooled below ambient temperature. Muntean's method is to spray that region with isopropyl alcohol followed by accelerated evaporation with a high-speed portable fan (video: initiation of the "cold challenge") [3]. The thermal imaging camera should be maintained at about a 70 cm distance from the subject while waiting at least 5 min after removal of any covering to allow the overall body temperature to balance with that of the room temperature [4].

Observed rewarming points or "hot spots" can be marked under direct camera visualization (Fig. 8.1a). Most easily accomplished in a few minutes as a bedside test in the office setting, the marked points will be a valuable guide to delineate where further pursuit for corroboration using the ubiquitous audible Doppler probe or even duplex ultrasound if warranted can best be achieved (video: initiation of the "cold challenge"). In the operating room itself, the "cold challenge" would be safer by covering the area with ice chips or preferably a moist towel soaked in ice water, but this is more difficult to get uniform regional coolness.

8.2.2 Intraoperative

High temperatures throughout the flap as assessed using the thermogram palette will assure adequate perfusion and usually total viability while the flap is in situ (Fig. 8.1c). This would be especially valuable to prove this for a local perforator flap where extensive subfascial dissection may have been done [14]. However, homogeneous darker colors throughout and particularly if involving only flap margins may represent coolness more likely due to environmental factors or something as simple as the use of local vasoconstrictors.

8.2.3 Postoperative

A viable flap implying maintained perfusion via a microanastomosis, when monitored postoperatively, should show little change in the thermogram spectrum over time (Fig. 8.1d). Cessation of arterial infusion will result in a cold flap with a dramatic darker color change, but venous congestion may be more difficult to perceive as some perfusion may persist, and thus there will still be some heat emission for an indeterminate time. Even a minor change in the color could imply flap circulatory embarrassment, yet it may be so subtle that is not recognized by the casual observer. The take-home message from this conundrum is that thermography so far remains not a good method for objective flap monitoring.

8.3 Discussion

Smartphone thermal digital imaging is now a cheap and more readily obtainable means for the preoperative identification of perforators than more conventional technologies that may be either too expensive or unavailable, whose attributes and detriments are better described elsewhere in this edition. Those indeed are reliable and sound alternatives, but in contrast to thermography, they are expensive and may require exposure to contrast media or ionizing radiation or be relatively time-consuming during their application [1, 15, 16].

As already inferred, the best indication for the use of thermography will be in the preoperative phase whenever a perforator-based flap is desirable, by not only for the identification of perforator location but sometimes over time the orientation of "true" anastomoses between perforasomes to allow creation of the best functional perforator angiosome [15, 17]. Intraoperative assistance mainly serves to reassure the presence of flap per-

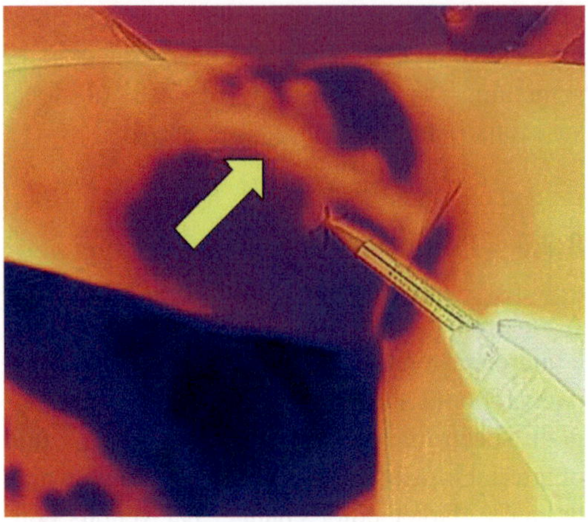

Fig. 8.2 At time of "cold challenge" of calf region, a medial sural artery perforator has been marked just posterior to a "heat line" (arrow) that corresponded to the greater saphenous vein

fusion, but visible alterations in monitoring postoperatively will not be rapid enough to allow an objective assessment that would reliably ensure a timely "take-back" if that prove to be essential.

Other limitations of thermography need also be recognized. The detection of ongoing physiological alterations in surface body temperature as directly correlated to perforators is possible, but not so is their morphology. As a consequence, thermography cannot recognize the origin or path of a perforator which could have an oblique course to the skin after penetrating the deep fascia or may sometimes diverge into multiple branches causing multiple "hot spots" from a single perforator that could not be so realized [3, 17]. Background thermal interference for a myriad of reasons and artifacts such as the presence of cutaneous veins or axial arteries that persist in spite of the "cold challenge," which Zhang [18] has termed "heat lines" (Fig. 8.2), may distort the appearance or recognition of true "hot spots."

8.4 Conclusion

The search for the perfect complementary, portable, accurate, and bedside vascular imaging tool in many ways can be fulfilled using thermography, but, realistically, accuracy in all operative phases is not truly possible. This modality should be recognized to be an inexpensive but expeditious adjunct for the preoperative evaluation of the cutaneous circulation, yet often it is still better employed to facilitate the use of other conventional methods of perforator identification.

References

1. de Weerd L, Mercer JB, Weum S. Dynamic infrared thermography. Clin Plast Surg. 2011;38(02):277–92.
2. de Weerd L, Weum S, Mercer JB. The value of dynamic infrared thermography (DIRT) in perforator selection and planning of free DIEP flaps. Ann Plast Surg. 2009;63(03):274–9.
3. Muntean MV, Strilciuc S, Ardelean F, Georgescu AV. Dynamic infrared mapping of cutaneous perforators. J Xiangya Med. 2018;3:16.
4. Pereira N, Valenzuela D, Mangelsdorff G, Kufeke M, Roa R. Detection of perforators for free flap planning using smartphone thermal imaging: a concordance study with computed tomographic angiography in 120 perforators. Plast Reconstr Surg. 2018;141(03):787–92.
5. Theuvenet WJ, Koeyers GF, Borghouts MH. Thermographic assessment of perforating arteries. A preoperative screening method for fasciocutaneous and musculocutaneous flaps. Scand J Plast Reconstr Surg. 1986;20(01):25–9.
6. Saint-Cyr M, Wong C, Schaverien M, Mojallal A, Rohrich RJ. The perforasome theory: vascular anatomy and clinical implications. Plast Reconstr Surg. 2009;124(05):1529–44.
7. Tenorio X, Mahajan AL, Elias B, et al. Locating perforator vessels by dynamic infrared imaging and flow Doppler with no thermal cold challenge. Ann Plast Surg. 2011;67(02):143–6.
8. Sheena Y, Jennison T, Hardwicke JT, Titley OG. Detection of perforators using thermal imaging. Plast Reconstr Surg. 2013;132(06):1603–10.
9. Hardwicke JT, Osmani O, Skillman JM. Detection of perforators using smartphone thermal imaging. Plast Reconstr Surg. 2016;137(01):39–41.
10. Muntean MV, Achimas-Cadariu PA. Detection of perforators for free flap planning using smartphone thermal imaging: a concordance study with computed tomographic angiography in 120 perforators. Plast Reconstr Surg. 2018;142(04):604e.
11. Pereira N. Reply: detection of perforators for free flap planning using smartphone thermal imaging: a concordance study with computed tomographic angiography in 120 perforators. Plast Reconstr Surg. 2018;142(04):605e.
12. de Weerd L, Mercer JB, Setså LB. Intraoperative dynamic infrared thermography and free-flap surgery. Ann Plast Surg. 2006;57(03):279–84.

13. Itoh Y, Arai K. Use of recovery-enhanced thermography to localize cutaneous perforators. Ann Plast Surg. 1995;34(05):507–11.
14. Pereira N, Hallock GG. Smartphone thermography for lower extremity local flap perforator mapping. J Reconstr Microsurg. 2021;37:59–66.
15. Chubb D, Rozen WM, Whitaker IS, Ashton MW. Images in plastic surgery: digital thermographic photography ("thermal imaging") for preoperative perforator mapping. Ann Plast Surg. 2011;66(04):324–5.
16. Hallock GG. Doppler sonography and color duplex imaging for planning a perforator flap. Clin Plast Surg. 2003;30(03):347–57. v–vi.
17. Chubb DP, Taylor GI, Ashton MW. True and 'choke' anastomoses between perforator angiosomes: part II. Dynamic thermographic identification. Plast Reconstr Surg. 2013;132:1457–64.
18. Zhang Y, Xiao W, Ng S, Zhou H, Min P, Xi W, Masia J, Blondeel P, Feng S. Infrared thermography-guided designing and harvesting of pre-expanded pedicled flap for head and neck reconstruction. J Plast Reconstr Aesthet Surg. 2021;74(9):2068–75.

Augmented Reality

9

Nicolás Pereira and Juan Pablo Camacho

9.1 Introduction

Augmented reality (AR) is the addition of artificial information to one or more senses, allowing the user to perform tasks more efficiently. This can be achieved by superimposing images, videos, or computer-generated models [1]. Other senses can even be enhanced through electrical impulses for taste, smell, or haptic feedback [2]. Azuma first reported AR in 1997 [3], proposing three elements in his definition: (a) a connection between the virtual world and the real world, (b) real-time interaction, and (c) 3D-based tracking and positioning.

The main difference between AR and virtual reality (VR) is that the latter occurs in a completely virtual world [4]. A third concept that is also used is "mixed reality" (MR), in which aspects of AR and VR are combined. There is an overlapping of information in the real environment (semi-immersive experience), with coexistence and interaction between them [5] (Table 9.1). In this chapter, we will talk about AR and MR indistinctly.

Supplementary Information The online version contains supplementary material available at https://doi.org/10.1007/978-981-97-7278-0_9.

N. Pereira (✉) · J. P. Camacho
Department of Plastic Surgery and Burns, Hospital del Trabajador, Santiago, Chile

Clínica Nea, Santiago, Chile

Table 9.1 Characteristics of augmented reality, virtual reality, and mixed reality

Augmented reality	Virtual reality	Mixed reality
Virtual objects are overlaid in a real environment in a passive way and without a chance to manipulate them	The objects and environment are complete virtual, offering a 100% immersive scene. The virtual objects can be manipulated in the virtual recreated world	Combines the characteristics of both AR and VR where virtual objects are layered over the real world and can interact between them and be manipulated by the user

9.2 Technical Aspects

The development of AR depends intrinsically on technological advances, with the last decade probably being the one with the greatest progress [4]. Despite the advancement and refinement of its components, basic necessary elements in AR are:

- Scene generator: Device or program responsible for rendering a scene.
- Tracking system: Allows to align the real objects with the virtual ones. In general, AR can be divided into two types based on the spatial registration method: marker-based (image recognition, object recognition) and marker-less (GPS, RFID, UWB, IMU, Wi-Fi, Bluetooth, etc.).

J. P. Hong et al. (eds.), *Imaging for Reconstructive Microsurgery*,
https://doi.org/10.1007/978-981-97-7278-0_9

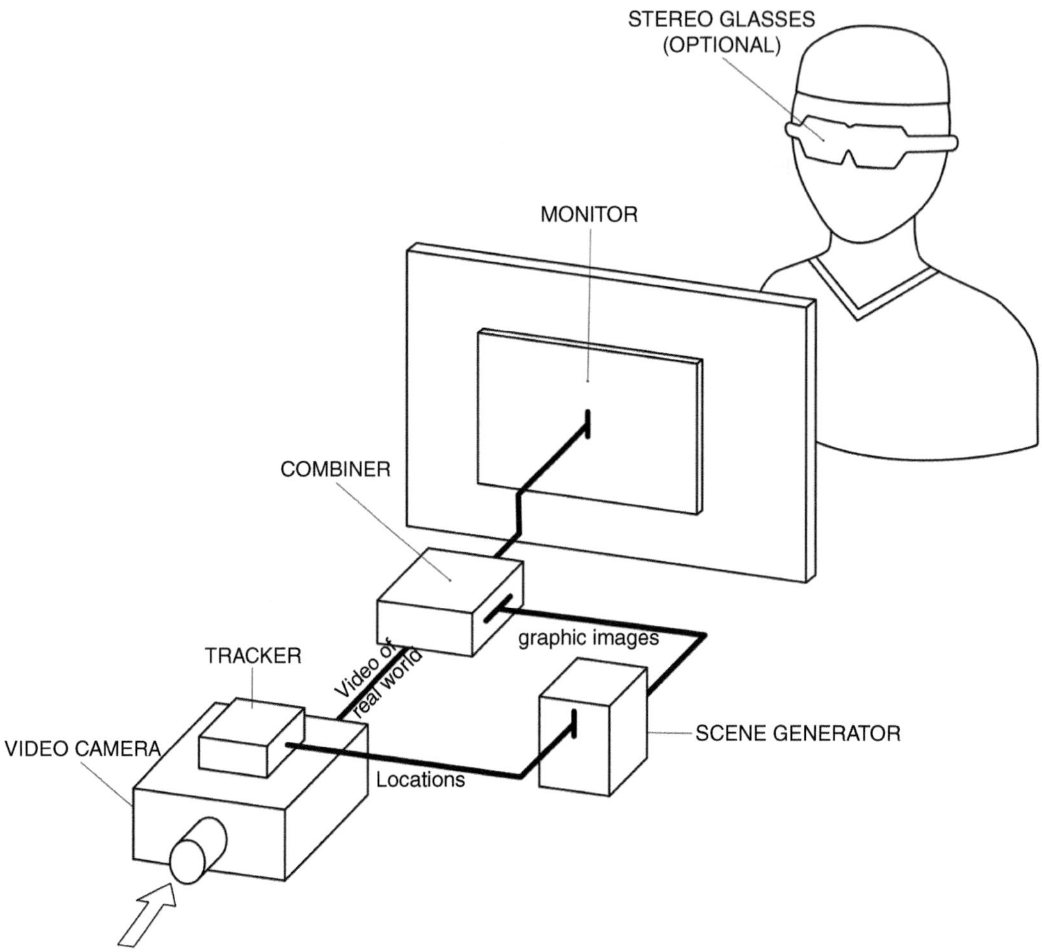

Fig. 9.1 Handheld device scheme

- Display: It is variable according to the use and is based on design decisions. Each type of screen has its benefits and cons.

In general terms, we can classify AR devices into the following types [3, 6]:

- Head-mounted devices (HMD)

  Information is displayed directly to the user on a screen (headpiece/visor/glasses). The user can use signs to direct the virtual environment. Some disadvantages are as follows: the cost, may depend on additional features (Wi-Fi, virtual software, etc.), may distract the user from the real environment, and may capture data that was not intended to be captured.
- Handheld devices (Fig. 9.1)

  Nonwearable technology. User uses his hands to manipulate and control. Accumulates digital information and transfers to a screen. Some disadvantages are as follows: the cost, may depend on additional features (Wi-Fi, virtual software, etc.), and user must hold the device.
- Spatial augmentation reality

  Technology that aims to enhance real-world experience but without a user-specific experience. May require projectors and/or monitors. Some disadvantages are as follows: the cost, may depend on additional features (Wi-Fi, virtual software, etc.), and could be a distractor to those on the surrounding environment who are performing another task.

The common limitation is that this technology is expensive to purchase and implement. However, given the latest advances in mobile technologies, we have introduced this innovation into our practice using the smartphone as a handheld device through an AR app [7].

9.3 Augmented Reality in Microsurgical Planning

AR surgical planning ranges from superficial perforator tracking to complex volumetric flap design [8, 9]. For perforator planning, Rozen et al. [10] were the first to introduce an image-guided stereotactic navigational system in DIEP flap for breast reconstruction [10]. Data was taken from 3D reconstruction of a computer tomography angiography (CTA) taken with fiducial markers on the bony landmarks of the hip and a reference on the thigh. Perforators were marked in the patient's abdominal wall on a scaled grid centered on the umbilicus. Then the information was processed by the navigation station, and after calibration, a wand was used to navigate through the patient's skin and mark the perforators. In 3D reconstruction based on CTA, all perforators were found with this technique, and this approach demonstrated a better correlation than the scanner only planning, with a distance within 0.2 cm of a distance seen at surgery vs 0.5 cm error margin in the classic approach. This work used a marker-based tracking system, with an external monitor to find the perforators. Even being one of the first works on this subject, its results were promising, and further development was made to overcome some problems and create new tools.

In order to create new tools, Hummelink et al. [11] described the handheld projection of perforators found in a 3D rendered CTA on a series of patient abdominal wall skin for DIEP planning compared to a Doppler technique. The umbilicus was the reference point, and a grid was overlaid to a ruler to assure scaling. The projector needed to be held by the user perpendicular to the surface to be displayed and in a proper distance to match size. Their preliminary results showed a greater number of correctly identified perforators (56.9% +/− 31.4% vs 84.3% +/− 25.8%; $p = 0.030$) and a shorter radius compared to US (7 +/− 4 mm vs 4 +/− 3 mm; $p = 0.009$). One of the benefits offered by this technique was the exact estimation of fascial perforator in the CTA vs the eventual skin detection on the ultrasound (US) detection. Despite their good results, one of the main problems they had was the correct calibration of the projector. Therefore, in 2019, they published a randomized controlled trial where they refine some previously described aspects [12]. The handheld projector had the ability to detect reference markers in the patient's skin, just like Rozen's navigational system previously mentioned, allowing to calibrate the image after recognition. Their results showed a greater number of perforators found (61.7 ± 7.3% vs 41.2 ± 8.2%; $p = 0.020$) and shorter harvest time, without major complication rates compared to US planning.

With the passage of time and the advent of new and more refined technologies, more and more detailed results have been achieved and allowed to dissect more tailored flaps for the specific needs of patients. An example of this was shown by Tang et al. [13] when, by using better CTA image acquisition and processing, a high-definition reconstruction of vascular tree was projected into the thigh of ALT flap patients. The need of special software and hardware makes it difficult to reproduce these methods.

To overcome these technical and cost constraints, since most plastic surgeons have a mobile phone, Pereira et al. [7] published their experience with a smartphone-based image superposition method. Information was taken from CTA and processed to manually identify and mark groin vascular anatomy and render them in a 3D abdominal wall reconstruction. This 2D photograph of a 3D render was exported to a smartphone, and with the help of a basic application (e.g., *Camera Lucida AR*), the image was faded to allow observation of both the picture and the patient in real time. With both images aligned, the vascular course was traced, and excellent correlation with handheld Doppler and surgical findings were obtained.

Even having technically improved some aspects, one of the main drawbacks was that the user needed to keep at least one hand busy, meaning less ability to perform other tasks and a constant tremor. In 2017, Bosc et al. [14] overcame this problem by using a see-through HMD (Moverio BT 200, Epson®, Nagano, Japan) to overlay perforators taken from a 3D reconstruction of a CTA preoperatively. By this technique, a hands-free stereoscopic image was represented over the abdominal wall for DIEP dissection. Tracking was made by image recognition in the umbilicus, like the other authors, and because the HMD made a real-time tracking, there was minimal tremor, and both hands were free to perform the tasks required. Twelve patients were studied, and all of them had a good correlation at surgical time. More interestingly, the 3D reconstruction permitted the evaluators to follow the vascular tree, even through the flap. One problem mentioned was that the LED lights of the operation room interfered with glass sensors, making it unstable. Also, with all the methods mentioned by now, images displayed were just static 2D projections of 3D reconstructions, not being able to adapt to the surfaces and movements. A solution to this problem was published by Nuri et al. [15], when a 3D reconstruction of a CTA was rendered to be used in a see-through HMD (HoloLens 1®, Microsoft Corp., Redmond, WA). After calibration, by aligning the anterior superior iliac spine and patella, a real-time, 3D image was overlaid to the thigh, allowing to see the perforators, muscles, and vascular tree in a more precise way than the US Doppler.

For lymphatic surgery, different approaches using AR exist. Hummelink et al. [16] used their in-house developed detector-projector to overlay CTA images with lymph nodes included in a DIEP flap to prevent lymphedema in breast reconstruction surgery. The lymph nodes related to the superficial circumflex iliac artery (SCIA), DIEP, and course were traced on multiple patients' skin preoperatively and compared to intraoperative dissection with good correlation. Pereira et al. reported in [17] technique for lymphovenous anastomosis planning where indocyanine green lymphography (ICG-L) with a near-infrared camera was performed preoperatively in a group of patients. Findings were marked, and standardized digital photographs were taken in different projections. With the same smartphone app previously used in perforator planning, on surgical day each patient's photos were superimposed preoperatively and traced over their skin (Fig. 9.2, Video 9.1). Suzuki et al. [18] performed a preoperative lymphovenous anastomosis planning by combining ICG-L and photoacoustic imaging (PAI). PAI sends lasers in specific wavelengths (797 and 835 nm), and then these rays are "caught" by venules and lymphatic vessels. Because lymph fluid is colorless, ICG is injected. The light is absorbed, and ultrasound waves are emitted. The waves are then captured and processed by the imaging system (PAI-05®; Luxonus, Kanagawa, Japan). This method allows to depict three-dimensional structures by using a bowl-shaped sensor to receive ultrasound waves emitted from the object at multiple points, including which run deeper. The processed images were exported to a see-through HMD (Moverio BT 30-E, Epson®, Nagano, Japan) and overlapped to the patient extremity to freehand track the images on their skin. Preoperative planning was consistent with intraoperative microscopic imaging and allowed to make incisions tailored to the point where lymphatic and venules cross each other. The main problems remain the same as perforator planning: there's the need to calibrate and align the images, which is sometimes difficult and time-consuming. Also, the image is a 2D picture overlaid in a 3D surface and does not adapt to movements.

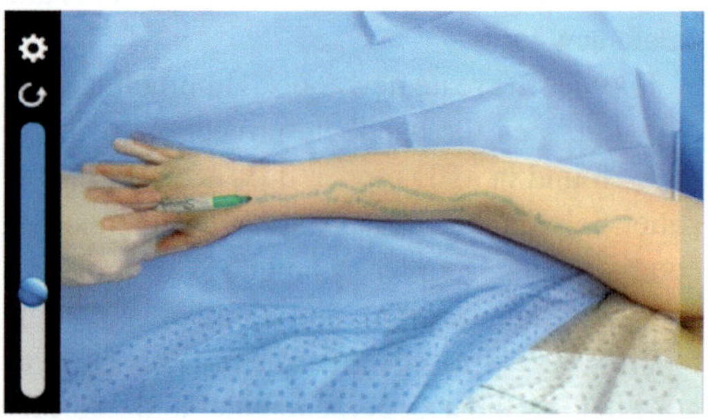

Fig. 9.2 Augmented reality microsurgical planning with a smartphone for lymphovenous anastomosis

The development of AR technology also can be applied to plan volumetric design of flaps. Hummelink et al. [19] used AR to obtain symmetric results in breast reconstruction by DIEP flap modeling. This was achieved by using a 3D stereophotogrammetry (3dMD Body, 3dMD LLC, Atlanta, USA) and a CTA reconstruction of the flap and perforators the same as their other publications [11, 12, 16]. The reference was the same breast or contralateral breast depending on timing. The volumetric design was trespassed to the 3D perforator render, and the flap positioned around the selected vessels. The preoperative planning resulted in good symmetry, and the volume harvested was almost identical to the estimated one (5 +/− 27 g difference).

9.4 How to Perform Augmented Reality Microsurgical Planning with a Smartphone (ARM-PS)

Using superficial circumflex iliac artery perforator (SCIP) flap as a model, AR microsurgical planning can be performed using a smartphone as a handheld device [7] (Fig. 9.3).

- Lower extremity CTA images are obtained using a 64-detector row helical CT system (Brilliance 64; Philips, Amsterdam, the Netherlands) with perforator protocol, maximum intensity projection, and 1-mm slice width.

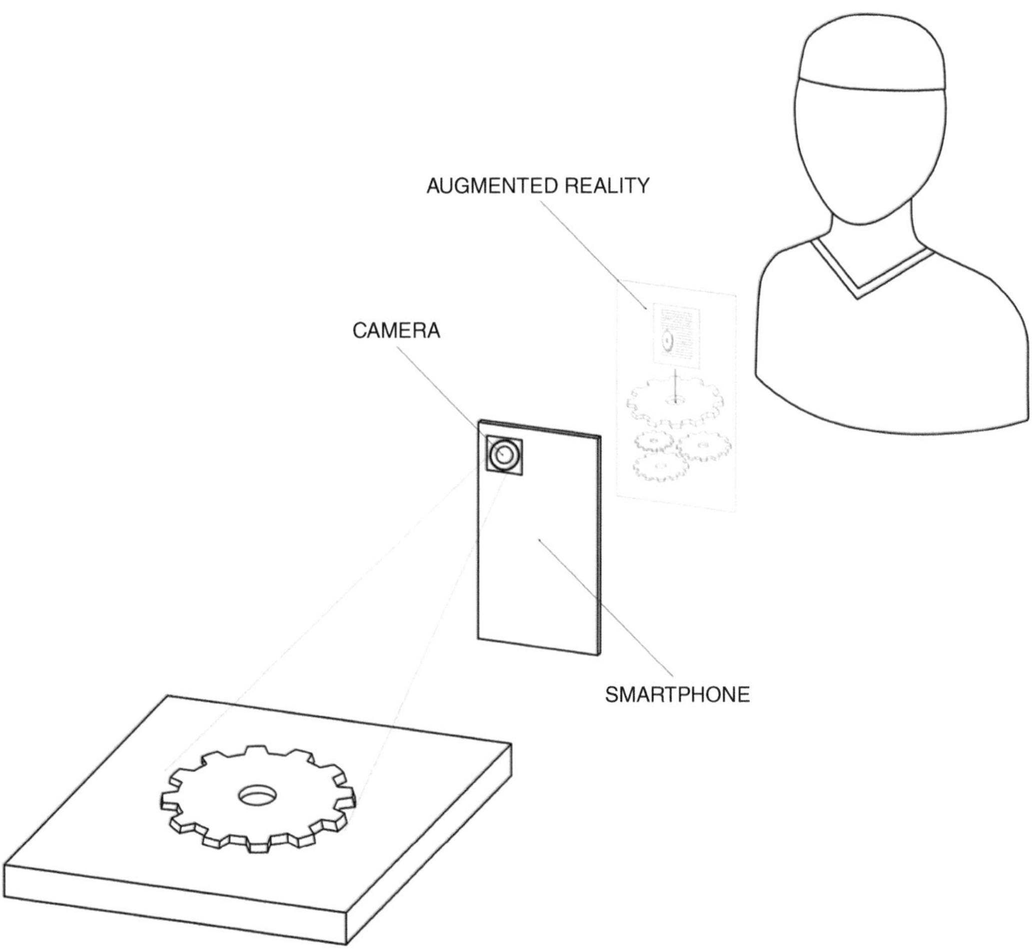

Fig. 9.3 Smartphone as a handheld device scheme

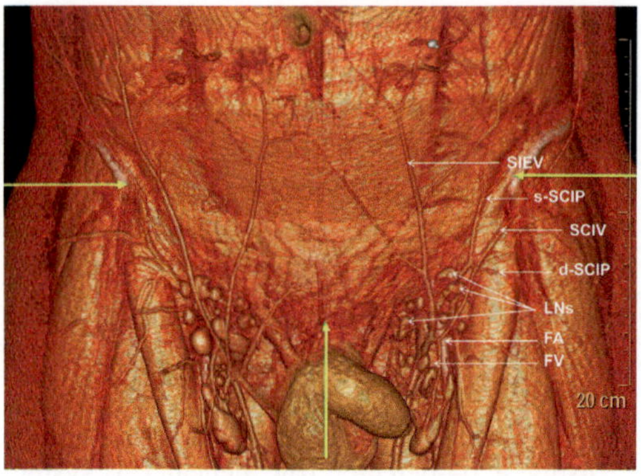

Fig. 9.4 3D reconstruction image of inguinal and lower abdomen vascular anatomy. Landmarks used are umbilicus and yellow arrows (both anterior superior iliac spines and superior border of pubic symphysis). (*SIEA* superficial inferior epigastric artery, *s-SCIP* superficial branch of superficial circumflex iliac artery perforator, *d-SCIP* deep branch of superficial circumflex iliac artery perforator, *LNs* lymph nodes, *FA* femoral artery, *FV* femoral vein)

- A three-dimensional (3D) reconstruction image of inguinal and lower abdomen vascular anatomy is obtained using multimodality advanced vessel analysis software (AVA) (Philips, Amsterdam, the Netherlands) to identify referential landmarks, i.e., umbilicus, both anterior superior iliac spines (ASIS) and superior border of pubic symphysis (PS) (Fig. 9.4).
- The 3D image obtained by CTA is reviewed online in a smartphone (Samsung Galaxy S21, Seoul, South Korea) and downloaded directly to the picture's gallery excluding sensitive information.
- The 3D image is imported from the smartphone's gallery to an AR app (*Camera Lucida AR*) to superimpose the image with the camera (Fig. 9.5).
- Freehand drawings are performed guided through the smartphone screen by fixing the image to the landmarks (umbilicus, both ASIS and PS) and identifying arteries and veins derived from the femoral vessels (superficial inferior epigastric [SIE], superficial branch of SCIP [s-SCIP], deep branch of SCIP [d-SICP]) and groin lymph nodes (Fig. 9.6, Video 9.2).
- Drawings performed with ARM-PS can be correlated with handheld Doppler and intraoperative findings (Fig. 9.7, Video 9.3).

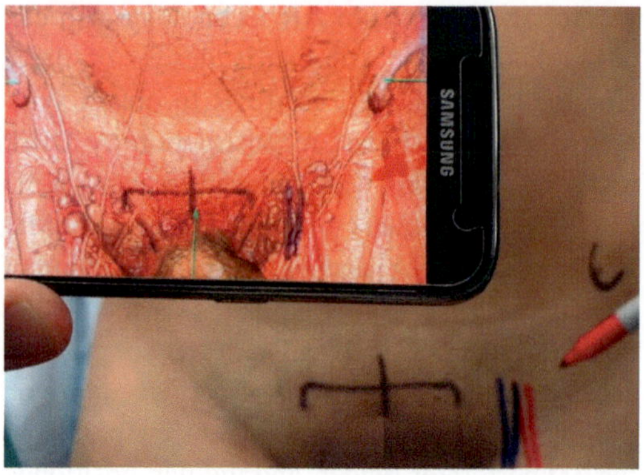

Fig. 9.5 Augmented reality microsurgical planning with a smartphone (ARM-PS). The 3D image of the groin vascular anatomy is imported to the augmented reality app to overlap the image with the smartphone camera

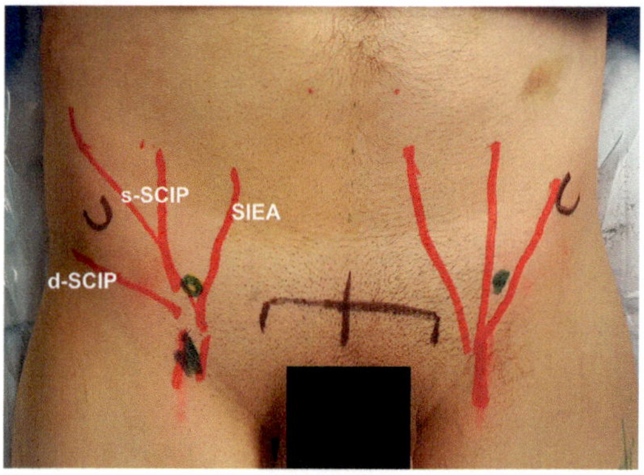

Fig. 9.6 Preoperative markings of the vascular anatomy of the left groin for SCIP flap using ARM-PS. (*d-SCIP* deep branch of superficial circumflex iliac artery perforator, *s-SCIP* superficial branch of superficial circumflex iliac artery perforator, *SIEA* superficial inferior epigastric artery)

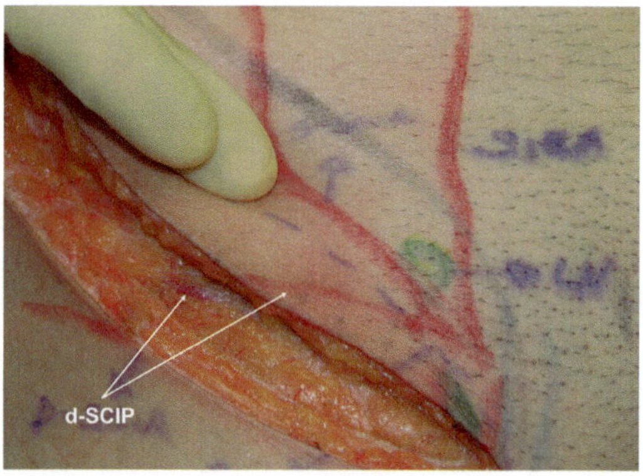

Fig. 9.7 Correlation of ARM-PS drawings with intraoperative findings of a left SCIP flap (same patient in Fig. 9.6)

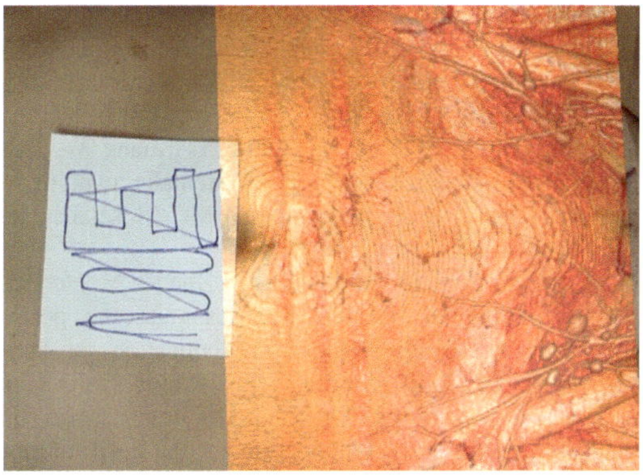

Fig. 9.8 ARM-PS using an anchor (second-generation app) for more accuracy

Recently, we have been using second-generation AR apps for high-end mobiles (e.g., *Da Vinci Eye* for Android, *Tracing Projector* for iOS). These allow us to lock the image to avoid user's tremor and alignment issues. These apps are based on the use of an anchor that allows the image to be fixed, so that it does not lose its alignment if inadvertent movements occur, allowing it to be more efficient and accurate (Fig. 9.8, Video 9.4).

9.5 Augmented Reality for the Intraoperative Microsurgery

Less advances have been made in this field, maybe because of the need to work in such small space as in microsurgical field. That is why most of studies are related to macroscopic structures as bones. Battaglia et al. [20] in 2019 and Lin et al. [21] in 2022 published their experience in mandible reconstruction with free fibula flaps by using AR for preparation but also harvest and navigation. Virtual osteotomy guides allowed to reconstruct in a more accurate way the new mandible, also preview its vessels related to the segment to dissect and avoid damaging it. This was achieved using smartphones or AR HMD. Pratt et al. [22] in 2018 used HoloLens1 (Microsoft Corporation, Redmond, WA, USA) to overlay a CTA 3D render over each patient leg and find the most useful perforator to design a flap. The operator first adjusts the image to the anatomical landmarks of each patient (principally bony prominences) and the, by hand gestures or voice commands, control the rotation and translation. Perforators were correctly found in comparison to US Doppler and intraoperative finding, and flaps dissected without any complication.

On a more specific topic related to microsurgery, Bigdeli et al. [23] in 2015 used AR to demonstrate intraoperatively free flap perfusion by near-infrared indocyanine green video angiography (ICG-NIR-VA). This technology uses an ICG angiography combined with white light visualization, with highlighted perfusion, including a color-coded perfusion flow scale for optimized anatomical understanding to provide HD resolution on visible and IR channels with a frame rate of 20–30 fps. The field of view is 14 × 11 cm^2 at a nominal working distance of 30 cm. The authors used flap dissection and inset to assess the correct perfusion. In some cases, congestion occurred, and after revision thrombus was found. It was evidenced by the absence of ICG clearance and translated to a color-fused image. In other cases, hypoperfusion was shown early after inset and ended in distal flap necrosis, acting as a predictor of flap survival. The ICG-NIR-VA system allowed a virtual view of flap perfusion anatomy by fusion imaging in real time, and the system improved decision-making for flap design and surgical decisions in some patients. It enabled an intuitive understanding of complex surgical perfusion scenarios during free flap surgery via an "augmented perfusion."

9.6 Conclusions

The use of augmented reality in microsurgery is a reality, especially in the planning and execution of microsurgical flaps. Although it has some limitations in terms of massive access to this technology, we have been able to see that the use of the AR for smartphones is an easy, noninvasive, and accurate method that provides a dissection route map, thereby standardizing flap harvesting, and shows a perfect correlation with intraoperative findings. It reduces operating time and may improve operative results, thereby decreasing donor site morbidity.

References

1. Khor WS, Baker B, Amin K, Chan A, Patel K, Wong J. Augmented and virtual reality in surgery—the digital surgical environment: applications, limitations and legal pitfalls. Ann Transl Med. 2016;4(23):454.
2. Reidsma D, Katayose H, Nijholt A, editors. Advances in computer entertainment: 10th international conference, ACE 2013 Boekelo, The Netherlands, November 12–15, 2013, proceedings. Berlin: Springer; 2013.
3. Azuma RT. A survey of augmented reality. Presence Teleoperators Virtual Environ. 1997;6:355–85.
4. Tan Y, Xu W, Li S, Chen K. Augmented and virtual reality (AR/VR) for education and training in the AEC industry: a systematic review of research and applications. Buildings. 2022;12:1529.
5. Lee GK, Moshrefi S, Fuertes V, Veeravagu L, Nazerali R, Lin SJ. What is your reality? Virtual, augmented, and mixed reality in plastic surgery training, education, and practice. Plast Reconstr Surg. 2021;147(2):505–11.
6. Al Omran Y, Abdall-Razak A, Sohrabi C, Borg TM, Nadama H, Ghassemi N, Oo K, Ghanem AM. Use of augmented reality in reconstructive microsurgery: a systematic review and development of the augmented reality microsurgery score. J Reconstr Microsurg. 2020;36(4):261–70.
7. Pereira N, Kufeke M, Parada L, Troncoso E, Bahamondes J, Sanchez L, Roa R. Augmented reality microsurgical planning with a smartphone (ARM-PS): a dissection route map in your pocket. J Plast Reconstr Aesthet Surg. 2019;72(5):759–62.
8. Vles MD, Terng NCO, Zijlstra K, Mureau MAM, Corten EML. Virtual and augmented reality for preoperative planning in plastic surgical procedures: a systematic review. J Plast Reconstr Aesthet Surg. 2020;73(11):1951–9.
9. Sayadi LR, Naides A, Eng M, Fijany A, Chopan M, Sayadi JJ, Shaterian A, Banyard DA, Evans GRD, Vyas R, Widgerow AD. The new frontier: a review of augmented reality and virtual reality in plastic surgery. Aesthet Surg J. 2019;39(9):1007–16.
10. Rozen WM, Ashton MW, Stella DL, Phillips TJ, Taylor GI. Stereotactic image-guided navigation in the preoperative imaging of perforators for DIEP flap breast reconstruction. Microsurgery. 2008;28(6):417–23.
11. Hummelink S, Hameeteman M, Hoogeveen Y, Slump CH, Ulrich DJ, Schultze Kool LJ. Preliminary results using a newly developed projection method to visualize vascular anatomy prior to DIEP flap breast reconstruction. J Plast Reconstr Aesthet Surg. 2015;68(3):390–4.
12. Hummelink S, Hoogeveen YL, Schultze Kool LJ, Ulrich DJO. A new and innovative method of preoperatively planning and projecting vascular anatomy in DIEP flap breast reconstruction: a randomized controlled trial. Plast Reconstr Surg. 2019;143(6):1151e–8e.
13. Tang Y, Guo Q, Li X, Huang Y, Kuang W, Luo L. Augmented reality-assisted systematic mapping of anterolateral thigh perforators. BMC Musculoskelet Disord. 2022;23(1):1047.
14. Bosc R, Fitoussi A, Pigneur F, Tacher V, Hersant B, Meningaud JP. Repérage des vaisseaux perforants par réalité augmentée: application au lambeau perforant d'artère épigastrique inférieure profonde [Identification of perforating vessels by augmented reality: Application for the deep inferior epigastric perforator flap]. Ann Chir Plast Esthet. 2017;62(4):336–9.
15. Nuri T, Mitsuno D, Iwanaga H, Otsuki Y, Ueda K. Application of augmented reality (AR) technology to locate the cutaneous perforator of anterolateral thigh perforator flap: a case report. Microsurgery. 2022;42(1):76–9. https://doi.org/10.1002/micr.30735. Epub 2021 Mar 31.
16. Hummelink S, Schultze Kool LJ, Ulrich DJ. Displaying inguinal lymph nodes before transplantation in a deep inferior epigastric perforator flap breast reconstruction using an innovative projection method. J Plast Reconstr Aesthet Surg. 2016;69(3):376–80.
17. Pereira N, Venegas J. Augmented reality microsurgical planning with a smartphone for lymphovenous anastomosis. Plast Reconstr Surg. 2019;144(5):955e–6e.
18. Suzuki Y, Kajita H, Watanabe S, Otaki M, Okabe K, Sakuma H, Takatsume Y, Imanishi N, Aiso S, Kishi K. Surgical applications of lymphatic vessel visualization using photoacoustic imaging and augmented reality. J Clin Med. 2021;11(1):194.
19. Hummelink S, Verhulst AC, Maal TJJ, Hoogeveen YL, Schultze Kool LJ, Ulrich DJO. An innovative method of planning and displaying flap volume in DIEP flap breast reconstructions. J Plast Reconstr Aesthet Surg. 2017;70(7):871–5.
20. Battaglia S, Badiali G, Cercenelli L, Bortolani B, Marcelli E, Cipriani R, Contedini F, Marchetti C, Tarsitano A. Combination of CAD/CAM and augmented reality in free fibula bone harvest. Plast Reconstr Surg Glob Open. 2019;7(11):e2510.
21. Lin QQ, Wang F, Sun JL, Zhang HZ, Xi Q. Accurate mandible reconstruction by mixed reality, 3D printing, and robotic-assisted navigation integration. J Craniofac Surg. 2022;33(6):1720–4.
22. Pratt P, Ives M, Lawton G, Simmons J, Radev N, Spyropoulou L, Amiras D. Through the HoloLens™ looking glass: augmented reality for extremity reconstruction surgery using 3D vascular models with perforating vessels. Eur Radiol Exp. 2018;2(1):2.
23. Bigdeli AK, Gazyakan E, Schmidt VJ, Hernekamp FJ, Harhaus L, Henzler T, Kremer T, Kneser U, Hirche C. Indocyanine green fluorescence for free-flap perfusion imaging revisited: advanced decision making by virtual perfusion reality in visionsense fusion imaging angiography. Surg Innov. 2016;23(3):249–60.

Imaging for Reconstructive Microsurgery: Indocyanine Green

10

P. Rastogi and David W. Chang

Since the start of the twenty-first century, the intraoperative use of fluorescence imaging has increased steadily, with published evidence demonstrating its effectiveness in a variety of surgical domains including ophthalmology, oncologic, gastrointestinal, and endocrine surgery [1–3]. This chapter aims to elucidate the expanding role of indocyanine green (ICG) lymphangiography within the sphere of microsurgery. The utility of ICG lymphangiography in the diagnostic evaluation and management of lymphedema, as well as its adjunctive role in evaluating tissue perfusion, will be considered.

10.1 ICG: Mechanism of Action and Administration

ICG is a water-soluble dye that binds to plasma proteins and fluoresces when exposed to near-infrared light (750–810 nm) [4]. The fluorophore can be injected systemically (intravenously) or locally (intradermally) to assess tissue perfusion or lymphatic flow, respectively. When activated by a laser- or light-emitting diode, ICG fluorescence is visualized with either handheld cameras or microscopes with an integrated near-infrared imaging system. The short half-life of ICG (3–5 min) confers an excellent safety profile and allows for repeated assessments if necessary [5]. Reported adverse effects of ICG (e.g., anaphylaxis) are rare (0.07–0.1%) [5, 6]. In a recently published consensus statement [7], a group of international experts agreed that ICG could be used in most patients, even those with known or suspected allergy to iodine. Similarly, in a recently published article reporting on patients with endometrial cancer receiving ICG for sentinel lymph node mapping ($n = 1414$), less than 5% of patients with a documented iodine or contrast allergy experienced any allergic reaction after ICG administration [8]. Nonetheless, the authors recognize that institutional practices for ICG use in patients with iodine or contrast allergies may vary.

10.2 ICG Lymphangiography and Lymphedema

Chronic lymphedema affects 250 million people worldwide, with cancer-related surgery being the major cause in developed countries [5]. Historically, lymphoscintigraphy has been considered the gold standard for the diagnosis and severity staging of lymphedema [9]. Despite this, lymphoscintigraphy is expensive, time-consuming, associated with poor image resolution

P. Rastogi · D. W. Chang (✉)
Section of Plastic and Reconstructive Surgery, Department of Surgery, The University of Chicago Medicine, Chicago, IL, USA
e-mail: Pratik.Rastogi@uchicagomedicine.org; dwchang@uchicagomedicine.org

J. P. Hong et al. (eds.), *Imaging for Reconstructive Microsurgery*,
https://doi.org/10.1007/978-981-97-7278-0_10

(no clear depiction of lymphatic vessels), and not suitable for real-time intraoperative use [9–12]. This ultimately limits a surgeon's ability to accurately predict potential lymphatic anastomotic sites, based on imaging alone.

10.2.1 Lymphedema Staging

In 2007, Ogata et al. [13] first reported the use of ICG to detect lymphatic pathways. In addition to the macroscopic identification of lymphatic vessels, ICG angiography has been increasingly utilized to stage the severity of lymphedema. In 2007, Unno et al. [14] first reported ICG lymphography findings such as *Milky Way sign, dermal backflow,* and *obstructed fluorescence image,* associated with secondary lower-limb lymphedema. In 2011, Yamamoto et al. [12, 15] proposed a formal classification system of ICG imaging findings according to lymphedema severity. The authors broadly categorized ICG lymphedema findings into linear and dermal backflow patterns [12]. The authors reported that the abnormal dermal backflow signs (*splash, stardust,* and *diffuse*) represented abnormal lymphatic circulation and correlated positively with an increase in clinical severity [12]. Moreover, the *splash* pattern was identified as the earliest finding on ICG lymphangiography of asymptomatic limbs in patients with secondary lower-limb lymphedema, even at a subclinical stage [10].

Presently, the diagnosis and severity staging of lymphedema is most often based on either the MD Anderson Cancer Center Scale (MDACCS) [16, 17] or the Dermal Backflow Scale (DBS) [15, 18], both of which have been validated and are reproducible [9] (Table 10.1). The MDACCS focuses on the visualization of patent lymphatic vessels in combination with the presence of DBF. In contrast, the DBS focuses on the proximal to distal extension of different DBF patterns (in order of severity: normal, splash, stardust, and diffuse) [9, 12, 15–18]. Figure 10.1 highlights representative images of lymphedema severity based on the MDACCS.

Notably, several studies have demonstrated poor to slight correlation between International Society of Lymphology (ISL) clinical stage (present gold standard), lymphedema volume, and the findings of ICG lymphangiography [17, 19, 20]. This observation further supports the belief that lymphedema severity depends mostly on the extent of intrinsic lymphatic damage, not on the duration or severity of lymphedema symptoms alone [17]. This further reinforces the utility of ICG lymphangiography in both the diagnostic and therapeutic management of patients with lymphedema.

10.2.2 ICG Lymphangiography and Lymphovenous Bypass

The senior author (D. W. Chang) has previously reported his technique for ICG lymphangiography in 100 consecutive lymphovenous bypass cases for the treatment of secondary extremity lymphedema [17] (Fig. 10.2). In this technique, lymphangiography is performed injecting ICG (0.01–0.02 mL) intradermally into each finger/toe web of the affected limb. ICG lymphangiog-

Table 10.1 MD Anderson Cancer Center and Dermal Backflow Scales: assessment of severity of lymphedema using ICG lymphangiography [15–19]

Stage	MD Anderson Cancer Center Scale	Dermal Backflow Scale
0	No dermal backflow	No dermal backflow
1	Many patent lymphatics and minimal dermal backflow	Splash pattern around the axilla
2	Moderate number of patent lymphatics and segmental dermal backflow	Stardust limited between olecranon and axilla
3	Few patent lymphatics with extensive dermal backflow	Stardust distal to olecranon
4	Dermal backflow involving the hand	Stardust involving the hand
5	ICG does not move proximal to injection site	Diffuse and stardust pattern involving the entire limb

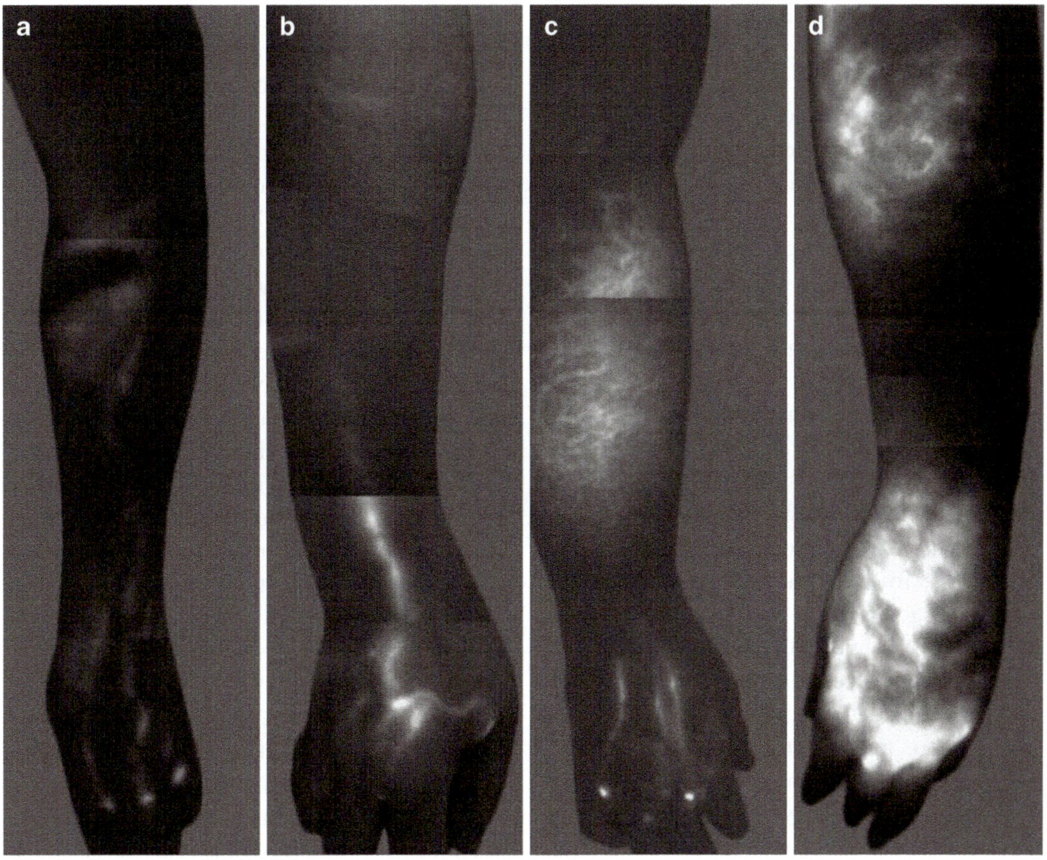

Fig. 10.1 M. D. Anderson lymphedema classification based on ICG findings. (**a**) Stage 1, (**b**) stage 2, (**c**) stage 3, and (**d**) stage 4 [17]. [*From:* Chang DW, Suami H, Skoracki R. A prospective analysis of 100 consecutive lymphovenous bypass cases for treatment of extremity lymphedema. Plastic and reconstructive surgery. 2013;132(5):1305–14]

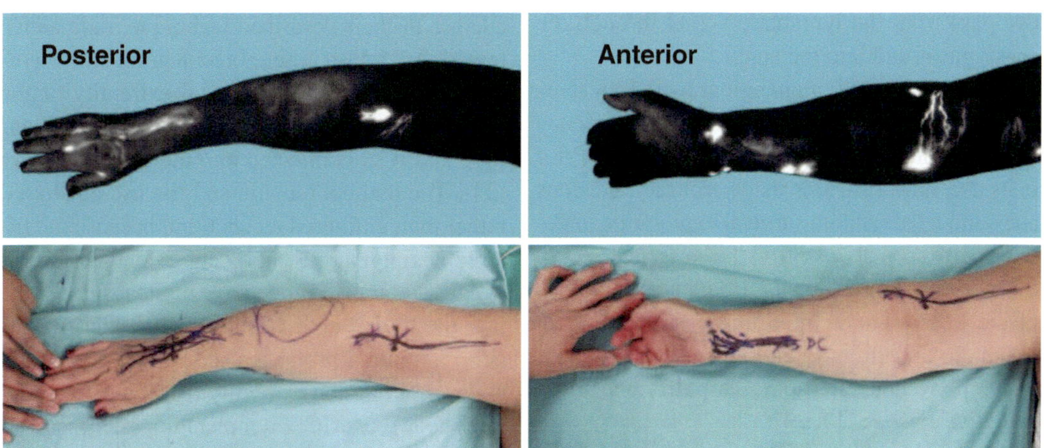

Fig. 10.2 ICG lymphangiography visualized using Hamamatsu Photodynamic Eye demonstrating aberrant lymphatic drainage and dermal backflow [17]. [*From:* Chang DW, Suami H, Skoracki R. A prospective analysis of 100 consecutive lymphovenous bypass cases for treatment of extremity lymphedema. Plastic and reconstructive surgery. 2013;132(5):1305–14]

raphy and lymphovenous bypass can be safely performed under local anesthesia or general anesthesia depending on the logistics and the setting [12, 21]. Nonetheless, soon after the ICG injections, a near-infrared camera is utilized to visualize fluorescent images of lymphatic vessels and/or dermal backflow stains. Visible lymphatic pathways are subsequently marked, and the incision sites for lymphovenous bypasses are planned. Bypass is not performed in cases of nearly normal-appearing lymphatics or in cases of severe lymphedema with extensive dermal backflow where no lymphatic channels can be identified [22].

The patient's limb is subsequently prepared for surgery. Local anesthetic with epinephrine (30 G needle) is used prior to incision to optimize hemostasis. To further help visualize superficial lymphatic vessels, isosulfan blue dye (0.1–0.2 mL) is injected intradermally into each finger/toe web space and/or 1–2 cm distal to each incision. Using a surgical microscope, 2–3 cm incisions are made at the predetermined sites based on the ICG mapping. The subdermal region is dissected to identify lymphatic vessels. A viable lymphatic vessel is subsequently anastomosed to an adjacent recipient venule to create the bypass (end-end, end-side, or side-end configuration) with 11–0 or 12–0 nylon sutures (30–50 μm needles). The patency of the bypasses is confirmed by observing ICG or isosulfan blue dye pass from the lymphatic vessel through the anastomosis and into the venule.

The use of ICG lymphangiography represents a significant advance in the technical efficiency of performing lymphovenous anastomoses. Prior to its use, most surgeons made arbitrary incisions and conducted random surgical exploration under the microscope to identify the vessels [17]. In theory, the improvements in identifying lymphatic vessels may limit unnecessary surgical trauma to an extremity and increase the number of lymphovenous anastomoses performed in an operative episode [17, 23].

10.2.3 ICG, Reverse Lymphatic Mapping, and Vascularized Lymph Node Transfer

Vascularized lymph node transplant (VLNT) has become an increasing popular option in the surgical armamentarium for lymphedema, particularly for patients with a paucity of functional lymphatics available for lymphovenous bypass [24, 25]. The exact mechanism of action of VLNT remains controversial, but theories about functional improvement with VLNT include the induction of spontaneous lymphangiogenesis as well as the ability of tissue to provide a local "pump action" or to rejuvenate a cicatrized surgical or radiotherapy bed [26]. Reported studies have demonstrated up to a 40% reduction in the volume component of limbs (fluid component) treated with VLNT [25–28]. Despite these potential benefits, the risk of donor site lymphedema remains a significant concern [29, 30].

To mitigate the risk of secondary donor site lymphedema, Dayan et al. [24] described their technique of reverse lymphatic mapping for vascularized lymph node transplant, a modification of Klimberg's technique of axillary reverse mapping [31] for sentinel lymph node biopsy. The combined use of ICG and radioactive tracer in this setting allows the surgeon to both confirm the presence of lymphatic tissue for VLNT and minimize the risk of secondary donor site lymphedema. In their described technique, radioactive tracer (0.2 mL of filtered technetium-sulfur colloid) is injected into the distal extremity of the donor site (first and second web space of finger/toe), and ICG is injected into the trunk centrally [24]. The authors recommend the use of filtered rather than unfiltered technetium, because the filtered variety has a more consistent molecular weight and transit time and exhibits faster uptake into the lymph node basin [24, 32]. During surgery, a gamma probe is used to identify lymph nodes draining the extremity (especially the sentinel node), and ICG lymphangiography is used to identify lymph nodes draining the trunk (which are harvested for vascularized lymph node transplant) [24]. The technique enables the surgeon to navigate the groin and axillary lymph node basin with real-time physiologic assessment of a patient's lymphatic anatomy and obviates the need to rely on static anatomic landmarks [24, 33].

10.3 Free Flap and Skin Perfusion Assessment

The adequate assessment of tissue viability and perfusion is the central dictum of reconstructive microsurgery. Flap perfusion is traditionally assessed using variables like temperature, color, capillary refill, turgor, and dermal edge bleeding. Despite the popular wisdom of "traditionalist" plastic surgeons, these methods are not infallible. For example, it has been shown that clinical assessment can miss up to 41% of cases of mastectomy skin flap ischemia [34, 35]. Moreover, a recent systematic review reported that rates of fat necrosis post deep inferior epigastric perforator flap breast reconstruction varied from 12 to 45% [36]. Appreciably, the intraoperative clinical assessment of fat necrosis risk or partial skin flap necrosis is not as tangible as the more arbitrary decision of whether a flap is absolutely viable or not.

ICG angiography images can be assessed both qualitatively and quantitatively. Qualitatively, as the perfusion increases, the fluorescence intensity increases. Although predicting perfusion in areas of high fluorescence intensity is easy, decision-making within the areas of lower intensity (the gray zones) can be more challenging [37]. The light detection device can quantitatively assess dye emission using various computer algorithms to calculate different parameters representing perfusion [38–40]. Absolute perfusion values are derived directly from the intensity of fluorescence or pixel values of the gray scale. Relative perfusion values are based on a reference region on the ICG image selected by the surgeon (standard for comparison to other regions) [38, 39]. Analysis systems can subsequently create a contour map over studied tissue, with contour lines representing areas of isofluorescence [38, 39]. Relative values and contour lines may vary with time, representing changes in signal intensity and perfusion. Furthermore, quantification systems can automatically calculate rates of arterial inflow and venous outflow during video surveillance, which may be graphically represented [40, 41]. Despite the different qualitative and quantitative methods, there is no gold standard method to measure perfusion in free tissue or skin flaps. Moreover, the rates of adoption of quantitative assessment of ICG angiography in clinical microsurgery remain poorly reported in the literature.

Several studies have supported the utility of ICG angiography in microsurgery. A recent systematic review conducted by Parmeshwar et al. [42], which investigated ICG angiography use during free flap breast reconstruction, reported that the odds of developing fat necrosis were 69% less in the ICG cohort than when perfusion assessment was based on clinical assessment alone. Notably, the study did not report any statistically significant difference for total or partial flap loss. Furthermore, anastomotic patency has been assessed with ICG angiography both intraoperatively and postoperatively, in other studies, leading to increased survival of flaps [43, 44]. Similarly, studies have also demonstrated that real-time visualization with ICG angiography is helpful in minimizing rates of mastectomy skin flap necrosis with up to 90% sensitivity when compared with clinical assessment alone [37, 45–48]. Despite these results, there is some concern that ICG angiography may overpredict poor perfusion zones [34, 49].

Despite its emerging utility, no formal guidelines exist to guide the use of ICG angiography in plastic and reconstructive surgery [7].

Table 10.2 Consensus recommendations [7] guiding use of ICG angiography

1. Recommended dose of ICG administration is 0.05 mg/kg
2. Perfusion assessment performed >20 s but <1 min after ICG administration
– Arterial perfusion usually becomes visible within seconds to, at most, minutes after ICG administration
3. Best camera angle (61°–90°) and distance (20–30 cm) from the target tissue
– Angle and distance may vary according to camera type
4. Ambient light, patient body temperature, and vasopressor/tumescence may affect perfusion assessments
– These factors should be considered dynamically when assessing ICG angiography images

Considerable variability continues to exist in ICG dosage and administration as well as optimal camera logistics (positioning, angle, and distance). The influence of other dynamic factors (ambient light, body temperature, vasopressor, and tumescence use) on perfusion assessment with ICG angiography is variably understood [7]. Table 10.2 highlights some preliminary recommendations, made by a panel of experts, to standardize ICG angiography practice [7]. Although these recommendations represent the consensus opinions of experts, they are the present best foundation for future guidelines.

10.4 Conclusion

The role of ICG in reconstructive microsurgery continues to evolve. In lymphedema, ICG lymphangiography has facilitated identification of lymphatic channels, improved staging of lymphedema severity, helped target optimal sites for lymphovenous bypass, and improved the fidelity of vascularized lymph node transfer procedures. ICG angiography has facilitated perfusion assessment (qualitative and quantitative), helping to mitigate skin and fat necroses. Further standardization will ensure that the scope of ICG utilization will continue to broaden and become more precise in the future.

References

1. Zaidi N, Bucak E, Okoh A, Yazici P, Yigitbas H, Berber E. The utility of indocyanine green near infrared fluorescent imaging in the identification of parathyroid glands during surgery for primary hyperparathyroidism. J Surg Oncol. 2016;113(7):771–4.
2. Zelken JA, Tufaro AP. Current trends and emerging future of indocyanine green usage in surgery and oncology: an update. Ann Surg Oncol. 2015;22(Suppl 3):S1271–83.
3. Keller DS, Ishizawa T, Cohen R, Chand M. Indocyanine green fluorescence imaging in colorectal surgery: overview, applications, and future directions. Lancet Gastroenterol Hepatol. 2017;2(10):757–66.
4. Reinhart MB, Huntington CR, Blair LJ, Heniford BT, Augenstein VA. Indocyanine green: historical context, current applications, and future considerations. Surg Innov. 2016;23(2):166–75.
5. Burnier P, Niddam J, Bosc R, Hersant B, Meningaud JP. Indocyanine green applications in plastic surgery: a review of the literature. J Plast Reconstr Aesthet Surg. 2017;70(6):814–27.
6. Cornelissen AJM, van Mulken TJM, Graupner C, Qiu SS, Keuter XHA, van der Hulst R, et al. Near-infrared fluorescence image-guidance in plastic surgery: a systematic review. Eur J Plast Surg. 2018;41(3):269–78.
7. Schols RM, Dip F, Lo Menzo E, Haddock NT, Landin L, Lee BT, et al. Delphi survey of intercontinental experts to identify areas of consensus on the use of indocyanine green angiography for tissue perfusion assessment during plastic and reconstructive surgery. Surgery. 2022;172(6S):S46–53.
8. Zammarrelli WA 3rd, Afonso AM, Broach V, Sonoda Y, Zivanovic O, Mueller JJ, et al. Sentinel lymph node biopsy in patients with endometrial cancer and an indocyanine green or iodinated contrast reaction—a proposed management algorithm. Gynecol Oncol. 2021;162(2):262–7.
9. van Heumen S, Riksen JJM, Bramer WM, van Soest G, Vasilic D. Imaging of the lymphatic vessels for surgical planning: a systematic review. Ann Surg Oncol. 2023;30(1):462–79.
10. Mikami T, Hosono M, Yabuki Y, Yamamoto Y, Yasumura K, Sawada H, et al. Classification of lymphoscintigraphy and relevance to surgical indication for lymphaticovenous anastomosis in upper limb lymphedema. Lymphology. 2011;44(4):155–67.
11. Pappalardo M, Lin C, Ho OA, Kuo CF, Lin CY, Cheng MH. Staging and clinical correlations of lymphoscintigraphy for unilateral gynecological cancer-related lymphedema. J Surg Oncol. 2020;121(3):422–34.
12. Yamamoto T, Narushima M, Doi K, Oshima A, Ogata F, Mihara M, et al. Characteristic indocyanine green lymphography findings in lower extremity lymphedema: the generation of a novel lymphedema severity staging system using dermal backflow patterns. Plast Reconstr Surg. 2011;127(5):1979–86.

13. Ogata F, Azuma R, Kikuchi M, Koshima I, Morimoto Y. Novel lymphography using indocyanine green dye for near-infrared fluorescence labeling. Ann Plast Surg. 2007;58(6):652–5.
14. Unno N, Inuzuka K, Suzuki M, Yamamoto N, Sagara D, Nishiyama M, et al. Preliminary experience with a novel fluorescence lymphography using indocyanine green in patients with secondary lymphedema. J Vasc Surg. 2007;45(5):1016–21.
15. Yamamoto T, Yamamoto N, Doi K, Oshima A, Yoshimatsu H, Todokoro T, et al. Indocyanine green-enhanced lymphography for upper extremity lymphedema: a novel severity staging system using dermal backflow patterns. Plast Reconstr Surg. 2011;128(4):941–7.
16. Nguyen AT, Suami H, Hanasono MM, Womack VA, Wong FC, Chang EI. Long-term outcomes of the minimally invasive free vascularized omental lymphatic flap for the treatment of lymphedema. J Surg Oncol. 2017;115(1):84–9.
17. Chang DW, Suami H, Skoracki R. A prospective analysis of 100 consecutive lymphovenous bypass cases for treatment of extremity lymphedema. Plast Reconstr Surg. 2013;132(5):1305–14.
18. Narushima M, Yamamoto T, Ogata F, Yoshimatsu H, Mihara M, Koshima I. Indocyanine green lymphography findings in limb lymphedema. J Reconstr Microsurg. 2016;32(1):72–9.
19. Jorgensen MG, Toyserkani NM, Hansen FCG, Thomsen JB, Sorensen JA. Prospective validation of indocyanine green lymphangiography staging of breast cancer-related lymphedema. Cancers (Basel). 2021;13(7):1540.
20. Garza RM, Ooi AS, Falk J, Chang DW. The relationship between clinical and indocyanine green staging in lymphedema. Lymphat Res Biol. 2019;17(3):329–33.
21. Yamamoto T, Narushima M, Yoshimatsu H, Seki Y, Yamamoto N, Oka A, et al. Minimally invasive lymphatic supermicrosurgery (MILS): indocyanine green lymphography-guided simultaneous multisite lymphaticovenular anastomoses via millimeter skin incisions. Ann Plast Surg. 2014;72(1):67–70.
22. Garza RM, Beederman M, Chang DW. Physical and functional outcomes of simultaneous vascularized lymph node transplant and lymphovenous bypass in the treatment of lymphedema. Plast Reconstr Surg. 2022;150(1):169–80.
23. Chang DW. Lymphaticovenular bypass for lymphedema management in breast cancer patients: a prospective study. Plast Reconstr Surg. 2010;126(3):752–8.
24. Dayan JH, Dayan E, Smith ML. Reverse lymphatic mapping: a new technique for maximizing safety in vascularized lymph node transfer. Plast Reconstr Surg. 2015;135(1):277–85.
25. Beederman M, Garza RM, Agarwal S, Chang DW. Outcomes for physiologic microsurgical treatment of secondary lymphedema involving the extremity. Ann Surg. 2022;276(4):e255–e63.
26. Raju A, Chang DW. Vascularized lymph node transfer for treatment of lymphedema: a comprehensive literature review. Ann Surg. 2015;261(5):1013–23.
27. Winters H, Tielemans HJP, Paulus V, Hummelink S, Slater NJ, Ulrich DJO. A systematic review and meta-analysis of vascularized lymph node transfer for breast cancer-related lymphedema. J Vasc Surg Venous Lymphat Disord. 2022;10(3):786–95 e1.
28. Ozturk CN, Ozturk C, Glasgow M, Platek M, Ashary Z, Kuhn J, et al. Free vascularized lymph node transfer for treatment of lymphedema: a systematic evidence based review. J Plast Reconstr Aesthet Surg. 2016;69(9):1234–47.
29. Azuma S, Yamamoto T, Koshima I. Donor-site lymphatic function after microvascular lymph node transfer should be followed using indocyanine green lymphography. Plast Reconstr Surg. 2013;131(3):443e–4e.
30. Vignes S, Blanchard M, Yannoutsos A, Arrault M. Complications of autologous lymph-node transplantation for limb lymphoedema. Eur J Vasc Endovasc Surg. 2013;45(5):516–20.
31. Klimberg VS. A new concept toward the prevention of lymphedema: axillary reverse mapping. J Surg Oncol. 2008;97(7):563–4.
32. Newman EA, Newman LA. Lymphatic mapping techniques and sentinel lymph node biopsy in breast cancer. Surg Clin N Am. 2007;87(2):353–64. viii.
33. Halvorson EG, Orgill DP. Discussion: reverse lymphatic mapping: a new technique for maximizing safety in vascularized lymph node transfer. Plast Reconstr Surg. 2015;135(1):286–8.
34. Phillips BT, Lanier ST, Conkling N, Wang ED, Dagum AB, Ganz JC, et al. Intraoperative perfusion techniques can accurately predict mastectomy skin flap necrosis in breast reconstruction: results of a prospective trial. Plast Reconstr Surg. 2012;129(5):778e–88e.
35. Phillips BT, Munabi NCO, Roeder RA, Ascherman JA, Guo L, Zenn MR. The role of intraoperative perfusion assessment: what is the current state and how can i use it in my practice? Plast Reconstr Surg. 2016;137(2):731–41.
36. Bhullar H, Hunter-Smith DJ, Rozen WM. Fat necrosis after DIEP flap breast reconstruction: a review of perfusion-related causes. Aesth Plast Surg. 2020;44(5):1454–61.
37. Moyer HR, Losken A. Predicting mastectomy skin flap necrosis with indocyanine green angiography: the gray area defined. Plast Reconstr Surg. 2012;129(5):1043–8.
38. Johnson AC, Colakoglu S, Chong TW, Mathes DW. Indocyanine green angiography in breast reconstruction: utility, limitations, and search for standardization. Plast Reconstr Surg Glob Open. 2020;8(3):e2694.
39. Mattison GL, Lewis PG, Gupta SC, Kim HY. SPY imaging use in postmastectomy breast reconstruction patients: preventative or overly conservative? Plast Reconstr Surg. 2016;138(1):15e–21e.

40. Holm C, Dornseifer U, Sturtz G, Basso G, Schuster T, Ninkovic M. The intrinsic transit time of free microvascular flaps: clinical and prognostic implications. Microsurgery. 2010;30(2):91–6.
41. Wang CY, Wang CH, Tzeng YS, Lin CT, Chou CY, Chiang IH, et al. Intraoperative assessment of the relationship between nipple circulation and incision site in nipple-sparing mastectomy with implant breast reconstruction using the SPY imaging system. Ann Plast Surg. 2018;80(2S Suppl 1):S59–65.
42. Parmeshwar N, Sultan SM, Kim EA, Piper ML. A systematic review of the utility of indocyanine angiography in autologous breast reconstruction. Ann Plast Surg. 2021;86(5):601–6.
43. Holm C, Mayr M, Hofter E, Dornseifer U, Ninkovic M. Assessment of the patency of microvascular anastomoses using microscope-integrated near-infrared angiography: a preliminary study. Microsurgery. 2009;29(7):509–14.
44. Hitier M, Cracowski JL, Hamou C, Righini C, Bettega G. Indocyanine green fluorescence angiography for free flap monitoring: a pilot study. J Craniomaxillofac Surg. 2016;44(11):1833–41.
45. Liu EH, Zhu SL, Hu J, Wong N, Farrokhyar F, Thoma A. Intraoperative SPY reduces post-mastectomy skin flap complications: a systematic review and meta-analysis. Plast Reconstr Surg Glob Open. 2019;7(4):e2060.
46. Munabi NC, Olorunnipa OB, Goltsman D, Rohde CH, Ascherman JA. The ability of intra-operative perfusion mapping with laser-assisted indocyanine green angiography to predict mastectomy flap necrosis in breast reconstruction: a prospective trial. J Plast Reconstr Aesthet Surg. 2014;67(4):449–55.
47. Yang CE, Chung SW, Lee DW, Lew DH, Song SY. Evaluation of the relationship between flap tension and tissue perfusion in implant-based breast reconstruction using laser-assisted indocyanine green angiography. Ann Surg Oncol. 2018;25(8):2235–40.
48. Newman MI, Samson MC, Tamburrino JF, Swartz KA. Intraoperative laser-assisted indocyanine green angiography for the evaluation of mastectomy flaps in immediate breast reconstruction. J Reconstr Microsurg. 2010;26(7):487–92.
49. Krishnan KG, Schackert G, Steinmeier R. The role of near-infrared angiography in the assessment of post-operative venous congestion in random pattern, pedicled island and free flaps. Br J Plast Surg. 2005;58(3):330–8.

Part III

Section C. Application for reconstructive surgery – *will review all applicable modalities for these flaps, which is the most valuable modality*

11 Evaluation of Overall Circulation of the Lower Limb

Feras Alshomer and Joon Pio Hong

11.1 Introduction

Lower extremity reconstruction still represents a challenging situation despite the recent advancements in reconstructive microsurgery. It begins with the moment of injury with factors related to zone of injury and its timing, the status of the wound especially the presence of infection, and vascularity status of the involved limb. These issues extends into the postoperative period with all these factors act collectively to dictate the healing and recovery phase [1]. With that, safety of lower extremity reconstruction has been established in several studies with high flap success rate. However, this requires meticulous anticipation of several variables that might hinder such success [2]. One of these factors is the vascularity status of the limb with its essential role in assuring successful reconstruction. This is absolutely essential in situations of limb trauma or chronic ischemia. This also extends to its relation to selecting potential flap perforators from the same limb in preparation of flap option or in selecting proper recipient vessels [3]. For that, a routine physical examination looking to assess the quality of soft tissue of the involved extremity together with checking for palpable pulse and limb temperature, as well as capillary refill with the potential adaptation of handheld Doppler examination, all may give a clue about the vascularity status of the limb. However, in situations of chronic limb ischemia or when physical examination results are inconclusive, additional investigative work is essential to show detailed examination of the limb vascularity prior to any surgical intervention [4]. In this chapter, a review of the different imaging modalities utilized in the evaluation of lower extremity vascular status will be presented, showcasing the essential role each modality has and its implications in preoperative planning of different reconstructive approaches as well as the intraoperative and postoperative utility.

11.2 Computed Tomography Angiography (CTA)

Radiologic lower extermity vascular assessment is usually indicated when there is loos of one or more peripheral pulses or when there is evidence of documented neurologic deficit or when deal-

F. Alshomer
Division of Plastic Surgery, Department of Surgery, King Abdulaziz Medical City, Ministry of National Guard—Health Affairs (MNG-HA), King Abdullah International Medical Research Center (KAIMRC), Riyadh, Saudi Arabia

Department of Plastic Surgery, Asan Medical Center, University of Ulsan, School of Medicine, Seoul, South Korea

J. P. Hong (✉)
Department of Plastic Surgery, Asan Medical Center, University of Ulsan, School of Medicine, Seoul, South Korea

J. P. Hong et al. (eds.), *Imaging for Reconstructive Microsurgery*,
https://doi.org/10.1007/978-981-97-7278-0_11

ing with compound fracture. However, the authors have shown that for lower extremity reconstruction related to various reasons that involves either trauma, post-oncologic resection or in relation to chronic wound condition, detailed vascularity assessment was indicated in about 75–80% of the cases [4]. One simple way to deliver such evaluation was seen with the use of CT angiography. This modality was described as fast and minimally invasive capable of providing detailed vascular assessment of the whole limb with visualization of tiny vascular structures as small as 1 mm [5]. Such utility was also proved effective in trauma cases as it allows for simultaneous assessment of vascularity and limb fractures. It also allows detailed three-dimensional (3D) assessment that can easily guide toward potential vascular obstruction site [6]. An example of the utility of 3D CTA with different clinical scenarios is shown in Fig. 11.1. Moreover, it has the potential for soft tissue and metallic hardware assessment and visualization of arteries and veins together with their diameter estimation [7]. The essential role of this modality was shown previously by work of Duymaz et al. in which they showed about 28.9% incidence of single-vessel occlusion in traumatic cases even with normal vascular examination of foot perfusion was found. They also pointed out that CTA-proven arterial occlusion was an independent risk factor for flap and limb loss in adult patients [8]. The efficacy of this modality in detecting vascular occlusive state was also beneficial in pediatric lower extremity traumatic cases with similar conclusion [9].

The role of CTA is not only limited to the assessment of limb vascularity but also extends to its essential role in planning the reconstructive approach. Among which is the role in preoperative flap perforator mapping as shown in Fig. 11.2 [10]. The authors also have shown previously the utility of CTA in the detailed analysis of the superficial (medial) perforator of superficial circumflex iliac artery perforator (SCIP) flap which showed 100% correlation to the surgical findings that includes the source of origin, course, and perforator penetration pattern to the fascia and the overlying skin [11]. This also applies to other flap types in which the utility of multidetector CTA allows detailed preoperative determination of proper donor perforator with detailed assessment that includes source vessel, diameter, location, and pathway through the muscle and fascia which decreases the operative time [12]. Moreover, direct analysis of limb vascular anomalies like in cases of fibula flap planning was also feasible. All of this enables surgeons to properly plan ahead with efficiency the decision for pedicle dissection and elevation thickness of the flap [11, 13, 14].

Furthermore, CTA is able to provide a detailed 3D evaluation of the limb vascularity in occlusive state. CTA has the capability of showing vessel calcification from atherosclerosis and/or occlusion. In such situation, collateral vessels may be the sole supply to the limb in which with this imaging modality such variation is clearly visualized (Fig. 11.1c). The importance of this finding resides in the fact that one may raise the flap with the collateral blood supply causing eventual limb ischemia. This is particularly true in diabetic patients with atherosclerosis in which common femoral artery (CFA) is frequently involved with eventual occlusion with limb vascularity dependent mainly on collateral blood supply from the deep femoral artery (DFA). The authors have investigated this phenomenon by reviewing several sets of CTA images and found a mean occlusion rate of the CFA to be around 15.6% with limb vascularity dependent on deep femoral artery (DFA) and lateral circumflex femoral artery collateral blood supply with about 0.6% of the screened patients having collateral only from the later source [15]. These findings are of great importance as one might not consider ipsilateral anterolateral thigh (ALT) flap as an option if limb vascularity was solely dependent on collateral supply and other options should be considered.

Additional advantages are the ease of contrast delivery which can be accessed through peripheral veins without the need for specialized teams for close monitoring. Additionally, CTA was shown to be more cost-effective for

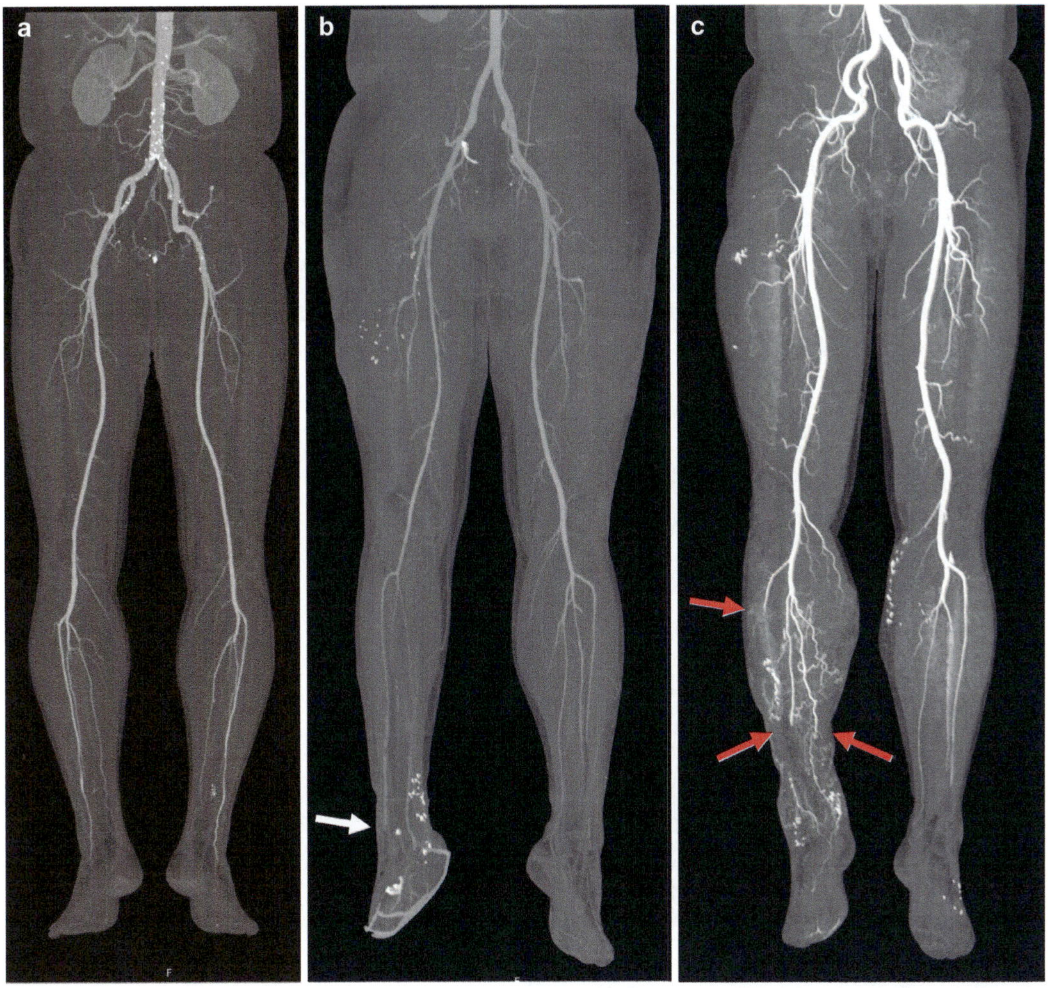

Fig. 11.1 The utility of computed tomography angiography (CTA) in lower limb vascular evaluation. (**a**) Normal lower extremity vascular assessment is shown in the 3D reconstructed CTA view. All lower limb major vessels (anterior tibial "ATA," posterior tibial "PTA," and peroneal arteries "PA") are clearly visualized with good patency. (**b**) An example of an abnormal lower limb CTA findings in which the ATA has a distal cutoff with occlusion at the right ankle level (white arrow) in addition to lower limb traumatic deformity. An additional example of the utility of CTA in lower limb vascular assessment is shown in (**c**) in which the right lower limb vascularity is totally dependent on collateral circulation "red arrows" with signal cutoff of all three vessels of the lower limb at the mid-leg level with scattered vascular calcifications

limb vascularity evaluation with less radiation as compared to conventional angiography. The use of CTA was shown to have a high sensitivity that reaches about 95.1% and a specificity of 98.7%. The use of this modality might be associated with false-positive findings in about 1.3% of the cases and is mostly related to contrast-induced vasospasm which can be alleviated with the simultaneous injection of vasodilators during the examination. Additionally, clear visualization might be hindered in cases of metallic implants with artifacts in which the need for other modalities like conventional angiography might be warranted [16].

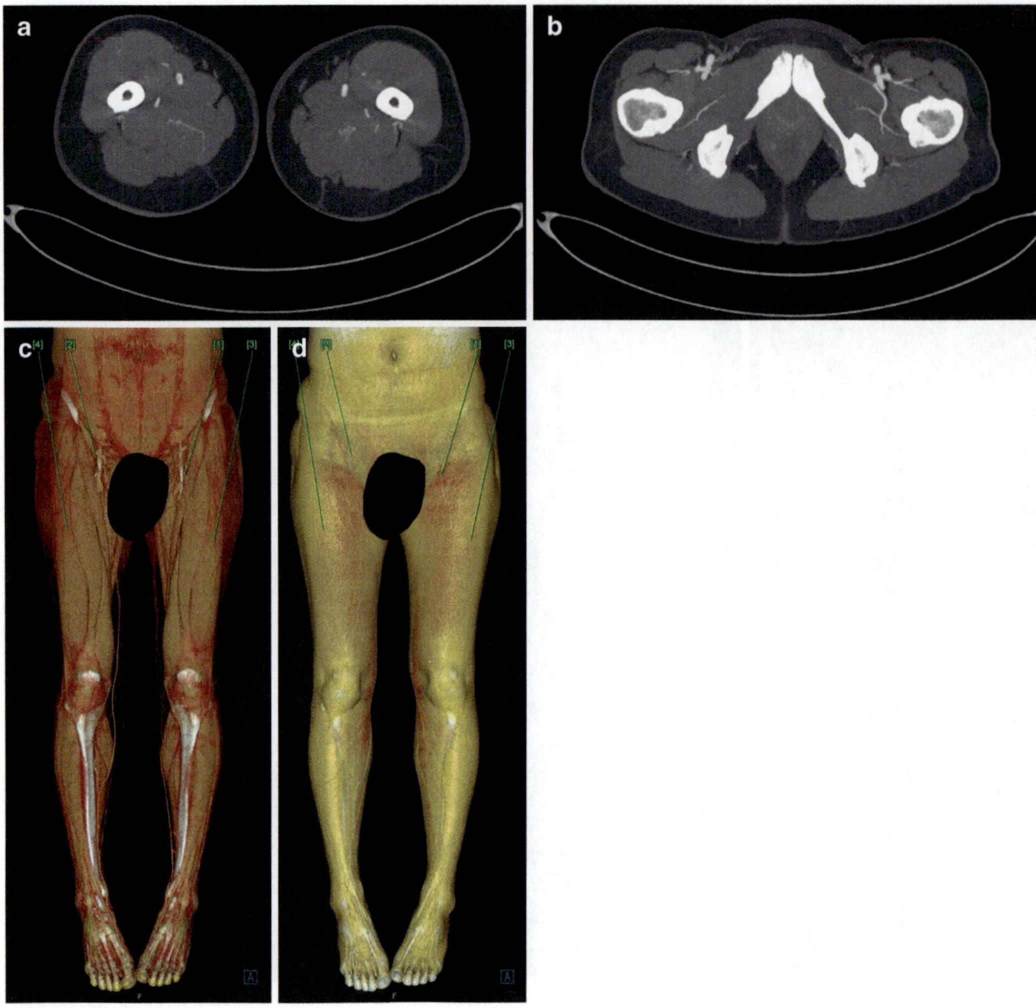

Fig. 11.2 Preoperative surgical planning with computed tomography angiography (CTA). Axial view of contrast-enhanced CTA in which the perforators of anterolateral thigh flap "ALT" are shown in (**a**) and the vascular pedicle of superficial circumflex iliac artery perforator flap (SCIP) is shown in (**b**); both are marked by red indicator. The course of the perforator fascial penetration point together with the thickness of the soft tissue can be clearly visualized. The view can be further enhanced with the use of three-dimensional volumetric reconstructed view as seen in (**c**) and (**d**) in which surface topography and the location of the perforators can be further localized with accuracy during preoperative planning

11.3 Digital Subtraction Angiography (DSA)

Among the additional modalities that can help in detailed evaluation of lower extremity vascular status is the use of angiography. In classical angiography, iodinated contrast is administered intra-arterially with live X-ray views being taken. This was later extended to DSA in which contrasted images are subtracted from pre-contrast mask pictures to create a two-dimensional images in two directions to show detailed vascular images with live view feature. The images obtained in this technique were said to provide a detailed intravascular anatomical assessment of the vascular structure in examination [17]. The role of

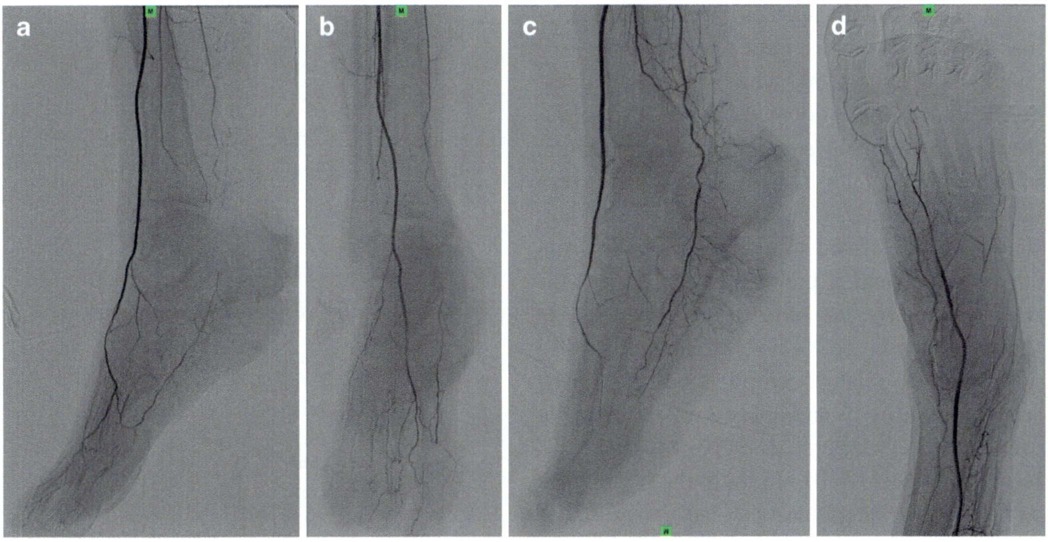

Fig. 11.3 Utility of digital subtraction angiograph (DSA) in foot revascularization. A case example that shows the status of foot vascularity in a diabetic patient. Preintervention photos show occlusion of the posterior tibial artery with retrograde flow in two views (anteroposterior and lateral) as shown in (**a**, **b**). The patient then underwent endovascular intervention with ballooning which managed to open the vessel the re-establishment of the flow as shown in (**c**, **d**)

this modality in lower extremity vascular assessment in light of other faster modalities like CTA may reside in cases where metallic hardware might obscure the image quality of CTA by artifacts with later implications on proper determination of limb vascularity. However, its routine use in extremity vascular assessment is controversial [4]. This is related to the nature of being an invasive modality with intervention access site-related complications like hematoma, pseudoaneurysm formation, the need for extended hospital stay with bed rest awaiting for access site healing. Moreover, high dose of radiation, the need for specialized team with associated cost, and contrast-related complications like renal injury, allergy, and direct vascular injury or contrast-related vasoconstriction might make vessel assessment and caliber estimation unreliable [17]. In free flap planning, the role of angiography was predominantly reported previously for fibula flap showing the continuity of three leg vessels and to rule out anomalies like peronea magna as well as atherosclerotic plagues [17].

The true utility however in lower extremity vascular assessment resides in the nature that it can allow direct endovascular intervention for optimal recipient vessel preparation and selection. A case example is shown in Fig. 11.3. Previous studies have shown the efficacy of this modality to diagnose and manage stenosis and occlusion preoperatively with high limb salvage and free flap success rate [18–21]. For such utility, the authors have shown in previous systemic review the different revascularization approaches utilized in previous literature in relation to diabetic foot ulcer with peripheral arterial disease. In one direction, foot revascularization was applied indirectly using the best collateral option, while in the other, direct revascularization of the main vessel supplying the area of interest was applied using the angiosome concept. The latter approach was popularized with the further understanding of foot vascularity and the description of the six angiosome zones of the foot each supplied by its own artery. However, data showed much debate between the two approaches with more favorable inclination toward the latter approach in diabetic patient population as they typically have poor collateral vessels [22].

An example of the application of this modality in ischemic foot reconstruction was shown by the authors' previous work which investigated the utility of angiosome-oriented preoperative percutaneous transluminal angioplasty in preparation of ischemic foot management. After the intervention, the transcutaneous oximetry level was shown to be elevated to about 40 mmHg from about 17–19 mmHg preintervention level. This was followed by flap reconstruction which also showed increased $TcPO_2$ level to about 60 mmHg with low flap-related complications [23]. The successful utility of angioplasty was also shown even if the revascularized artery was used as a recipient vessel [18–20]. In the authors' previous work, balloon angioplasties and intravascular stents are usually performed as a first-line modality when dealing with ischemic foot; however, frequent restenosis is a common complication in a way that was reported in previous literature to reach about 45–84% with the odds ratio of flap failure being significantly high (17.59, "$p < 0.001$") in those who had a history of angioplasty [24]. In that series, five cases of flap lost were encountered for which all were doing well for a period of 2 weeks postoperatively after which flap compromise occurs and repeated CT angiography shows complete occlusion with restenosis of the pedicle and all cases need repeated intervention. For that, strict vigilance in postoperative flap monitoring in this patient population is needed. Moreover, multidisciplinary team approach with the reconstructive surgeon working closely with interventional radiologist to ensure timely delivered management is needed for restenosis to occur. This can include the need for immediate repeated angioplasty which has been described previously in the literature with interventions that include ballooning and/or thrombolytics to ensure endovascular revascularization with eventual flap salvage with high success rate [19, 21, 25]. In our institution, we have adopted a similar approach in which we have incorporated an operative theater with direct and close access to interventional radiology (IR) procedure room allowing for an immediate revascularization when condition implies with close collaboration and coordination with IR team as a hybrid approach (Fig. 11.4).

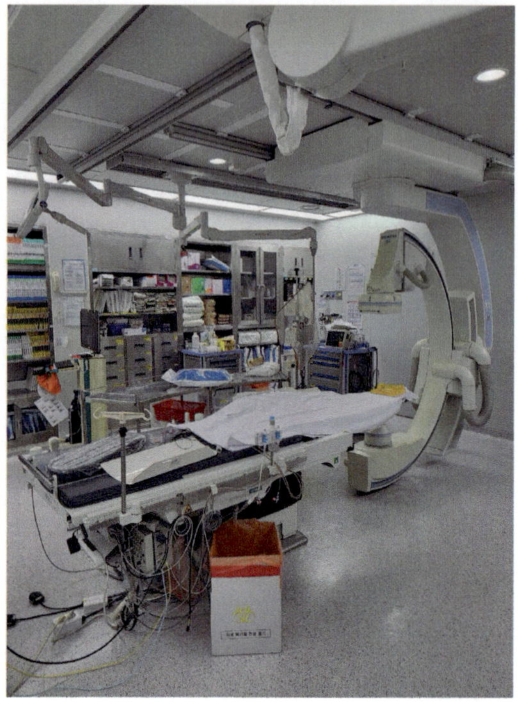

Fig. 11.4 Hybrid operative room with direct access to interventional radiology (IR) setup. The photo shows our IR room setup with a direct access to the operative room theater allowing for hybrid approach with interventional radiology (IR) procedures for an immediate revascularization intervention when needed in collaboration with IR team

A sound logic approach regarding the utility of this modality in lower extremity vascular evaluation was mentioned as an essential part of the management guidelines related to diabetic foot ulcer with peripheral arterial disease in which it was recommended to obtain urgent vascular imaging with potential revascularization if patients had an ankle pressure of <50 mmHg, an ankle/brachial index (ABI) of <0.5, a toe pressure of <30 mmHg, or a transcutaneous oximetry ($TcPO_2$) of <25 mmHg. Additionally, imaging with possible intervention should be considered if diabetic foot ulcer was not healing within 4–6 weeks despite optimal management [26].

11.4 Color Duplex Ultrasonography (CDU)

With the evolution of reconstructive surgery and the introduction of super-microsurgery, many advancements and adaptation of ultrasound technology became an essential tool in the hand of reconstructive surgeons. The utility of ultrasound machine to display real-time color-coded image of the vascular structures being evaluated in certain area is notable. Different linear array transducers with variable frequencies can be used that ranged from high-frequency (>20 MHz) all the way to ultrahigh-frequency (about 70 MHz) probes and utilized with variable application profiles in lower extremity vascular examination with artery is usually shown in red color while the vein is shown in blue color depending on the flow pattern and direction of the blood vessels to the transducer [27]. With higher frequency, better resolution is encountered for small vascular structures, but it has the limitation of less penetration depth, for which 20 MHz transducers can give a good balance and great resolutions for applications related to skin vascularity pattern but not that great for recipient vessel assessment. Perhaps one of the classic applications of this imaging modality was in its essential role for initial screening for deep vein thrombosis as adjunct to other clinical and radiological modalities [28]. This was also incorporated previously for preoperative planning of extremity flap reconstruction with great impact on the success rate optimizing recipient vessel selection [29]. In our institution, we routinely utilized linear array high-frequency CDU for various applications related to lower extremity reconstruction to a point that it represents an integral part of our practice in which the examiner can set and examine the velocity of flow, tissue characteristics, flap perforator size and course, recipient vessel characteristics, location, diameter, source vessel in case of perforator anastomosis, and to differentiate pedicle vasculature from surrounding vessels especially for buried flaps all were valid anatomical information provided through CDU assessment [30]. An example of such was in the authors' previous work that showed the utility of this modality in a step-by-step fashion for ALT flap mapping. What is so special in this example is related to the variability of the perforator pattern that is either musculocutaneous or septocutaneous course with tedious dissection in the former compared to direct dissection in the latter. Moreover, in case of multiple perforators, CDU can guide in selecting proper one with the easiest dissection course saving the operative time [31]. In similar approach, the same concepts can be applied to recipient vessels with identifications of potential superficial vessels near or within the defect with ease. This can be truly applied for local flap options around extremity defect, for which perforators are marked and checked for their flow velocity, fascial penetration point, and axiality with vertical orientation as the best options related to extremity local flap option [32]. Not only recipient arteries are potentially screened by CDU, but also recipient veins that are either superficial or deep can also be screened in similar fashion. Also, in case of flap having superficial vain as dominant outflow that is far away from the pedicle, this can also be anticipated preoperatively prior to flap elevation. All of these parameters, in conjunction with the information provided by other modalities like CTA, also can be utilized to control the thickness of raised flap in which thin flap elevation is possible after knowing the course, direction, and fascial penetration points of the flap perforator with eventual ease in flap elevation as described earlier [33–35]. An example of SCIP flap CDU planning is shown in Fig. 11.5.

All previously mentioned information represents detailed anatomic mapping of the area of interest the CDU imaging can provide. Additionally, different physiologic information can also be obtained with this modality that includes flow velocity and flow volume of recipient artery with the velocity representing an essential indicator of recipient vessel fitness [36]. The normal range of the velocity of the recipient vessels will help to determine its adequacy in which

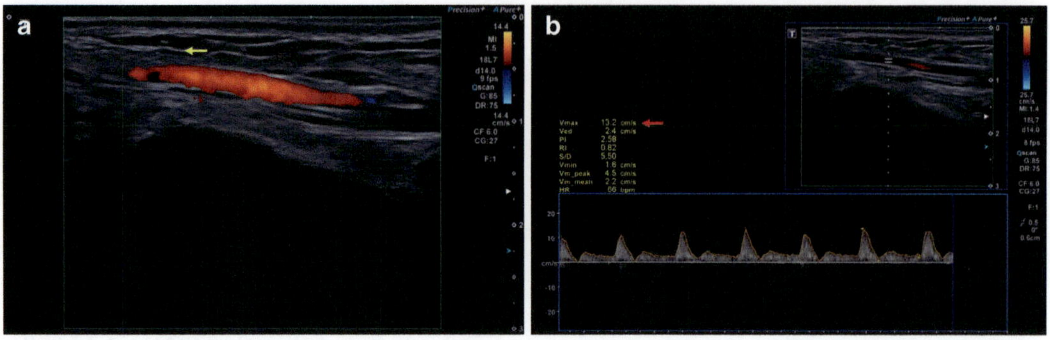

Fig. 11.5 Preoperative mapping of superficial circumflex iliac artery perforator (SCIP) flap with the use of color duplex ultrasonography (CDU). The case example shows the utility of CDU in the preoperative marking of SCIP flap. The pedicle is visualized with its path under the superficial fascia as indicated by the yellow arrow in (**a**). Further assessment of the pedicle flow velocity was done with a flow velocity about 13.2 cm/s (red arrow) as shown in (**b**)

the velocity of the axial arteries in the leg (anterior tibial, posterior tibial, and peroneal arteries) were shown to have a peak arterial velocity of about 55 +/− 10 cm/s. When assessing perforators as potential recipient vessels, previous work of the author showed that perforators with velocity over 15–20 cm/s can be safely used as a potential recipient in ischemic diabetic foot reconstruction [36]. For any abnormalities or deviations from these reference parameters, it is advisable to look for alternative recipient options or to apply trial to fix the underlying issue to optimize the outcome with other modalities like interventional angioplasty. One classic example for such approach is when to assess potential recipient vessels near or within the zone of injury, for that assessment of flow velocity and tissue characteristics like scarring and fibrosis might give a hint about the suitability of such vessels prior to surgical exploration. Furthermore, the authors have analyzed the effect of ankle position on the flow volume of recipient vessels and showed that for dorsalis pedis artery the flow velocity changes from 19.81 ± 3.88 mL/min in dorsiflexion position, to 11.71 ± 4.72 mL/min in relaxed position, to 3.47 ± 1.41 mL/min in plantar flexion position. Similarly, for posterior tibial artery flow, it changes from 9.08 ± 8.25 mL/min in dorsiflexion position, to 14.78 ± 2.45 mL/min in relaxed position, to 19.03 ± 5.03 mL/min in plantar flexion position. For that, the authors recommended to put the patient in ankle dorsiflexion whenever anterior tibial artery was used as a recipient vessel and ankle plantar flexion whenever posterior tibial artery was utilized as a recipient vessel [37]. A clinical case example of the utility of CDU and velocity assessment implication in flap monitoring is shown in Fig. 11.6.

Additionally, when deciding for intraoperative vein grafting, CDU can be quite helpful to look for proper donor vein with good size match and quality, all of which shortens the operative time. Among the other applications of this imaging technique is flap monitoring. The authors have shown previously the efficacy of this modality as a very useful adjunct to clinical monitoring for early detection of flap compromise. The use of CDU provided anatomic and hemodynamic information of the vascular status of the flap anastomosis prior to clinical signs of flap failure. The use of this modality as a monitoring tool had a 100% positive predictive value with the detection capacity of vessels that are less than 0.5 mm with 100% accuracy in detecting flap perfusion loss for various pedicle depths that ranged between 0.5 and 7 cm in noninvasive fashion [38]. Among the recent advancements that involved the use of CDU in extremity vascular evaluation was the introduction of superb microvascular imaging (SMI), in which the CDU sig-

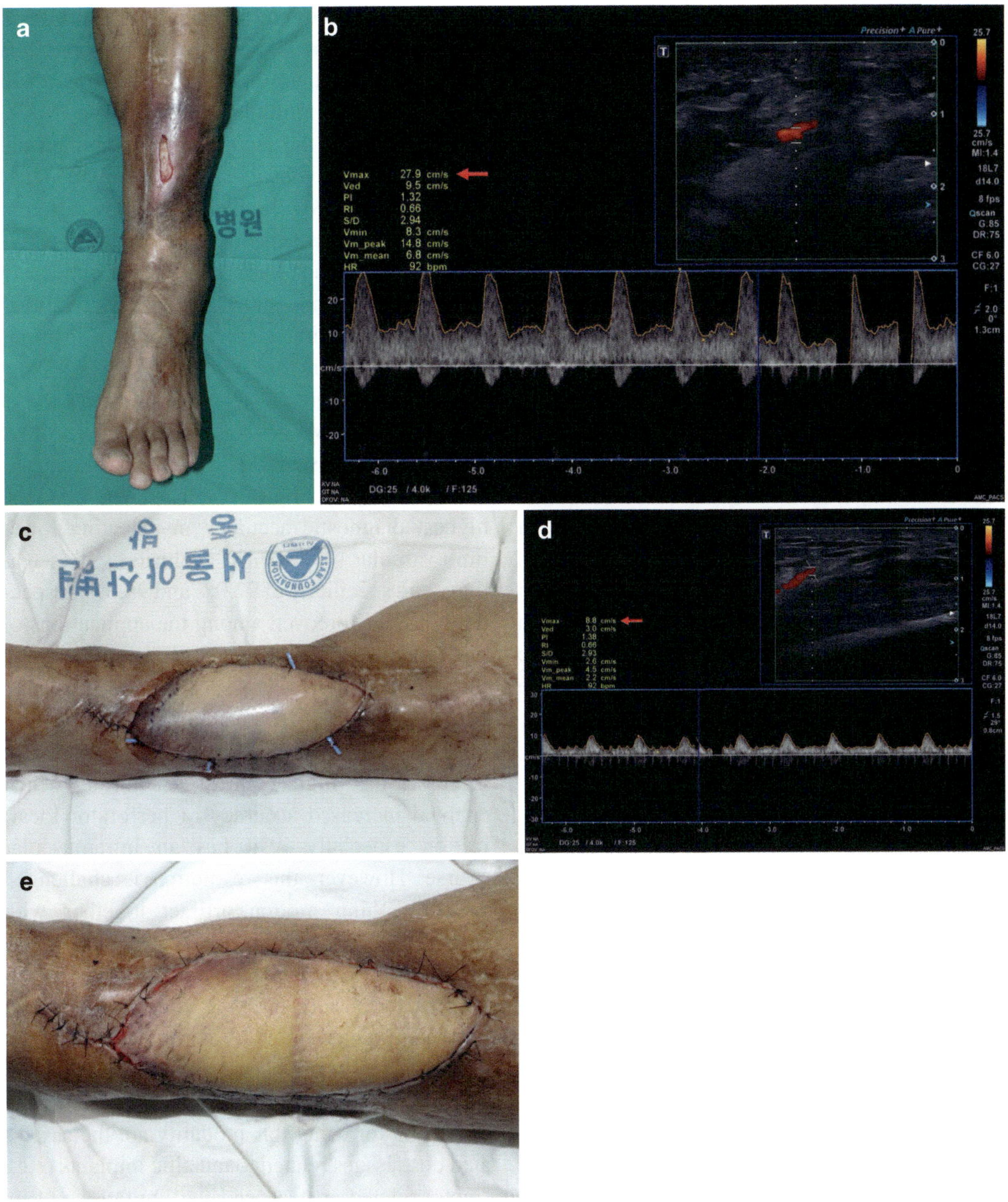

Fig. 11.6 Clinical example of the utility of color duplex ultrasonography (CDU) in flap monitoring. Preoperative view of a patient's left lower limb with anterior distal third of the leg ulcer after history of trauma and chronic osteomyelitis is shown in (**a**). The patient was planned for wound debridement and SCIP flap coverage with anastomosis to anterior tibial artery collateral vessels. Preoperatively, the CDU was utilized to measure the flow velocity of the recipient vessel which was about 27.9 cm/s as shown in (**b**) (red arrow). The procedure was performed, and on day 2 postoperatively the flap was noticed to except sings of compromise as shown in (**c**). CDU was repeated and the pedicle was noticed to have decreased velocity as shown in (**d**) (red arrow). Flap was salvaged non-operatively with ankle position adjustment and staring heparin infusion which recovered without any compromise as shown in (**e**)

nal is further enhanced to allow the visualization of very low flow velocity with filtration of signal artifact and enhanced frame rate, resolution, and sensitivity. Suto et al. have shown the utilization of this technique in assessing foot minute angiosome perfusion with detailed quantification through a measurable vascular index (VI) in chronic limb ischemia patients with plantar SMI-VI having the highest diagnostic performance of limb ischemia with sensitivity of 88.6% and specificity of 95.6% [39]. Although the use of CDU provides various advantages as described earlier, however, this technique has some limitations in that it has a steep learning curve that requires frequent familiarity with the ultrasound machine and the different transducers as well as the scanning modes and their applications in regard to vascularity assessment, all of which reflects on the proficiency of the operator and on the quality of the information gained from such imaging. Additionally, the high cost of these devices makes their availability such a challenge [28, 36, 38].

11.5 Magnetic Resonance Angiography (MRA)

With the recent advancements in the field of magnetic resonance (MR) and particularly MR angiography (MRA), different applications of this imaging modality have shown its great utility in extremity vascular evaluation. This modality is capable of providing high-quality assessment that includes ischemia related to peripheral vascular disease in addition to different vascular anomalies with the potential of dynamic visualization of the anomaly in different anatomical positions without the need for ionizing radiation [40]. Perhaps one of the difficulties associated with its widespread use is the various options of imaging and postprocessing protocols, some of which are quite complex depending on different vendors [41]. Among the protocols specific for vascular imaging are time-of-flight (TOF), ramped flip angle TOF, multiple slab acquisition TOF, phase contrast, balanced steady-state free precession, fast spin echo, and fluoro-triggered contrast-enhanced and time-resolved protocol. For the image postprocessing, different protocols also existed that are specific for angiographic data and include multiplanar reformation (MPR) which will show the acquired images in multiple planes for easier visualization, maximum intensity projection (MIP) which will show different image projections depending on the highest signal intensity, and lastly volumetric rendering (VR) which will show the data in three-dimensional fashion, all of which can be manipulated with different thresholding to properly show the lesion of interest [41]. When it comes to the case utility of MRA when compared to other modalities in vascularity evaluation like DSA, CTA, and CDU, contrast-enhanced MRA had the highest diagnostic accuracy in detecting lower limb vascular stenosis and occlusion with sensitivity and specificity of 92.0% and 96.5%, respectively [42]. Moreover, among the applications of this modality that showed increased interest was the perforator flap mapping. It has been pointed out that although MRA has lower spatial resolution when compared to other modalities like CTA, it has high contrast resolution which enabled increased accuracy of perforator localization especially if it has an intramuscular course. However, this resolution is challenged with breathing motion artifact together with extended scanning time [43]. For perforator marking and because of the issue of using metallic pins for surface marking with magnetism, it has been pointed out that vitamin E capsule can be utilized by being placed as surface landmarks for easier perforator localization [41]. Among the criticisms for using this modality are the associated cost, issues related to metallic implants (e.g., stents) related artifact, and the limitations of its use in patients with pacemaker or patients with claustrophobia [40].

11.6 Indocyanine Green (ICG) Angiography

Despite the great utility of the previously described modalities to assess limb vascular status, still there remains a challenge related to assessing the minute microvascular circulation of the extremity with its great implications on wound assessment. For that different modalities were described for their potential role in that purpose and include percutaneous oxygen saturation and fluorescein dye angiography but with several limitations. The use of indocyanine green (ICG) angiography was presented as a novel solution that can obviate the limitations encountered in other modalities with real-time visualization of microvascular blood flow. After the injection of the ICG dye peripherally, the dye will be exited, and then it will reflect the near-infrared light at the end of the spectrum at 805 nm and 835 nm which can be read by any photometer that will show the dye distribution in the soft tissue and especially subdermal vasculature due to the penetration depth of about 2 mm with eventual guide of tissue perfusion [44]. Different utilities of ICG angiography in plastic surgery literature were mentioned with special emphasis on perfusion assessment post-reconstruction. Perhaps of the important utilization of this technique in lower extremity vascular evaluation in addition to its essential role post-flap reconstruction is in the assessment of native tissue perfusion. Den Hoven et al. have shown the great utility of this technique in predicting postoperative skin necrosis postamputation in patients with chronic limb ischemia [45]. Moreover and in similar approach, Wilke et al. showed that the use of ICG angiography was associated with high negative predictive value and positive predictive value to anticipate wound complications related to hypoperfusion in the lower extremity after sarcoma resection. This allowed the surgeons to change the wound management plan like the method of closure or suture technique to decrease postoperative wound complications [46]. The use of this technique was associated with accurate assessment of tissue perfusion and the microcirculation near the wound, with potential multiple assessment points due to the short half-life of the dye without the need for radiation and with high safety profile [47]. Clinical example of the utility of ICG angiography is shown in Fig. 11.7.

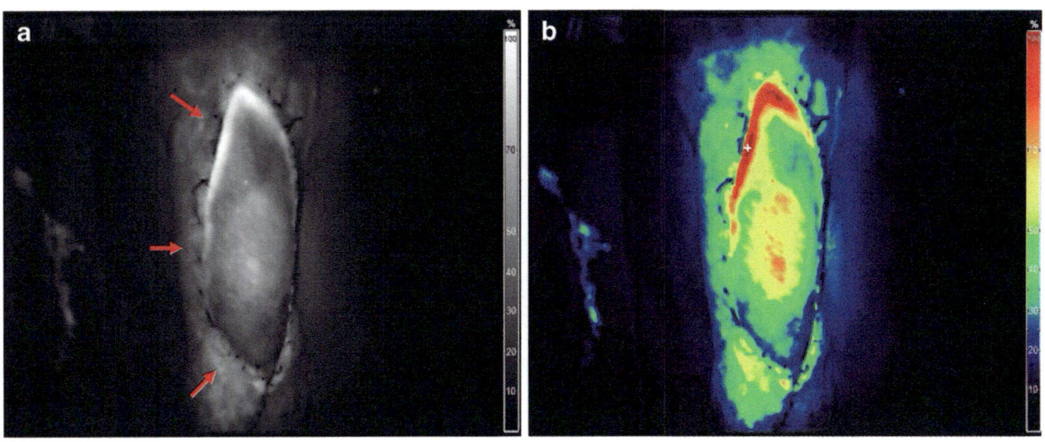

Fig. 11.7 Utility of indocyanine green (ICG) angiography in perfusion assessment. The utility of ICG in perfusion assessment is shown in relation to the same clinical scenario mentioned in Fig. 11.6. After peripheral infusion of ICG dye, perfusion assessment can be easily identified for different parameters that first include the assessment of surrounding native tissue after wound debridement which showed intact vascularity as indicated by red arrows in both grayscale (**a**) and colored map (**b**) images. Next, flap perfusion is also assessed after the dye reaches the flap which shows also intact vascular perfusion in both images

11.7 Conclusion

After reviewing the different imaging modalities described above, it is clear that a sound logic approach is needed when investigating a lower extremity vascularity in which a combined utility of different modalities might be applied to reach a proper clinical diagnosis and to plan future therapeutic interventions. Each of these modalities has their own pros and cons in which proper understanding and case-based application is needed when selecting each imaging modality. Table 11.1 summarizes the advantages and potential challenges associated with each modality described.

Table 11.1 Comparative assessment of different imaging modalities described

	Computed tomography angiography (CTA)	Digital subtraction angiography (DSA)	Color duplex ultrasonography (CDU)	Magnetic resonance angiography (MRA)	Indocyanine green (ICG) angiography
Applications	• Limb vascularity assessment • Perforator flap planning • Flap selection in limb vascular occlusive state • Flap soft tissue thickness planning • Simultaneous assessment of soft tissue and bone	• Limb vascularity assessment • Utility in revascularization interventions	• Limb vascularity assessment and flow velocity quantification • Perforator flap planning • Flap thickness planning • Postoperative flap monitoring	• Limb vascularity assessment • Perforator flap planning	• Soft tissue vascular perfusion assessment • Flap vascular perfusion assessment
Advantages	• Fast • Minimally invasive • Capable of providing detailed vascular assessment of the whole limb • Capable of providing three-dimensional (3D) reconstructed view of the limb vascular structure for easier visualization	• Simultaneous assessment of limb vascularity and revascularization procedure when needed	• Allow real-time utility preoperatively, intraoperatively, and postoperatively • Portable • Provides numerical values for easier assessment • Provides detailed assessment of minute vascularity	• High resolution • Potential for contrast-free scanning	• Direct visualization of perfusion assessment • Portable • Easy to interpret

(continued)

Table 11.1 (continued)

	Computed tomography angiography (CTA)	Digital subtraction angiography (DSA)	Color duplex ultrasonography (CDU)	Magnetic resonance angiography (MRA)	Indocyanine green (ICG) angiography
Disadvantages	• Need for contrast agent • Potential contrast-related complications • Issues related to radiation • Lack of clarity in cases of metallic implant with artifacts	• Need for specialized team and associated cost • More invasive nature • Contrast-related complications • More radiation and procedure time requiring special precautions and monitoring	• The high cost of the devices limits its widespread application • Need for steep learning curve with frequent familiarity with the different scanning modes and device interface • Limited perpetration depth depending on the frequency of scanning transducers • Operator dependent	• Resolution is affected by motion artifact • Extended scanning time • Contrast-related complications if it was used • Various scanning protocols depending on device manufacturer	• ICG dye-related complications and contraindications • Limited penetration depth of up to 1.5–2 cm

The table summarizes the potential applications of different imaging modalities reviewed and compares the advantages and disadvantages of each technique

References

1. Gottlieb LJ, Krieger LM. From the reconstructive ladder to the reconstructive elevator. Plast Reconstr Surg. 1994;93:1503.
2. Xiong L, Gazyakan E, Kremer T, et al. Free flaps for reconstruction of soft tissue defects in lower extremity: a meta-analysis on microsurgical outcome and safety. Microsurgery. 2016;36(6):511–24.
3. Abdelfattah U, Power HA, Song S, Min K, Suh HP, Hong JP. Algorithm for free perforator flap selection in lower extremity reconstruction based on 563 cases. Plast Reconstr Surg. 2019;144(5):1202–13.
4. Hong JP, Park CJ, Suh HP. Importance of vascularity and selecting the recipient vessels of lower extremity reconstruction. J Reconstr Microsurg. 2021;37(01):083–8.
5. Prokop M. Multislice CT angiography. Eur J Radiol. 2000;36(2):86–96.
6. Sung YD, Kim HH. Usefullness with 3D CT angiography in microsurgical reconstruction. Arch Plast Surg. 2006;33(2):175–80.
7. Rieger M, Mallouhi A, Tauscher T, Lutz M, Jaschke WR. Traumatic arterial injuries of the extremities: initial evaluation with MDCT angiography. Am J Roentgenol. 2006;186(3):656–64.
8. Duymaz A, Karabekmez FE, Vrtiska TJ, Mardini S, Moran SL. Free tissue transfer for lower extremity reconstruction: a study of the role of computed angiography in the planning of free tissue transfer in the posttraumatic setting. Plast Reconstr Surg. 2009;124(2):523–9.
9. Hsu CS, Hellinger JC, Rubin GD, Chang J. CT angiography in pediatric extremity trauma: preoperative evaluation prior to reconstructive surgery. Hand. 2008;3(2):139–45.
10. Lee JW, Kim HK, Kim SR, Han YS, Park JH. Preoperative identification of a perforator using computed tomography angiography and metal clip marking in perforator flap reconstruction. Arch Plast Surg. 2015;42(01):78–83.
11. Suh HSP, Jeong HH, Choi DH, Hong JPJ. Study of the medial superficial perforator of the superficial circumflex iliac artery perforator flap using computed tomographic angiography and surgical anatomy in 142 patients. Plast Reconstr Surg. 2017;139(3):738–48.
12. Hong JP, Choi DH, Suh H, et al. A new plane of elevation: the superficial fascial plane for perforator flap elevation. J Reconstr Microsurg. 2014;30(07):491–6.
13. Kim EK, Kang BS, Hong JP. The distribution of the perforators in the anterolateral thigh and the utility of multidetector row computed tomography angiography in preoperative planning. Ann Plast Surg. 2010;65(2):155–60.
14. Smit JM, Dimopoulou A, Liss AG, et al. Preoperative CT angiography reduces surgery time in perforator flap reconstruction. J Plast Reconstr Aesthet Surg. 2009;62(9):1112–7.
15. Suh HP, Kim Y, Suh Y, Hong J. Multidetector computed tomography (CT) analysis of 168 cases in diabetic patients with total superficial femoral artery

occlusion: is it safe to use an anterolateral thigh flap without CT angiography in diabetic patients? J Reconstr Microsurg. 2018;34(01):065–70.
16. Soto JA, Múnera F, Morales C, et al. Focal arterial injuries of the proximal extremities: helical CT arteriography as the initial method of diagnosis. Radiology. 2001;218(1):188–94.
17. Smit JM, Klein S, Werker PM. An overview of methods for vascular mapping in the planning of free flaps. J Plast Reconstr Aesthet Surg. 2010;63(9):e674–82.
18. Huang CC, Chang CH, Hsu H, et al. Endovascular revascularization and free tissue transfer for lower limb salvage. J Plast Reconstr Aesthet Surg. 2014;67(10):1407–14.
19. Hahn HM, Jeong YS, Hong YS, et al. Use of revascularized artery as a recipient in microvascular reconstruction of the lower leg: an analysis of 62 consecutive free flap transfers. J Plast Reconstr Aesthet Surg. 2017;70(5):606–17.
20. Janhofer DE, Lakhiani C, Kim PJ, et al. The utility of preoperative arteriography for free flap planning in patients with chronic lower extremity wounds. Plast Reconstr Surg. 2019;143(2):604–13.
21. Kim JY, Choi HG, Uhm KI, Kim SH, Kim CK, Shin DH. Salvage of a free flap using postoperative percutaneous angioplasty in patients with diabetic foot ulcers. Arch Plast Surg. 2014;41(06):788–90.
22. Hinchliffe RJ, Brownrigg J, Andros G, et al. Effectiveness of revascularization of the ulcerated foot in patients with diabetes and peripheral artery disease: a systematic review. Diabetes Metab Res Rev. 2016;32:136–44.
23. Kwon JG, Cho M-J, Pak CJ, Suh HP, Hong JP. A retrospective case series on free flap reconstruction for ischemic diabetic foot: the nutrient flap further explained. Plast Reconstr Surg. 2022;149(6):1452–61.
24. Oh TS, Lee HS, Hong JP. Diabetic foot reconstruction using free flaps increases 5-year-survival rate. J Plast Reconstr Aesthet Surg. 2013;66(2):243–50.
25. Lee SY, Seong IH, Park BY. Percutaneous transluminal ballooning angioplasty for flap salvage in a complex lower extremity reconstruction. Plast Reconstr Surg Glob Open. 2020;8(9):e3077.
26. Hinchliffe RJ, Forsythe RO, Apelqvist J, et al. Guidelines on diagnosis, prognosis, and management of peripheral artery disease in patients with foot ulcers and diabetes (IWGDF 2019 update). Diabetes Metab Res Rev. 2020;36:e3276.
27. Hallock GG. Color duplex imaging for identifying perforators prior to pretransfer expansion of fasciocutaneous free flaps. Ann Plast Surg. 1994;32(6):595–601.
28. Frisbie J, Cuff R. Role of duplex ultrasound screening/surveillance in high-risk deep vein thrombosis patients. In: Noninvasive vascular diagnosis: a practical textbook for clinicians. Springer; 2021. p. 1–11.
29. Janhofer DE, Lakhiani C, Kim PJ, et al. The utility of preoperative venous testing for lower extremity flap planning in patients with lower extremity wounds. Plast Reconstr Surg. 2020;145(1):164e–71e.
30. Cho M-J, Kwon JG, Pak CJ, Suh HP, Hong JP. The role of duplex ultrasound in microsurgical reconstruction: review and technical considerations. J Reconstr Microsurg. 2020;36(07):514–21.
31. Kehrer A, Sachanadani NS, da Silva NPB, et al. Step-by-step guide to ultrasound-based design of alt flaps by the microsurgeon—basic and advanced applications and device settings. J Plast Reconstr Aesthet Surg. 2020;73(6):1081–90.
32. Hong JP, Hur J, Kim HB, Park CJ, Suh HP. The use of color duplex ultrasound for local perforator flaps in the extremity. J Reconstr Microsurg. 2022;38(03):233–7.
33. Kwon JG, Brown E, Suh HP, Pak CJ, Hong JP. Planes for perforator/skin flap elevation—definition, classification, and techniques. J Reconstr Microsurg. 2022;39:179.
34. Jeong HH, Hong JP, Suh HS. Thin elevation: a technique for achieving thin perforator flaps. Arch Plast Surg. 2018;45(04):304–13.
35. Visconti G, Bianchi A, Hayashi A, et al. Thin and superthin perforator flap elevation based on preoperative planning with ultrahigh-frequency ultrasound. Arch Plast Surg. 2020;47(04):365–70.
36. Hong JP, Kim HB, Park CJ, Suh HP. Using duplex ultrasound for recipient vessel selection. J Reconstr Microsurg. 2022;38(03):200–5.
37. Suh YC, Kim HB, Brown E, Hong JP, Suh HP. Maximizing the flap inflow in a foot reconstruction: ultrasonographic evaluation of artery flow in accordance with the angle of the ankle. Plast Reconstr Surg. 2021;148(2):258e–61e.
38. Gonzalez J, Gardikiotis I, Ruiz-Moya A, et al. Duplex echography as an adjuvant tool to clinical examination to detect early postoperative free flap vascular compromise. Microsurgery. 2021;41(2):109–18.
39. Suto Y, Sato W, Yamanaka T, et al. Utility of superb microvascular imaging in the assessment of foot perfusion in patients with critical limb ischemia. Diagnostics. 2022;12(11):2577.
40. Dhaliwal J, Hecht EM, Roditi G, Douglas P. MR angiography series: MR angiography of the extremities. Radiographics. 2022;42(4):E132–3.
41. Kuo AH, Nagpal P, Ghoshhajra BB, Hedgire SS. Vascular magnetic resonance angiography techniques. Cardiovasc Diagn Ther. 2019;9(Suppl 1):S28.
42. Edgerley D, Rahi A. TH4.1 Systematic review of preoperative magnetic resonance angiography, computed tomography angiography and duplex ultrasonography for diagnosis and planning of surgical, endovascular or hybrid procedures for lower limb revascularisation. Br J Surg. 2022;109(Supplement_5):znac248.
43. Agrawal MD, Thimmappa ND, Vasile JV, et al. Autologous breast reconstruction: preoperative magnetic resonance angiography for perforator flap vessel mapping. J Reconstr Microsurg. 2015;31(01):001–11.

44. Dzurinko VL, Gurwood AS, Price JR. Intravenous and indocyanine green angiography. Optometry. 2004;75(12):743–55.
45. Van Den Hoven P, Van Den Berg SD, Van Der Valk JP, et al. Assessment of tissue viability following amputation surgery using near-infrared fluorescence imaging with indocyanine green. Ann Vasc Surg. 2022;78:281–7.
46. Wilke BK, Schultz DS, Huayllani MT, et al. Intraoperative indocyanine green fluorescence angiography is sensitive for predicting postoperative wound complications in soft-tissue sarcoma surgery. J Am Acad Orthop Surg. 2021;29(10):433–8.
47. Shibata R, Takeda S, Takahashi H, Kurahashi S, Yamauchi K-I. Usefulness of indocyanine green fluorescence angiography for the urgent decision of the level of limb amputation. JPRAS Open. 2022;33:119–21.

12 Recipient Vessel Selection in Reconstructive Surgery

Changsik John Pak

12.1 Introduction

Reconstructive surgery has made significant progress since the early 1960s, with the introduction of axial vessels as a fundamental concept. The initial generations of axial pattern flaps relied on well-known vessels described in anatomy books, such as the radial artery for the radial forearm flap and the thoracic vessel for the latissimus dorsi flap. At that time, harvesting these flaps was considered revolutionary but is now relatively simple due to their consistent anatomy. Further exploration of vascular structures is typically recommended only if the vessel has been damaged by previous surgery or trauma.

In the past two decades, notable advancements in flap design have emerged, leading to the utilization of perforated vessels branching off from the main vessel. These perforators can be traced back to well-known vessels and help reduce donor site morbidity. However, the exact location of these perforators can vary significantly. Preoperative vascular mapping techniques have been introduced to identify the predominant perforator and pathways, facilitating skin harvesting.

Several methods are employed for this purpose, with the most commonly used techniques being handheld Doppler (HHD), color duplex sonography (CDS), digital subtraction angiography (DSA), computed tomography angiography (CTA), and magnetic resonance angiography (MRA). HHD was first reported for localizing donor and beneficiary vessels in facial reconstruction in 1975. During the same period, angiography (later replaced by DSA) was primarily introduced to assess the vascular anatomy of flaps in the lower extremities. CDS emerged as a means of planning flaps in the 1980s and became the standard mapping method in the 1990s. Significant progress has been made in applying CTA and MRA in the last decade.

This overview aims to describe various vascular mapping systems, including their advantages and limitations, to assist novice microsurgeons in planning free flaps. Other mapping methods, such as indocyanine green and near-infrared imaging, exist but are primarily used for intraoperative flap design. Therefore, they are outside the scope of this overview.

12.2 Handheld Doppler (HHD)

Handheld Doppler (HHD) utilizes a pencil-like Doppler probe to emit and receive reflected ultrasound waves, enabling red blood cell movement detection. The choice of probe frequency depends on the depth and diameter of the vessel being investigated, with commonly used frequencies

C. J. Pak (✉)
Department of Plastic and Reconstructive Surgery, Seoul Asan Medical Center, Seoul, South Korea

J. P. Hong et al. (eds.), *Imaging for Reconstructive Microsurgery*,
https://doi.org/10.1007/978-981-97-7278-0_12

being 8 MHz and 10 MHz, offering peak sensitivities of 20 mm and 15 mm, respectively. To enhance ultrasound conduction between the probe and skin, it is recommended to apply ultrasound gel. When searching for a perforator, it is advised to vary the pressure applied by the Doppler probe on the skin surface; when the detected sound corresponds to the perforator running directly toward the HHD, increasing pressure results in a decrease in the magnitude of the pulsating sound.

HHD offers several advantages, including noninvasiveness, small machine size, low cost, portability, and ease of examination. Additionally, the unique probe can be sterilized and used intraoperatively to assist in planning and confirming vascular pulsation during surgery.

However, the most commonly used Doppler probe (8 MHz) has some limitations. These include a limited detection depth of 20 mm and an inability to determine the specific vessel generating the Doppler signal detected by the HHD. As a result, detecting the perforator's emergence through the fascia becomes unreliable when the thickness of the skin and subcutaneous tissue is less than 20 mm. Furthermore, HHD does not provide three-dimensional (3D) images of vascular structures and surrounding anatomy that can be stored and retrieved later.

HHD has been primarily employed for identifying perforators on the trunk and extremities.

The use of HHD has been reported with varying success rates. For instance, a study by Yu and Youssef [1] compared the HHD signal location of 8 MHz and 10 MHz probes with intraoperative results in 100 patients undergoing ALT (anterolateral thigh) reconstruction. The 8 MHz probe exhibited a positive predictive value of 89% with no false negative effects, while the 10 MHz probe showed a positive predictive value of 94% and a negative predictive value of 43%. Another study by Shaw et al. [2] assessed HHD findings in 30 patients who underwent ALT reconstruction and found a considerable range of underestimation (30%) to overestimation (150%) in HHD outcomes. When combining DIEP (deep inferior epigastric perforator) and SGAP (superior gluteal artery perforator) flaps, a study of 32 deep lower abdominal perforator (DIEP) and eight superior temporal artery perforator (SGAP) flaps comparing HHD findings with intraoperative outcomes showed a positive predictive power of only 52.4%.

12.3 Color Duplex Sonography (CDS)

Color duplex sonography (CDS) operates on the same principle as HHD, detecting vascular blood flow by recording Doppler frequency shifts relative to blood flow velocity. In addition, CDS offers the advantage of displaying different speeds and directions of blood flow in color duplex mode, providing information on internal vessel diameter, course, and 3D visualization of the perivascular anatomy. Like HHD, CDS employs gel to enhance ultrasound conduction between the skin interface and the probe.

CDS, like HHD, is a noninvasive technique. However, it surpasses HHD in its ability to provide detailed information about vessel anatomy and the perforator in relation to the surrounding tissue. CDS can also perform quantitative analysis to determine the dominant perforator (Fig. 12.1).

One limitation of CDS is that it requires skilled personnel familiar with the anatomy of the free flap to perform the investigation. Furthermore, CDS must be reproducible under real-world dynamics. Another drawback, compared to other imaging techniques such as CTA, MRA, and DSA, CDS, like HHD, does not generate 2D or 3D images of the entire vascular anatomy available to the surgeon during flap design or reconstruction.

CDS has been successfully used for the preoperative evaluation of flaps in head, neck, trunk, and limb reconstructions. For example, Tsukino et al. conducted a reliability study of CDS on ten patients before performing ALT (anterolateral thigh) flaps, showing 100% concordance between CDS findings and intraoperative observations [3]. The reliability of CDS was also confirmed in

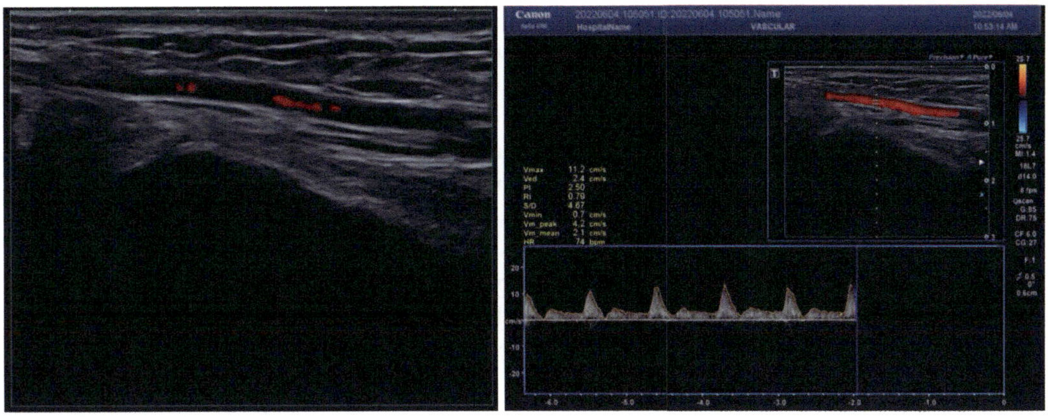

Fig. 12.1 Color duplex sonography (CDS) mapping for recipient vessel

separate reports involving six cases of DIEP (deep inferior epigastric perforator) flaps. CDS can provide valuable information on vascular flow, assessing potential damage to perforated vessels after liposuction surgery. Additionally, CDS is beneficial when minimizing radiation exposure is desired, as in the case of CTA.

12.4 Digital Subtraction Angiography (DSA)

Digital subtraction angiography (DSA) is a technique used to visualize vascular anatomy by administering an iodine-containing contrast agent into arteries while capturing X-ray images. In DSA, contrast-enhanced images are digitally subtracted from pre-contrast mask X-rays to create detailed depictions of vascular structures. This technique typically generates 2D images and often requires imaging in multiple directions to capture the entire vascular anatomy.

DSA offers several advantages, including the visualization of intraluminal vascular anatomy and the ability to assess atherosclerotic changes. However, there are some drawbacks associated with DSA. It is a time-consuming and invasive procedure involving iodinated contrast agents, which can potentially cause vascular or renal damage and allergic reactions. There is also a concern regarding radiation exposure. The vasoconstrictive effect of contrast agents can make accurate measurements of vessel diameter and assessment of small-bore vessels unreliable. Patients often need to maintain an upright position for several hours after the procedure to allow the puncture site to heal, which may require hospital admission. Additionally, DSA is relatively expensive, and there is a reported probability of 4.5% for developing pseudoaneurysms at the puncture site.

DSA has primarily been reported for nasal flaps in the context of free flap planning. In these cases, assessing the continuity of the three descending vessels, the branching level of the tibiofibular shaft, and the presence of atherosclerotic plaques is crucial. Angiography has been found to provide a more accurate assessment of vessel patency compared to conventional examinations such as the ankle-brachial index and HHD examination (Fig. 12.2).

DSA has also been used for planning abdominal dermal flaps based on the transverse and rectus abdominis muscles. Furthermore, it has been reported to be used intraoperatively to visualize the vasculature of the flap, aiding the surgeon in identifying the connection between the flap perforator and the axial flap vessel. This facilitates safe thinning and separation of the flap during secondary procedures. However, it is essential to note that using DSA for this purpose is relatively rare [4].

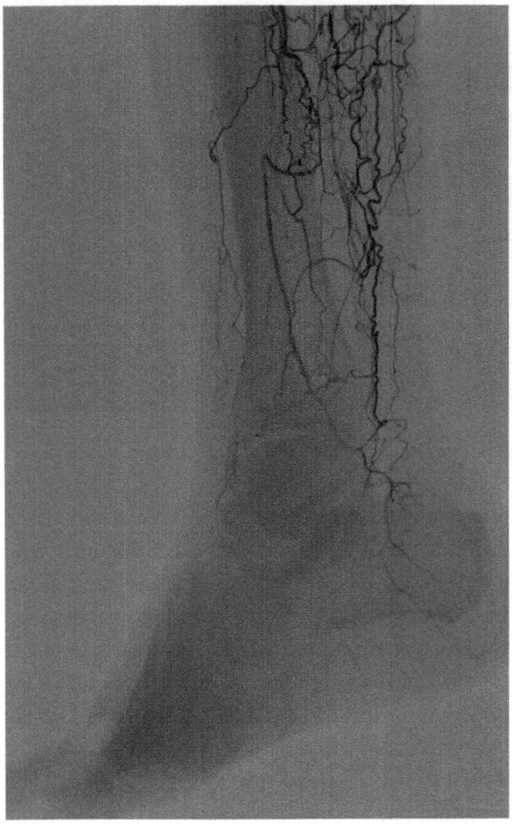

Fig. 12.2 Digital subtraction angiography (DSA) of lower extremity

12.5 Computed Tomography Angiography (CTA)

Computed tomography angiography (CTA) combines X-rays and computerized 3D analysis to produce detailed images of the vascular anatomy. The scanning speed and level of detail achievable depend on the number of detector rows in the CT scanner. Various studies have utilized CT scanners with different numbers of multiple detector rows, ranging from 4 to 64, to generate thin sections of approximately 1 mm or less. Fast injection of a venous contrast agent is performed to enhance the visualization of blood vessels during scanning.

The acquired data from the scan are processed using specialized software to generate maximum intensity projections and 3D volume rendering reconstructions. This post-processing step can take up to 30 min for perforated flaps. The resulting images provide precise visual details of vessel caliber, pathways, and their relationship to the surrounding anatomy. This enables surgeons to plan preoperative dissection strategies and select the appropriate perforator for safer and more efficient procedures [5].

CTA offers the advantage of providing detailed and accurate images of the vascular anatomy, aiding in preoperative planning, and facilitating rapid ablation. However, there are several considerations to keep in mind. CTA involves radiation exposure, with a reported dose of approximately 5.6 mSv. Using iodinated contrast agents introduces potential risks, including allergic reactions and renal or vascular damage. The vasoconstrictive effect of contrast agents can pose challenges in evaluating small-bore vessels. Additionally, CTA is unsuitable for repeated or long-term monitoring due to the cumulative radiation dose and the limitations associated with contrast agent administration (Fig. 12.3).

CTA is primarily employed in planning perforator flaps for breast reconstruction, particularly the deep inferior epigastric artery perforator (DIEP) and superior gluteal artery perforator (SGAP) flaps. It has also been used to assess the anterolateral thigh (ALT) vasculature and fibular flaps. Studies have reported a high correlation between CTA findings and intraoperative observations, including perforator location and size.

CTA provides valuable information for preoperative planning in reconstructive surgery involving perforator flaps. However, caution must be exercised considering the radiation dose and the potential risks associated with contrast medium administration.

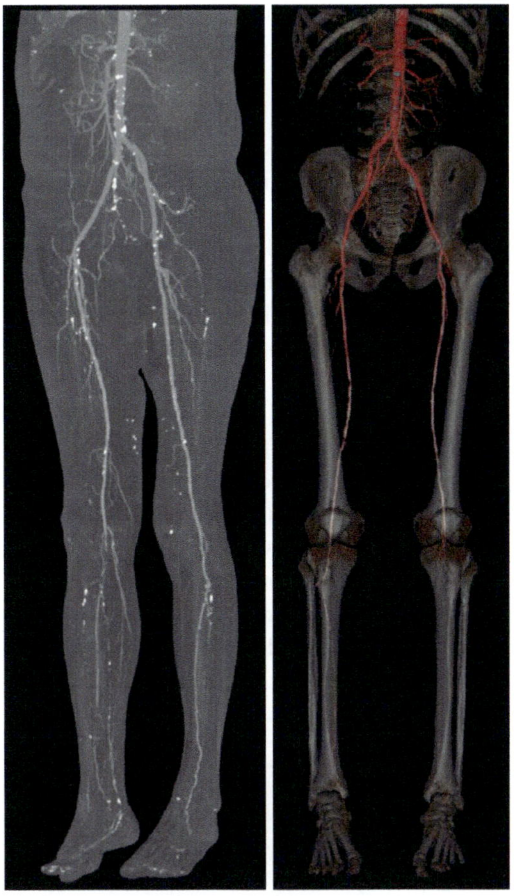

Fig. 12.3 Computed tomography angiography (CTA)

12.6 Magnetic Resonance Angiography (MRA)

Magnetic resonance angiography (MRA) utilizes strong magnetic fields and radiofrequency pulses to generate detailed images of internal body structures. A paramagnetic contrast agent, such as gadolinium, is injected to enhance the visualization of blood vessels in the images. Unlike computed tomography angiography (CTA), MRA does not involve radiation exposure, making it a safer patient procedure.

MRA can provide 3D images that enable surgeons to accurately assess the course, diameter, and relationships of surrounding structures and vessels before surgery. The procedure can be performed in both supine and prone positions, and images can be obtained without distortion due to pressure on flat surfaces. Additionally, MRA can visualize blood vessels without contrast agents, although with lower resolution.

The advantages of MRA include its nonradioactive nature, the potential to be performed without iodinated contrast agents, and its ability to produce 3D images. However, there are some limitations to consider. MRA is relatively expensive and may not be suitable for claustrophobic patients or those with implants containing ferrous metals. Compared to CTA, MRA may have limitations in accurately delineating smaller perforators, as CTA typically provides better resolution for vessels smaller than 1.0 mm [6].

MRA is primarily used in planning free fibula flaps and, more recently, for perforator mapping in breast reconstruction. Study focusing on the fibular skin flap demonstrated the potential of MRA to provide comprehensive information about the vasculature, including septal skin perforators that cannot be visualized with other tests such as Doppler and conventional angiography. The study reported a high correlation between MRA findings and intraoperative observations for DIEP flap procedures. However, for fibular flaps, the available literature regarding the predictive value of MRA should be more extensive and conclusive [7].

MRA is essential in providing preoperative information for reconstructive surgery involving perforator flaps due to its non-radiographic imaging advantages and the ability to visualize 3D vascular anatomy. However, its limitations must be considered, and careful patient selection and image interpretation are crucial factors to ensure its efficacy.

12.7 Discussion

There are several important considerations regarding preoperative mapping methods for flap planning. The studies reviewed in this overview primarily consist of large case series with low levels of evidence, which limits the ability to draw definitive conclusions. However, specific results offer clear guidance for clinical practice.

The authors emphasize the critical role of anatomical knowledge in successful flap harvesting and advocate for the use of preoperative mapping methods as a supplement to surgery. It is crucial to have a backup plan and be mindful of potential limitations in detecting discrepancies between perforated arteries and donor's veins with specific mapping methods.

The study environment should be considered, as the results may only be replicated in specialized units where specific mapping methods are available. Collaboration between radiologists and surgeons is essential to leverage the potential of advanced preoperative mapping fully.

CTA and MRA are emerging as the preferred methods for generating high-quality 3D images of vessels and surrounding structures in specialized settings. CTA is the preferred method for scanning perforator flaps due to its high accuracy in delineating small vessels and perforators. MRA offers advantages such as avoiding ionizing radiation and potentially nephrotoxic contrast agents.

Despite its limitations, portable Doppler (HHD) remains essential in clinical practice due to its portability, cost-effectiveness, ease of use, and availability during surgery. It may require improved accuracy in identifying perforators compared to CDS and CTA. However, it can serve as a default mapping device for thin flaps or as a complementary tool to CTA or MRA when planning specific flaps.

When selecting the appropriate preoperative mapping method for flap planning, it is important to adopt an individualized decision-making process. Factors such as available resources, practitioner expertise, and the specific requirements of each case should be carefully considered. The importance of ongoing research and development in refining mapping techniques and determining the optimal approaches for various flap scenarios cannot be overstated.

CDS (color Doppler sonography) is a noninvasive mapping device in vascular units. It provides some information about the 3D anatomy surrounding the vasculature but requires skilled staff with knowledge of flap surgery to perform and interpret the examination. CDS is considered suitable as a primary mapping option when CTA and MRA are contraindicated or when the intravascular flow is of particular interest.

Digital subtractive angiography (DSA) is becoming less favored as the primary mapping device due to its invasive nature, radiation exposure, and reliance on iodinated contrast agents. DSA produces 2D images and carries the risk of pseudoaneurysms.

For diabetic foot reconstruction, simple X-rays also can give information about the recipient vessel calcifications. Both posterior and anterior tibial artery status can be visualized in lateral and AP foot views (Fig. 12.4). We can get overall simplified information about the recipient's vessel. Also, using a color duplex ultrasonogram, we can see calcified walls on the gray

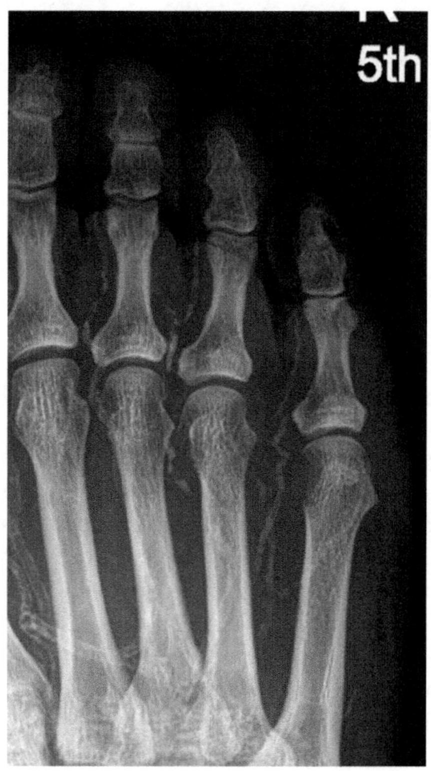

Fig. 12.4 Simple foot X-ray with calcification of the vessels

image setting, which should be informative for planning the site of free flap anastomosis.

The future development of free flap planning should focus on reducing reliance on invasive testing with potentially complicating contrast agents while improving 3D reconstruction. MRA holds significant potential, especially if it becomes as accurate as CTA with further advancements. However, portable Doppler (HHD) devices are always included in flap planning due to their ease of use and availability during surgery.

The authors suggest that future studies compare different mapping methods and prospectively assess diagnostic test results against intraoperative findings. Presently, CTA and MRA are considered the best methods for mapping the vasculature of perforator-dependent skin lamina. HHD is preferred for thin, simple, short anatomical structures and intraoperative skin assessments. DSA is being phased out, and CDS can be used as an alternative when other methods are contraindicated.

References

1. Yu P, Youssef A. Efficacy of the handheld Doppler in preoperative identification of the cutaneous perforators in the anterolateral thigh flap. Plast Reconstr Surg. 2006;118(4):928–33.
2. Shaw RJ, et al. Preoperative Doppler assessment of perforator anatomy in the anterolateral thigh flap. Br J Oral Maxillofac Surg. 2010;48(6):419–22.
3. Tsukino A, et al. Preoperative color Doppler assessment in planning of anterolateral thigh flaps. Plast Reconstr Surg. 2004;113(1):241–6.
4. Ohjimi H, et al. Analyzing the vascular architecture of the free TRAM flap using intraoperative ex vivo angiography. Plast Reconstr Surg. 2005;116(1):106–13.
5. Alonso-Burgos A, et al. Preoperative planning of deep inferior epigastric artery perforator flap reconstruction with multislice-CT angiography: imaging findings and initial experience. J Plast Reconstr Aesthet Surg. 2006;59(6):585–93.
6. Rozen WM, et al. Advances in the pre-operative planning of deep inferior epigastric artery perforator flaps: magnetic resonance angiography. Microsurgery. 2009;29(2):119–23.
7. Fukaya E, et al. Magnetic resonance angiography to evaluate septocutaneous perforators in free fibula flap transfer. J Plast Reconstr Aesthet Surg. 2010;63(7):1099–104.

Thinning the Flaps: Superthin, Ultrathin, and Pure Skin Flaps

13

Hidehiko Yoshimatsu

13.1 Introduction

The use of free flap transfer has revolutionized the ability to cover defects in hard-to-reach areas of the body that are not amenable to local flaps. This is especially beneficial in the treatment of malignant tumors where extensive removal is required. Despite the availability of many surgical options, bulky flaps remain a significant challenge in reconstruction. Microsurgeons have developed methods for flap thinning to address this problem, whether to use a very thin flap in areas such as the hand or dorsum of the foot or to obtain a flap from an obese patient. Extremely thin flaps are often necessary in the hands to avoid contracture when a skin graft is not appropriate or to cover defects in irradiated fields where skin grafts are less likely to succeed. This chapter will delve into the anatomy of perforators to the dermis, preoperative imaging for flap thinning, and various strategies for achieving ultrathin flaps.

13.2 Flap Design

The location of the pure skin perforator (PSP) or an arterial branch entering the dermis plays a crucial role in flap dissection, whether it is identified preoperatively using ultrasonography or intraoperatively through surgical dissection under a microscope. In an ideal scenario, the PSP should be situated in the center of the skin paddle, as in other perforator flaps. However, our experience suggests that there is no significant difference in flap survival rate and flap size whether the PSP is placed centrally or peripherally [1, 2]. The maximum extent of a PSP flap is presently unknown, but based on our experience, a single PSP can perfuse up to 10 cm from its entrance site. Flap size based on a single PSP can range from 3 to 60 cm^2, while flap size based on two or three PSPs can vary from 16 to 90 cm^2 and 22.75 to 90 cm^2, respectively. To prevent postoperative malperfusion of the flap, indocyanine green (ICG) angiography can be performed as it can detect both flap congestion and ischemia [3].

Supplementary Information The online version contains supplementary material available at https://doi.org/10.1007/978-981-97-7278-0_13.

H. Yoshimatsu (✉)
Department of Plastic and Reconstructive Surgery, Cancer Institute Hospital of the Japanese Foundation for Cancer Research, Tokyo, Japan

J. P. Hong et al. (eds.), *Imaging for Reconstructive Microsurgery*,
https://doi.org/10.1007/978-981-97-7278-0_13

13.3 Preoperative Imaging Modalities for Ultrathin and Pure Skin Flaps

The present gold standard for planning perforator flap elevation is computed tomography angiography (CTA), but its resolution limitation of around 0.5 mm makes it difficult to visualize pure skin perforators (PSPs) precisely. Color duplex ultrasonography can be useful for identifying the terminal branches of the SCIA in regions suitable for ultrathin flaps [4]. However, the use of color duplex mode decreases image resolution, making it impossible to visualize PSPs precisely. To overcome this limitation, an ultrasound device with an ultrahigh frequency of up to 70 MHz is needed to observe small arteries and veins entering the dermis layer, allowing for precise identification of PSPs [5]. When using ultrahigh frequency ultrasonography, the distal portion of the SCIA should first be identified using a probe with lower frequency around the anterior superior iliac spine (ASIS) (Fig. 13.1). Then, the ultrahigh frequency probe should be used to trace down the SCIA distally, looking for small branches entering the dermis (Fig. 13.2).

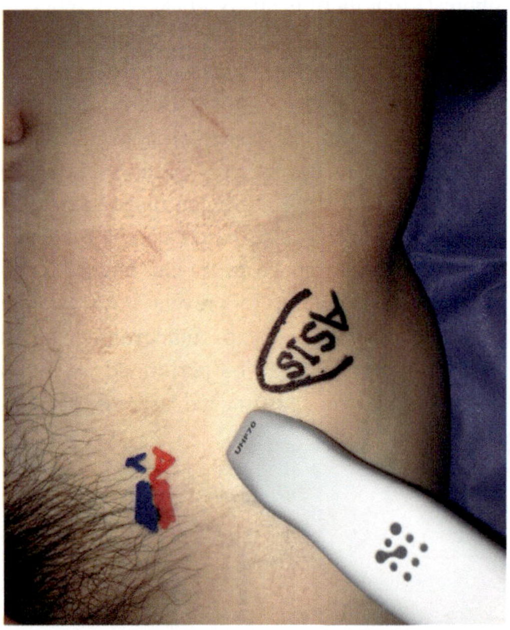

Fig. 13.1 When using ultrahigh frequency ultrasonography, the distal portion of the SCIA should first be identified using a probe with lower frequency around the anterior superior iliac spine

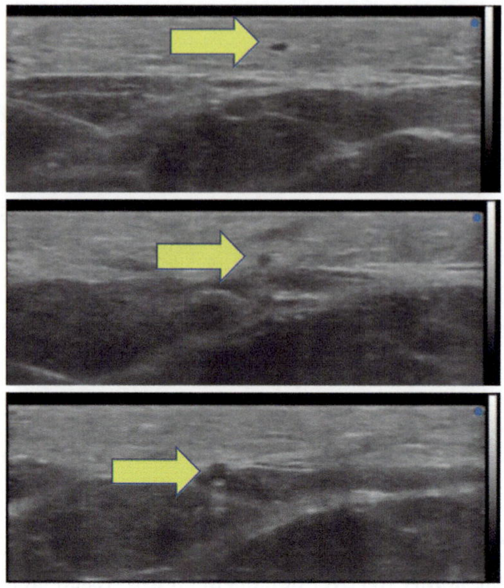

Fig. 13.2 The PSP (yellow arrow) can be visualized entering the dermis using an ultrahigh frequency ultrasonography

13.4 Flap Thinning

The dermal entry point of the artery is located in the center of the skin paddle's design. First, the superficial branch of the SCIA is identified according to the method described in a previous report, and the flap is then elevated above the superficial fascia [6]. To "unfloor" the pedicle (not "unroof" since the flap was now upside-down), the flap was turned over while still connected to the femoral artery (Fig. 13.3). Using a surgical microscope, the terminal branch of the superficial branch of the SCIA is then exposed and traced down to the site of dermal entry. The whole course of this terminal branch is marked with a pen, and any adipose tissues in other regions are removed until the dermis is visible using a pair of scissors (Fig. 13.4; Video 13.1).

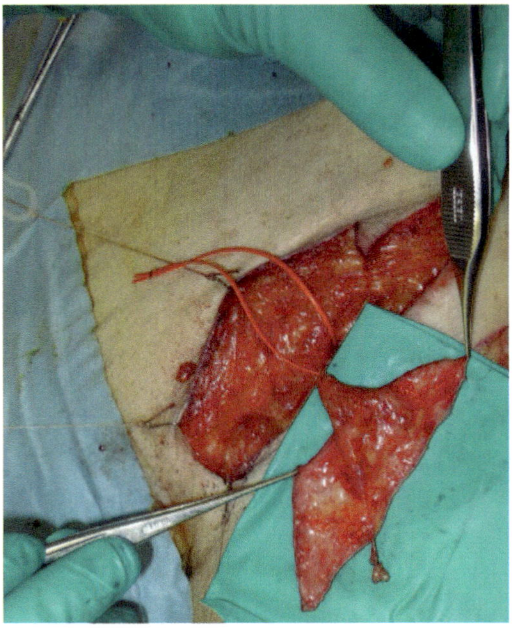

Fig. 13.3 After elevation of the flap above the superficial fascia, it is turned upside-down for further thinning

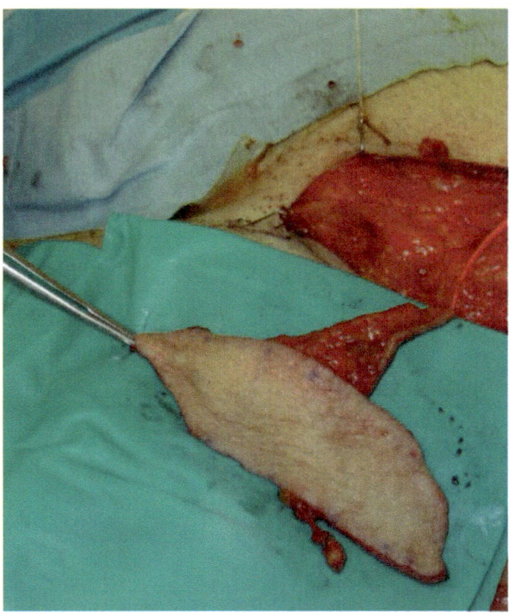

Fig. 13.4 After ultrathinning of the SCIP flap

References

1. Narushima M, Yamasoba T, Iida T, Yamamoto T, Yoshimatsu H, Hara H, Oshima A, Koshima I. Pure skin perforator flap for microtia and congenital aural atresia using supermicrosurgical techniques. J Plast Reconstr Aesthet Surg. 2011;64(12):1580–4.
2. Narushima M, Yamasoba T, Iida T, et al. Pure skin perforator flaps: the anatomical vascularity of the superthin flap. Plast Reconstr Surg. 2018;142(3):351e–60e.
3. Yoshimatsu H, Karakawa R, Scaglioni MF, Fuse Y, Tanakura K, Yano T. Application of intraoperative indocyanine green angiography for detecting flap congestion in the use of free deep inferior epigastric perforator flaps for breast reconstruction. Microsurgery. 2021;41(6):522–6.
4. Kehrer A, Sachanadani S, Batista P, da Silva S, Lonic D, Heidekrueger P, Taeger CD, Klein S, Jung EM, Prantl L, Hong JP. Step by step guide to ultrasound-based design of alt flaps by the microsurgeon—basic and advanced applications and device settings. J Plast Reconstr Aesthet Surg. 2020;73(6):1081–90.
5. Yoshimatsu H, Hayashi A, Yamamoto T, Visconti G, Karakawa R, Fuse Y, Iida T. Visualization of the "intradermal plexus" using ultrasonography in the dermis flap: a step beyond perforator flaps. Plast Reconstr Surg Glob Open. 2019;7(11):e2411.
6. Yoshimatsu H, Yamamoto T, Hayashi A, Iida T. Proximal-to-distally elevated superficial circumflex iliac artery perforator flap enabling hybrid reconstruction. Plast Reconstr Surg. 2016;138(4):910–22.

References

Imaging in the Postoperative Period

14

Shannon R. Garvey, Amy Chen, Asha D. Nanda, John B. Park, Frances Rodriguez Lara, Oluwaseun D. Adebagbo, Bernard T. Lee, and Ryan P. Cauley

14.1 Introduction

Imaging in the postoperative period allows for rapid diagnosis and management of complications. In particular, ultrasound is a safe and noninvasive imaging modality with broad procedural and diagnostic applications within plastic and reconstructive surgery. Given more recent technological advancements, high-resolution ultrasound devices are now readily available at the bedside to provide dynamic, real-time imaging at a much lower cost than other available imaging modalities. Here, we discuss the postoperative applications of ultrasound and other imaging modalities in reconstructive microsurgery.

S. R. Garvey · A. Chen · A. D. Nanda · J. B. Park
F. R. Lara · O. D. Adebagbo · B. T. Lee
R. P. Cauley (✉)
Division of Plastic and Reconstructive Surgery, Department of Surgery, Beth Israel Deaconess Medical Center, Harvard Medical School, Boston, MA, USA
e-mail: sgarvey1@bidmc.harvard.edu; achen29@bidmc.harvard.edu; bp373@rwjms.rutgers.edu; frances2@bu.edu; seun.adebagbo@tufts.edu; blee3@bidmc.harvard.edu; rcauley@bidmc.harvard.edu

14.2 Postoperative Flap Monitoring

Autologous free tissue transfer is a safe and reliable technique in reconstructive microsurgery with free flap loss rates ranging from 1 to 9%, depending on the type of reconstruction [1]. This is due in part to modern technological advances allowing for rapid detection and management of vascular compromise. Though relatively rare, flap thrombosis remains a devastating complication in microsurgery; however, studies have shown that continuous postoperative monitoring is associated with a decreased time to diagnosis, reexploration, and an increased rate of flap salvage [2]. Ultrasound has since emerged as an important tool for flap monitoring in the postoperative period. Though fluorescent indocyanine green (ICG) angiography is typically reserved for intraoperative assessment of anastomotic patency and flap perfusion, it can be used in the postoperative setting to confirm patency if a complication is suspected with other modalities.

14.2.1 Handheld Acoustic Doppler Sonography

Handheld acoustic Doppler, paired with clinical exam, is a commonly used method for postoperative flap monitoring. The major disadvantage of the handheld surface Doppler is that it allows

J. P. Hong et al. (eds.), *Imaging for Reconstructive Microsurgery*,
https://doi.org/10.1007/978-981-97-7278-0_14

only for an intermittent assessment of venous and arterial blood flow, rather than continuous monitoring. Further, the reliability of handheld acoustic Doppler is dependent on the experience of staff and ability of staff to correlate to clinical findings. In this way, it is a less objective measure of postoperative flap monitoring with lower inter-user reliability [3]. Despite disadvantages, the handheld acoustic Doppler is both cost-effective and easily obtained; thus, it remains a mainstay option for postoperative flap monitoring and is often employed in conjunction with other flap monitoring methods to ensure accuracy.

14.2.2 Implantable Doppler

Implantable continuous Doppler monitoring offers an alternative to handheld acoustic Doppler, with a higher overall flap-compromise detection rate [4]. Much like handheld acoustic Dopplers, implantable Dopplers should be utilized in the context of a thorough clinical exam. However, implantable Dopplers are of particular benefit in cases for which the clinical exam of the flap may not be possible, as is the case with buried flaps [5]. The use of an implantable continuous Doppler results in increased operating time, which is a notable disadvantage of this flap monitoring method [4]. Studies show that the overall sensitivity and specificity of implantable Doppler monitoring is high with arterial monitoring having significantly greater specificity than venous monitoring [6].

A flow coupler is an end-to-end anastomotic coupler with a removable Doppler attached. Coupler placement is a required step in most microvascular procedures; the use of a flow coupler therefore eliminates the increased operative time associated with other implantable Dopplers. When compared to other implantable Dopplers (i.e., Cook–Swartz Doppler), flow couplers were shown to be equivalent in monitoring blood flow to free flaps [7].

14.2.3 Laser Doppler Flowmetry

Laser Doppler flowmetry is a noninvasive technique utilizing a low-power laser that provides live feedback to the fibers of the probe. Different movements of red blood cells produce different electrical signals causing Doppler (frequency) shift in proportional to erythrocyte velocity [8]. The device ultimately produces quantitative outputs expressed as RPU (relative perfusion unit) or BPI (blood perfusion index). Laser Doppler flowmetry has been used for its noninvasive nature, feasibility, and its ability to measure blood flow in real time. Moreover, it has demonstrated its effectiveness in assessing microcirculation, allowing users to measure blood flow in small vessels that are miniscule to be visualized with traditional imaging techniques. Rothenberger et al. showed its ability to successfully detect arterial and venous occlusions in perforator flaps [9].

14.2.4 Color Duplex Ultrasonography

Color duplex ultrasonography is another noninvasive technique that incorporates color-enhanced Doppler and B-mode images producing real-time, color differentiated structures that allow users to easily identify abnormal flow (Fig. 14.1) [11]. It has been demonstrated to have multiple roles in the postoperative setting. Microvascular flow has been successfully quantified using color duplex ultrasound in different anatomic locations including the breast, head,

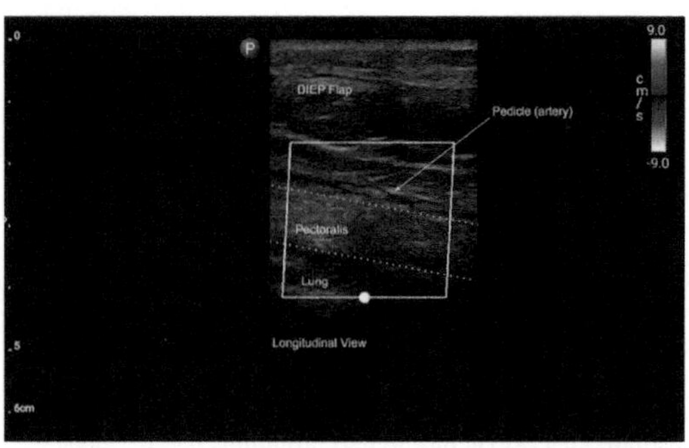

Fig. 14.1 Color Doppler ultrasound view of a deep inferior epigastric perforator (DIEP) flap pedicle, which demonstrates patent arterial flow. (This figure is quoted from Long et al. published in Journal of Reconstructive Microsurgery by Thieme Medical Publishers Inc., copyright 2022. Reprinted with permission from George Thieme Verlag KG [10])

neck, and extremities [12]. Its main advantage lies in its ability to provide precise, quantitative vascular inflow and outflow. The use of color duplex ultrasonography may reduce unnecessary flap revisions [13]. The technique has also been commended for its feasibility with successful use at bedside by surgeons [14]. Additionally, color duplex ultrasonography has the ability to differentiate between arterial and venous complications [14]. Furthermore, its use with scheduled time intervals or in conjunction with implantable laser Doppler has shown to achieve excellent salvage rates [15].

14.2.5 Flap Monitoring Protocols

Flap monitoring is a crucial aspect of postoperative care in reconstructive surgery, as it helps identify and manage complications such as flap ischemia and venous occlusions [16]. When occlusion of arterial or venous flow is detected, revision of the thrombosis can lead to successful flap salvage. Diagnosing flap ischemia in a timely manner is thus vital for successful flap transfer, as ischemia can become irreversible due to the no-reflow phenomenon [17]. Venous insufficiency of flaps can lead to microvascular lesions that become irreversible within 6–8 h [16].

Well-designed postoperative flap monitoring protocols can help avoid complications and salvage thrombosed flaps. Presently, there are no established, universal flap monitoring protocols. Flap monitoring involves clinical assessment such as physical examination and objective parameters using imaging and monitoring technologies [18]. Physical examination includes ensuring flap color, temperature, turgor, and capillary refill. Needle prick and skin incision to observe bleeding have also been described as physical examination components in flap monitoring [19]. Among the technologies used for objective parameters, tissue oximetry, handheld Doppler, implantable Doppler, laser Doppler flowmetry, and color duplex ultrasonography have demonstrated their effectiveness.

Studies have shown that monitoring flaps in the postoperative setting is critical, and monitoring frequency depends on the type of flap used and the surgeon's preference. An institution demonstrated that using implantable Dopplers and hourly external Doppler checks by nursing and resident physicians to check flaps in the postoperative ICU setting could help detect most vascular-related compromises within 24 h, with data suggesting that q2–4 h is appropriate after 72 h [20]. Jallali et al. conducted a study that showed that selected UK plastic surgeons most commonly used flap monitoring frequency that followed hourly checks for the first 24-h period, followed by every 1–2 hourly checks for the second 24-h period and then every 4-h checks for the third 24-h period [21]. The study also demonstrated higher flap viability rates when ultrasonographic technology such as handheld Doppler and laser Doppler flowmetry was used [20]. Finally, Shinomiya et al. implemented color ultrasonography in addition to conventional clinical examination of free flap transfers. They monitored flaps with clinical assessment every 2 h for the first postoperative day, every 4 h for the next 2 days, and every 6 h until day 7. Abnormal findings were reassessed with color duplex ultrasound to evaluate the need for reexploration, which was shown to reduce unnecessary exploration when conventional, physical examination of the flap was found to be abnormal [22].

While there are many different protocols implemented by plastic surgeons and institutions, and a universal monitoring algorithm is yet to be established, we introduce our algorithm that incorporates ultrasonography in flap monitoring in Fig. 14.2.

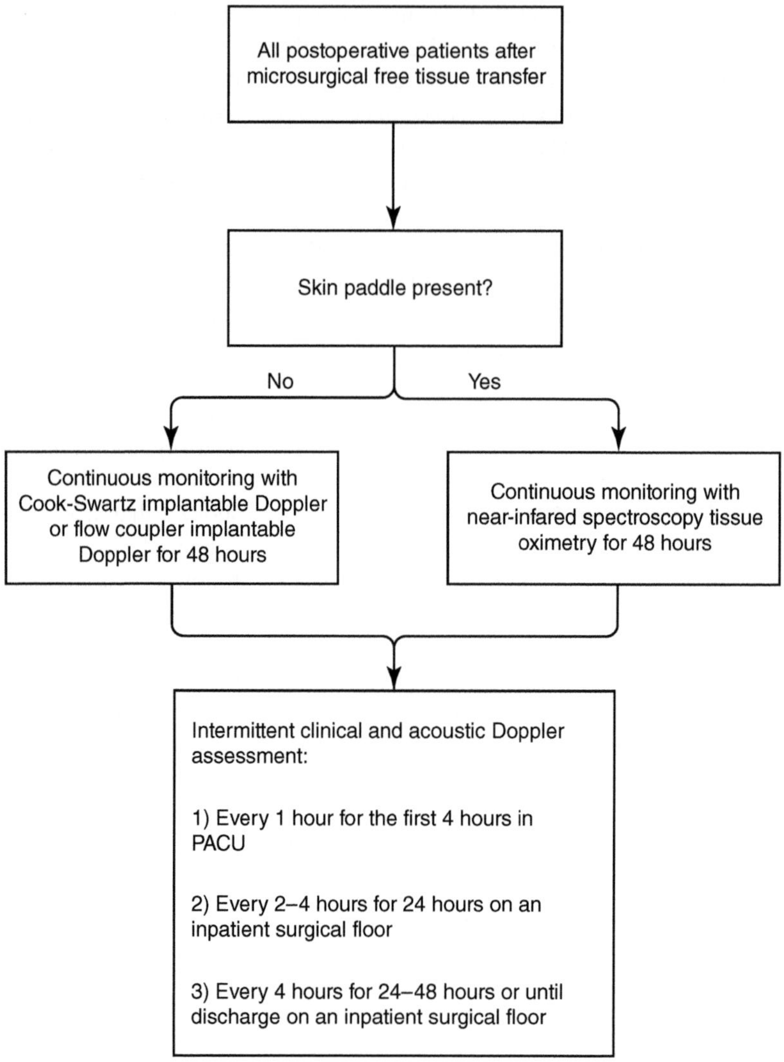

Fig. 14.2 Flap monitoring algorithm

14.3 Diagnosis and Management of Postoperative Complications

Widely available in a variety of clinical settings, point-of-care ultrasound (POCUS) allows for quick, cost-effective examination of many organ systems and can be used as a minimally invasive imaging modality in postoperative patients. Beyond flap monitoring, ultrasound is also the primary tool for diagnosis of complications such as hematoma, seroma, and soft tissue infection. Routine use of ultrasound can direct further management of complications in the postoperative period.

14.3.1 Hematoma

Detection of hematoma or seroma is often dependent on ultrasound. While the sonographic appearance of fluid is not always uniform, it is a reliable method for determining the presence of abnormal fluid collections. The shape of hematomas viewed on ultrasound can range from ovoid/spheroid to lentiform depending on the location. They are differentiated from seromas by the presence of wall irregularities and internal echoes, the latter of which are more frequently seen in more acute presentations. Septations may also be present but are not specific to hematomas [23]. Subacute and chronic hematomas are characterized by more well-defined margins, development of hypoechoic regions from liquefaction, and marginal hyperemia on color Doppler ultrasound. Sonographic appearance alone may not be enough to distinguish hematomas from abscesses, in which case ultrasound-guided percutaneous aspiration is necessary [24].

Clinically significant hematomas are often managed with evacuation in the operating room. Percutaneous drainage is usually only successfully performed for hematomas that have undergone liquefaction, which occurs 6–7 days after initial formation of the hematoma. Ultrasound-guided evacuation using a vacuum-assisted breast biopsy system (e.g., EnCor™ Breast Biopsy System [BD Bard, Tempe, AZ, USA]) in post-breast biopsy and postsurgical patients has been recently described. However, further study is required on the efficacy of this treatment modality, especially with respect to the extent of evacuation of larger and hardened clots, before it becomes more widely adopted [25].

14.3.2 Seroma

Seromas are characterized on imaging with low echogenicity or anechoic regions surrounded with little to no discernable wall (Fig. 14.3). They commonly occur after breast reconstruction, abdominoplasty, and hernia repair [26–28]. Although physical examination alone may be sufficient to diagnose asymptomatic seromas, radiological imaging should be obtained in cases of chronic unresolved seromas or when the diagnosis is uncertain. Delayed detection or inadequate treatment of seromas can result in the development of a fibrous pseudocapsule that can be observed on ultrasonography [29].

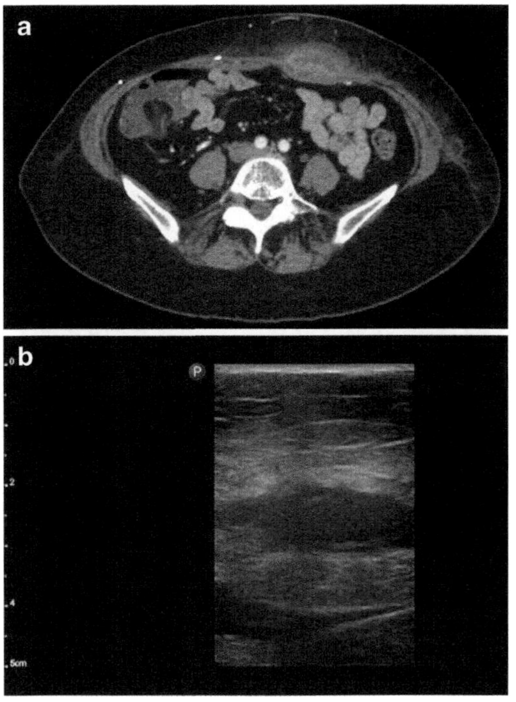

Fig. 14.3 Computed tomography image (**a**) and portable ultrasound image (**b**) of a donor site abdominal wall seroma following a deep inferior epigastric perforator (DIEP) flap. (This figure is quoted from Long et al. published in Journal of Reconstructive Microsurgery by Thieme Medical Publishers Inc., copyright 2022. Reprinted with permission from George Thieme Verlag KG [10])

With the exception of chronic encapsulated seromas requiring capsulectomy, large and/or symptomatic seromas are usually aspirated at bedside or in clinic, which may be done under ultrasound guidance.

14.3.3 Skin and Soft Tissue Infections

Ultrasonography can be an important tool for the diagnosis of skin and soft tissue infections, especially for cases that are not clinically evident based on physical exam alone [30, 31]. Cellulitis is characterized by hyperechoic subcutaneous tissue with anechoic striations from edema, which together impart a cobblestone appearance on ultrasonography (Fig. 14.4). The presence of hyperemia on color Doppler can help differenti-

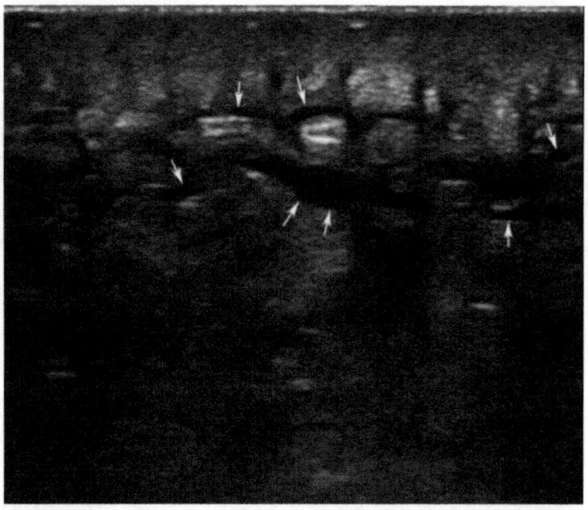

Fig. 14.4 Ultrasound appearance of cellulitis with areas of hypoechoic fluid within subcutaneous tissue forming a cobblestone pattern (arrows). (This figure is quoted from Adhikari et al. published in Journal of Ultrasound in Medicine by the American Institute of Ultrasound in Medicine, copyright 2012. Reprinted with permission from John Wiley and Sons [32])

ate infectious inflammation from other edematous states. It is especially important for clinical suspicion of cellulitis to be radiologically investigated, as the differential includes cellulitic superficial changes that accompany infection of deeper structures, such as abscesses and necrotizing fasciitis.

The accuracy of ultrasound for necrotizing fasciitis is limited by resolution at higher depth and has not been evaluated by data-driven studies, likely due to rarity of cases. POCUS can still be useful if hallmark signs can be observed that differentiate necrotizing fasciitis from cellulitis. Signs such as fascial thickening and peri-fascial gas locules with acoustic shadowing may indicate deep soft tissue infection necessitating further imaging with computed tomography [33].

Abscesses vary in appearance depending on location, content, and involvement of surrounding tissue. Echogenicity is especially subject to great variation because it is dependent on the maturity of the abscess [34]. More specific signs on ultrasound include posterior acoustic enhancement, internal debris, septations, and wall hyperemia from increased vascularity [34, 35].

14.4 Postoperative Pain Management

Postoperative pain management has been shown to reduce complications, postanesthesia care unit stays, and readmission rates. Multimodal anesthesia regimens are often a combination of nerve block techniques and non-opioid analgesics (e.g., NSAIDs, acetaminophen, and gabapentinoids) [36–38]. Ultrasound-guided thoracic paravertebral block, pectoral nerve block, and erector spinae block are commonly used for pain management in breast cancer surgeries [39]. Other common nerve blocks utilized in reconstructive microsurgery are available in Table 14.1. A common type of nerve block in abdominal reconstructive surgery is the transabdominal plane (TAP) block performed in procedures such as DIEP flaps. TAP blocks following DIEP reconstruction can help reduce postsurgical interval morphine requirements and length of hospital stay [49, 60]. The TAP block technique will depend on the approach utilized to localize the transversus abdominis plane between the transversus abdominis and internal oblique muscles. The plane can be identified in one of three ways: landmark-guided, using the Petit triangle, laparoscopic-guided, or ultrasound-guided [61–63].

Ultrasound-guided nerve blocks allow for sonographic anatomy visualization, improved accuracy, and safety. Ultrasound-guided imaging provides direct visualization of the relevant anatomy—the three muscle layers (external oblique, internal oblique, and transversus abdominis), the peritoneum, and intraperitoneal structures—as well as the advancing needle and the injected fluid [64]. Accurate target of the TAP compartment can be approached in three ways: subcostally (anterior abdominal wall, beneath the costal margin), laterally (lateral abdominal wall), and posteriorly (the anterolateral aspect of the quadratus lumborum muscle or at the level of the lumbar triangle of Petit). In most of these approaches, the patient should be in supine position [61]. The block could be administered intra-

Table 14.1 Nerve blocks in reconstructive microsurgery

Surgical site	Type of block	Targeted nerves	Landmarks	Probe orientation	Injection plane	Region of analgesia	Complications	Special considerations
Breast and chest wall	Intercostal nerve block [40]	Anterior cutaneous branches of intercostal nerves	Inferior edge of targeted rib	Probe longitudinal to the sternum at the angle of the rib	Between the internal intercostal muscle and innermost intercostal muscle	Lateral trunk and upper abdomen at the ipsilateral individual intercostal levels	Pneumothorax and systemic toxicity	Fourth intercostal nerve has the largest suprapleural approach to the breast
	Transversus thoracic muscle plane block [41]	Anterior cutaneous terminal branches of the intercostal nerves	At the level of third and fourth ribs, lateral to the lateral border of sternum	Probe parasagittal between the intercostal muscle and transversus thoracic muscle	Between the intercostal muscle and transversus thoracic muscle	Medial and parasternal areas of the chest wall	Pneumothorax and systemic toxicity	Can be performed bilaterally
	Paravertebral block [42, 43]	Nerve root at level of spinal cord	Spines of ipsilateral targeted vertebral bodies, often C7–T5	Probe parasagittal lateral to the spine of the vertebral bodies	Needle advanced until transverse process found and then walked off into paravertebral space	Individual ipsilateral thoracic dermatomes	Inadvertent vascular puncture, hypotension, and hematoma	Can also be used for abdominal and inguinal analgesia
	Interpectoral plane block (Pecs I) [44, 45]	Lateral and medial pectoral nerves	Pectoralis major muscle, pectoralis minor muscle, and the pectoral branch of the thoracoacromial artery	Probe paramedian orientation, rotated 90 degrees, and toward the lateral chest wall	Between the pectoralis major muscle and pectoralis minor muscle	Anterior chest wall	Hematoma	Performed in combination with the Pecs II block
	Interpectoral plane + pecto-serratus block (Pecs II) [44, 46]	Pectoral nerves, intercostobrachial nerve, intercostal nerves 3–6, thoracodorsal nerve, and long thoracic nerve	Second rib towards the third rib, visualize the pectoralis minor muscle, the insertion of the pectoralis major muscle, and serratus anterior muscle	Probe linear under the lateral third of the clavicle	Between the pectoralis minor muscle and serratus anterior	Anterior chest wall and axilla	None reported	Two injections are needed, theoretically providing wider breast coverage
	Erector spinae plane block [44, 47, 48]	Dorsal and ventral rami of the thoracic spinal nerves	T5 spinous process, trapezius muscle, transverse process, rhomboid major muscle, and erector spinae muscles	Probe 3 cm lateral to the midline of the T5 spinous process	Between the rhomboid major muscle and erector spinae muscles	T2–T9 between the midclavicular line and 3 cm lateral to midline	Pneumothorax	There is a thoracic and a lumbar block
Abdomen	Transversus abdominis plane block [49, 50]	Nerves from the anterior rami of thoracolumbar spinal nerves T6–L1	The bilateral rectus abdominis muscles lateral to the lateral border of the rectus muscle	Probe transverse to the anterolateral abdominal wall and moved posterolaterally across the mid-axillary line over the iliac crest	Between the transversus abdominis muscle and internal oblique muscle	Anterolateral abdominal wall	Abdominal wall hematoma, inadvertent peritoneal puncture, and possible visceral injury	The subcostal technique is an alternative approach (not described here)

(continued)

Table 14.1 (continued)

Surgical site	Type of block	Targeted nerves	Landmarks	Probe orientation	Injection plane	Region of analgesia	Complications	Special considerations
Upper extremity	Brachial plexus—supraclavicular block [51, 52]	Brachial plexus at the level of the trunk	Above the clavicle, subclavian artery, and the brachial plexus at the level of the trunks and divisions	Probe transverse over the posterior mid-neck	Lateral to medial at the level of the brachial plexus trunk, above the clavicle	Distal two-thirds of the upper extremity	Pneumothorax and hoarseness	Incidence of pneumothorax is as high as 6%
	Median nerve block [53, 54]	Median nerve	Lateral to flexor palmaris longus tendon, 2 cm distal to antecubital crease	Probe transverse over the proximal volar forearm	Between the tendons of the flexor palmaris longus and flexor carpi radialis muscle	Radial aspect of the palmar hand, palmar surface of the thumb, index and middle fingers, and radial aspect of the third digit	Intravascular injection and nerve injury	To identify the flexor palmaris longus tendon, have the patient oppose the thumb and fifth digit with the wrist flexed
	Ulnar nerve block [54, 55]	Ulnar nerve	Ulnar artery at medial side of volar forearm, superficial at level of wrist crease, and the radial and ulnar nerves	Probe horizontal over the medial forearm, distal to epicondyle of the humerus	Between the flexor carpi ulnaris and flexor digitorum profundus muscles	Ulnar aspect of the hand, including the small finger, fifth digit, and ulnar aspect of the fourth digit	Intravascular injection, nerve injury, and intramuscular hematoma	Anatomical structures at the level of the wrist may alter technique
	Radial nerve block [54, 56]	Radial nerve	Proximal to the styloid process of the radius, brachioradialis muscle, and brachialis muscle	Probe radially over the antecubital fossa, 45 degrees to the arm	Adjacent to the radial nerve, between the brachialis muscle and brachioradialis muscle	Radial aspect of the dorsal wrist, including the first, second, and third digits and radial aspect of the third digit	Intravascular injection and nerve injury	The radial nerve is difficult to visualize
Lower extremity	Popliteal nerve block [57, 58]	Sciatic nerve	Popliteal artery and vein in popliteal crease, semimembranosus, semitendinosus, and biceps femoris muscles	Probe transverse over the posterior mid-thigh	Between the sciatic nerve, biceps femoris muscle, and the vastus lateralis muscle	Below the knee, including the tibial and peroneal nerves	Motor nerve injury (foot drop)	For procedures on the medial aspect of the ankle, a saphenous block may be required
	Femoral nerve block [57–59]	Femoral nerve	Inguinal crease, superficial to the iliopsoas muscle group and deep to the fascia lata and fascia iliac	Probe linear over the femoral artery and vein	Lateral to the femoral nerve in the inguinal crease	Anterior and medial thigh down to and including the knee, medial leg, and foot	Motor nerve injury and hematoma	The three-injection method has higher efficacy than the single-injection technique

operatively, prior to closure of the abdomen, using a sterile ultrasound probe applied directly onto the abdominal fascia [65]. Ultrasound guidance provides accurate needle–nerve contact and confirmation of appropriate local anesthetic (LA) spread, making it advantageous over other landmark-guided methods whose success rates are unpredictable [61]. Under sonographic guidance, the surgeon can perform an aspiration test to avoid intravascular placement of the anesthetic agent. As the LA is injected, the TAP compartment will separate, pushing the transverse abdominis down. Following the block, the fascia of the transverse abdominis muscle should appear distended by the echolucent lens-shaped puddle of local anesthetic injected [49].

Intraoperative ultrasound-guided TAP blocks following DIEP reconstruction are not only efficient but have been shown to be safe and reproducible. Nerve block-related complications include vascular puncture, intravascular injection, intraneural injection, unpredictable spread of LA with potential motor block, bowel perforation, hematoma, local anesthetic systemic toxicity, and intrahepatic injection [61, 66]. The efficacy of the block is dependent on the spread of LA across the TAP compartment. Direct visualization allows for the use of minimum effective volume (15 mL) needed to produce adequate analgesia without compromising the success rates or block duration, reducing the risk of systemic local anesthetic toxicity and unintentional blockade of adjacent nerves [61, 66]. Complications, such as vascular puncture, intravascular injection, and intraneural injection, are not always preventable, as they are operator dependent. The absence of visible LA spread may be an indicator of intravascular injection, and nerve expansion is indicative of intraneural injection. Ultrasound use can facilitate early recognition of these potential issues [66].

Detailed knowledge of anatomy with adequate training and experience can enhance the efficiency and reduce complications associated with ultrasound-guided peripheral nerve blocks.

However, compared with traditional landmark techniques, even less experienced practitioners can achieve greater than 90% success rate in less time and fewer attempts because of the ability to visualize anatomy and target structures, needle, and local anesthetic spread via ultrasound guidance [66, 67].

14.5 Alternative Uses of Ultrasound

Given its ease of access and operator use, additional postoperative diagnostic and therapeutic uses for ultrasound in reconstructive microsurgery have been described. In particular, ultrasound may allow the plastic surgeon to expedite patient diagnosis and treatment or improve the safety of subsequent procedures.

14.5.1 Palpable Nodules

Fat necrosis is a relatively common complication in reconstructive microsurgery with potential aesthetic and imaging implications that can be particularly distressing for patients who undergo autologous breast reconstruction following mastectomy. Ischemia of the flaps' subcutaneous adipose tissue results in adipocyte necrosis and the formation of scar tissue (fat necrosis) or a fluid-filled sac (oil cyst) [68]. Clinically, this manifests as a palpable nodule that can mimic breast cancer recurrence, a concern of patients and plastic surgeons alike.

Therefore, ultrasound can be a valuable first step in the workup of a patient who presents with a palpable nodule. The ultrasonic characteristics of fat necrosis are varied and can range from classically benign features to those suspicious for malignancy [68]. Typical benign findings of fat necrosis include a regular, well-circumscribed mass that is hypoechoic or mixed echogenicity without vascularity on Doppler flow [69]. Soo et al. report echogenic internal bands that shift in orientation with changes in patient position to be a specific sonographic indicator of fat necrosis (Fig. 14.5) [71]. Similarly, oil cysts may present as regular, well-circumscribed masses that are anechoic without vascularity (Fig. 14.6). However, ultrasonic findings that may mimic or

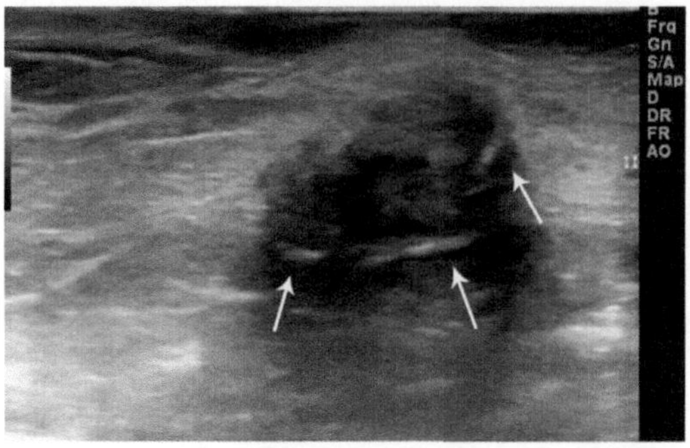

Fig. 14.5 Ultrasound image demonstrates an area of fat necrosis notable for echogenic internal bands (arrows), which may change with patient position. (This figure is quoted from Atasoy et al. published in Journal of Clinical Ultrasound by Wiley Periodicals Inc., copyright 2013. Reprinted with permission from John Wiley and Sons [70])

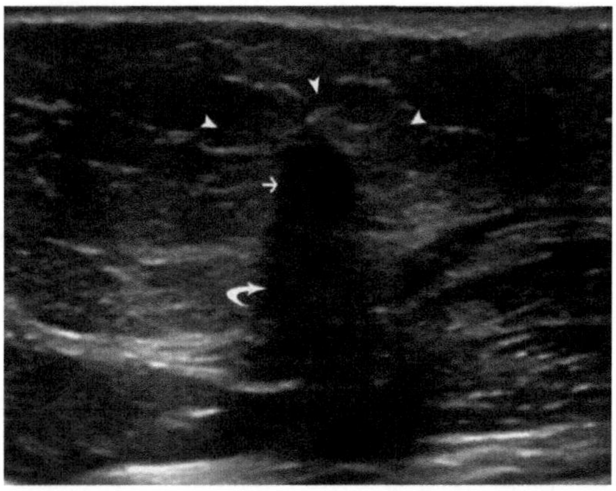

Fig. 14.6 An ultrasound image of a regular-shaped anechoic mass (arrows) with posterior acoustic enhancement (curved arrow) consistent with an oil cyst. (This figure is quoted from Atasoy et al. published in Journal of Clinical Ultrasound by Wiley Periodicals Inc., copyright 2013. Reprinted with permission from John Wiley and Sons [70])

otherwise be concerning for malignancy include large, irregular, and poorly circumscribed masses with vascularity [69].

If ultrasound examination demonstrates clear fat necrosis, the patient can be immediately reassured with continued clinical monitoring. However, masses with indeterminate features warrant further confirmatory testing, including mammography and biopsy. Furthermore, areas of fat necrosis with a fluid component that are painful or of cosmetic concern may be drained in the clinic under ultrasound guidance [72].

14.5.2 Deep Vein Thrombosis Screening

Deep vein thrombosis (DVT) is a frequent yet potentially costly complication following many surgical procedures. Duplex venous ultrasonography is a widely available and minimally invasive technology with a sensitivity and specificity for proximal DVT exceeding 95% [73]. Therefore, it remains the gold standard for the evaluation of DVT. A duplex venous ultrasound measures both venous compressibility (B-mode) and venous flow (Doppler). An incompressible vein on B-mode is diagnostic for DVT (Fig. 14.7). While diminished or absent flow on Doppler US is suggestive of a partial or totally occlusive thrombus, only venous incompressibility is required for a definitive diagnosis [75].

Though Swanson et al. report success with routine outpatient ultrasound screening for DVT in postoperative plastic surgery patients, the decision to proceed with imaging should be evaluated on a case-by-case basis considering both individual risk assessment and clinical judgment [76–78]. We recommend that in clinic ultrasound screening for DVT be considered in patients deemed high risk by Wells' criteria to aid in timely diagnosis and initiation of treatment but should not supersede a formal diagnostic ultrasound.

14.5.3 Postoperative Revision

Finally, ultrasound can be a valuable tool to aid in postoperative revision. In cases of contour deformity or volume deficiency, in particular following microsurgical breast reconstruction, autologous fat grafting may be indicated. Ultrasound guidance for autologous fat grafting may allow for better control of the injection plane and decrease risk of injury surrounding structures, such as the pleura or a previously placed implant [79]. Additionally, ultrasound guidance

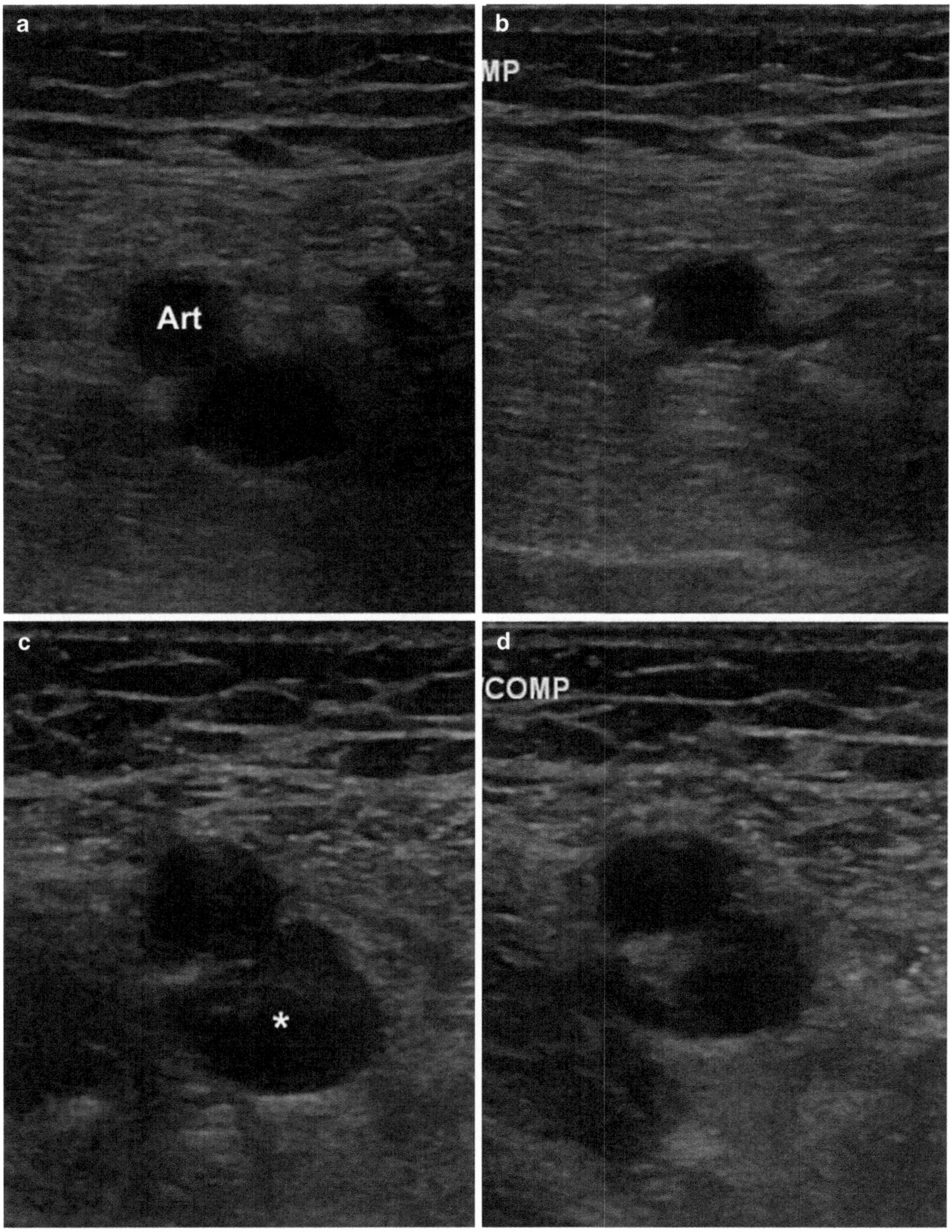

Fig. 14.7 Ultrasound imaging of a normal artery (Art) and vein (**a**) that compresses normally (**b**). Ultrasound imaging of a femoral vein thrombosis (*) without (**c**) and with (**d**) compression, demonstrating noncompressibility. (This figure is quoted from *Needleman* et al. published in *Circulation* by American Heart Association Inc., copyright 2018. Reprinted with permission from Wolters Kluwer Health, Inc. [74])

has been described as a tool for scar release to identify areas of tethering and improve safety when performing release in anatomically sensitive areas [80].

14.6 Other Imaging Modalities

New modalities for imaging have emerged that may potentially become integrated into regular use for postoperative wound and flap monitoring. Infrared thermography, which detects variations in temperature by measuring emitted electromagnetic radiation, has recently been proposed in several proof-of-concept studies as a relatively inexpensive alternative for detecting flap perfusion [81–83]. Further studies with larger patient samples, especially for less expensive nonmedical grade thermal cameras, are needed to compare the accuracy and effectiveness of thermal imaging with more established modalities such as ultrasound [84].

Oxygen perfusion imaging, which utilizes near-infrared spectroscopy to detect changes in oxygenated hemoglobin content in subcutaneous tissue, has also been introduced as a potential modality for monitoring postoperative flap perfusion [85–87]. Compared to thermal imaging, oxygen perfusion imaging is better suited for differentiating between arterial and venous perfusion [88]. However, its accuracy is impacted by perturbations of the skin surface, such as eschar, edema, and radiation-induced atrophy [89]. While many devices utilizing these technologies have become commercially available in recent years, it is unclear how individual differences between manufacturers impact the replicability of measurements. Further studies are needed to define how these emerging technologies can be best utilized in the clinical setting.

14.7 Conclusion

Imaging is particularly important for the postoperative care of patients who undergo reconstructive microsurgery. Ultrasound is a tool that is particularly suited as it allows for a real-time and cost-effective means of diagnosing and treating surgical complications. Importantly, ultrasound allows for postoperative flap monitoring and rapid detection of flap thrombosis improving time to reexploration and ultimately rates of flap salvage. Finally, ultrasound has demonstrated utility in the management of postoperative pain and has been described as a tool for postoperative revision. Newer imaging modalities have been proposed in the literature, such as infrared thermography and oxygen perfusion imaging, that may aid in the identification and management of postoperative wound and flap monitoring; however, these warrant future study.

References

1. Wong AK, Joanna Nguyen T, Peric M, Shahabi A, Vidar EN, Hwang BH, et al. Analysis of risk factors associated with microvascular free flap failure using a multi-institutional database. Microsurgery. 2015;35(1):6–12. https://doi.org/10.1002/micr.22223.
2. Lin SJ, Nguyen MD, Chen C, Colakoglu S, Curtis MS, Tobias AM, et al. Tissue oximetry monitoring in microsurgical breast reconstruction decreases flap loss and improves rate of flap salvage. Plast Reconstr Surg. 2011;127:1080–5.
3. Mericli AF, Wren J, Garvey PB, Liu J, Butler CE, Selber JC. A prospective clinical trial comparing visible light spectroscopy to handheld Doppler for postoperative free tissue transfer monitoring. Plast Reconstr Surg. 2017;140(3):604–13. https://doi.org/10.1097/PRS.0000000000003600.
4. Schmulder A, Gur E, Zaretski A. Eight-year experience of the Cook-Swartz Doppler in free-flap operations: microsurgical and reexploration results with regard to a wide spectrum of surgeries. Microsurgery. 2011;31(1):1–6. https://doi.org/10.1002/micr.20816.
5. Dunklebarger MF, McCrary H, King B, Carpenter P, Buchmann L, Hunt J, et al. Success of implantable Doppler probes for monitoring buried free flaps. Otolaryngol Head Neck Surg. 2022;167(3):452–6. https://doi.org/10.1177/01945998221082533.
6. Chang EI, Ibrahim A, Zhang H, Liu J, Nguyen AT, Reece GP, et al. Deciphering the sensitivity and specificity of the implantable Doppler probe in free flap monitoring. Plast Reconstr Surg. 2016;137(3):971–6. https://doi.org/10.1097/01.prs.0000480016.20326.8f.
7. Um GT, Chang J, Louie O, Colohan SM, Said HK, Neligan PC, et al. Implantable Cook-Swartz Doppler probe versus synovis flow coupler for the postoperative monitoring of free flap breast reconstruction. J Plast Reconstr Aesthet Surg. 2014;67(7):960–6. https://doi.org/10.1016/j.bjps.2014.03.034.

8. Micheels J, Alsbjorn B, Sorensen B. Laser Doppler flowmetry. A new non-invasive measurement of microcirculation in intensive care? Resuscitation. 1984;12(1):31–9. https://doi.org/10.1016/0300-9572(84)90056-x.
9. Rothenberger J, Amr A, Schaller HE, Rahmanian-Schwarz A. Evaluation of a non-invasive monitoring method for free flap breast reconstruction using laser Doppler flowmetry and tissue spectrophotometry. Microsurgery. 2013;33(5):350–7. https://doi.org/10.1002/micr.22096.
10. Long E, Maselli A, Barron S, Morgenstern M, Comer CD, Chow K, et al. Applications of ultrasound in the postoperative period: a review. J Reconstr Microsurg. 2022;38(3):245–53. https://doi.org/10.1055/s-0041-1740959.
11. Cho MJ, Kwon JG, Pak CJ, Suh HP, Hong JP. The role of duplex ultrasound in microsurgical reconstruction: review and technical considerations. J Reconstr Microsurg. 2020;36(7):514–21. https://doi.org/10.1055/s-0040-1709479.
12. Yano K, Hosokawa K, Nakai K, Kubo T, Hattori R. Monitoring by means of color Doppler sonography after buried free DIEP flap transfer. Plast Reconstr Surg. 2003;112(4):1177. https://doi.org/10.1097/01.PRS.0000077214.89627.23.
13. Khalid AN, Quraishi SA, Zang WA, Chadwick JL, Stack BC Jr. Color Doppler ultrasonography is a reliable predictor of free tissue transfer outcomes in head and neck reconstruction. Otolaryngol Head Neck Surg. 2006;134(4):635–8. https://doi.org/10.1016/j.otohns.2005.11.031.
14. Jacob DD, Kwiecien GJ, Cakmakoglu C, Moreira A. Color duplex ultrasound for localization of vascular compromise in microsurgical breast reconstruction. Plast Reconstr Surg. 2020;145(3):666e–7e. https://doi.org/10.1097/PRS.0000000000006600.
15. Stone CA, Dubbins PA, Morris RJ. Use of colour duplex Doppler imaging in the postoperative assessment of buried free flaps. Microsurgery. 2001;21(5):223–7. https://doi.org/10.1002/micr.1043.
16. Boissiere F, Gandolfi S, Riot S, Kerfant N, Jenzeri A, Hendriks S, et al. Flap venous congestion and salvage techniques: a systematic literature review. Plast Reconstr Surg Glob Open. 2021;9(1):e3327. https://doi.org/10.1097/GOX.0000000000003327.
17. May JW Jr, Chait LA, O'Brien BM, Hurley JV. The no-reflow phenomenon in experimental free flaps. Plast Reconstr Surg. 1978;61(2):256–67. https://doi.org/10.1097/00006534-197802000-00017.
18. Jones BM. Monitors for the cutaneous microcirculation. Plast Reconstr Surg. 1984;73(5):843–50. https://doi.org/10.1097/00006534-198405000-00025.
19. Jacobson A, Cohen O. Review of flap monitoring technology in 2020. Facial Plast Surg. 2020;36(6):722–6. https://doi.org/10.1055/s-0040-1721105.
20. Cornejo A, Ivatury S, Crane CN, Myers JG, Wang HT. Analysis of free flap complications and utilization of intensive care unit monitoring. J Reconstr Microsurg. 2013;29(7):473–9. https://doi.org/10.1055/s-0033-1345434.
21. Jallali N, Ridha H, Butler PE. Postoperative monitoring of free flaps in UK plastic surgery units. Microsurgery. 2005;25(6):469–72. https://doi.org/10.1002/micr.20148.
22. Shinomiya R, Sunagawa T, Nakashima Y, Kodama A, Hayashi Y, et al. Monitoring vascular compromise using ultrasound after free tissue transfer. J Ultrasound Med. 2020;39(6):1213–22. https://doi.org/10.1002/jum.15210.
23. Wicks JD, Silver TM, Bree RL. Gray scale features of hematomas: an ultrasonic spectrum. AJR Am J Roentgenol. 1978;131(6):977–80. https://doi.org/10.2214/ajr.131.6.977.
24. O'Rourke K, Kibbee N, Stubbs A. Ultrasound for the evaluation of skin and soft tissue infections. Mo Med. 2015;112(3):202–5.
25. Almasarweh S, Sudah M, Joukainen S, Okuma H, Vanninen R, Masarwah A. The feasibility of ultrasound-guided vacuum-assisted evacuation of large breast hematomas. Radiol Oncol. 2020;54(3):311–6. https://doi.org/10.2478/raon-2020-0041.
26. Turner EJ, Benson JR, Winters ZE. Techniques in the prevention and management of seromas after breast surgery. Future Oncol. 2014;10(6):1049–63. https://doi.org/10.2217/fon.13.257.
27. Kaafarani HM, Hur K, Hirter A, Kim LT, Thomas A, Berger DH, et al. Seroma in ventral incisional herniorrhaphy: incidence, predictors and outcome. Am J Surg. 2009;198(5):639–44. https://doi.org/10.1016/j.amjsurg.2009.07.019.
28. Salari N, Fatahi B, Bartina Y, Kazeminia M, Heydari M, Mohammadi M, et al. The global prevalence of seroma after abdominoplasty: a systematic review and meta-analysis. Aesthetic Plast Surg. 2021;45(6):2821–36. https://doi.org/10.1007/s00266-021-02365-6.
29. Goldman A, Wollina U, França K, Tchernev G, Lotti T. Chronic encapsulated seroma persisting for three years after abdominoplasty and a successful surgical solution. Open Access Maced J Med Sci. 2018;6(1):82–4. https://doi.org/10.3889/oamjms.2018.051.
30. Marin JR, Dean AJ, Bilker WB, Panebianco NL, Brown NJ, Alpern ER. Emergency ultrasound-assisted examination of skin and soft tissue infections in the pediatric emergency department. Acad Emerg Med. 2013;20(6):545–53. https://doi.org/10.1111/acem.12148.
31. Gottlieb M, Avila J, Chottiner M, Peksa GD. Point-of-care ultrasonography for the diagnosis of skin and soft tissue abscesses: a systematic review and meta-analysis. Ann Emerg Med. 2020;76(1):67–77. https://doi.org/10.1016/j.annemergmed.2020.01.004.
32. Adhikari S, Blaivas M. Sonography first for subcutaneous abscess and cellulitis evaluation. J Ultrasound Med. 2012;31(10):1509–12. https://doi.org/10.7863/jum.2012.31.10.1509.

33. Tso DK, Singh AK. Necrotizing fasciitis of the lower extremity: imaging pearls and pitfalls. Br J Radiol. 20181;91(1088):20180093. https://doi.org/10.1259/bjr.20180093.
34. Loyer EM, DuBrow RA, David CL, Coan JD, Eftekhari F. Imaging of superficial soft-tissue infections: sonographic findings in cases of cellulitis and abscess. AJR Am J Roentgenol. 1996;166(1):149–52. https://doi.org/10.2214/ajr.166.1.8571865.
35. Arslan H, Sakarya ME, Bozkurt M, Unal O, Dilek ON, Harman M. The role of power Doppler sonography in the evaluation of superficial soft tissue abscesses. Eur J Ultrasound. 1998;8(2):101–6. https://doi.org/10.1016/s0929-8266(98)00065-2.
36. Pavlin DJ, Chen C, Penaloza DA, Buckley FP. A survey of pain and other symptoms that affect the recovery process after discharge from an ambulatory surgery unit. J Clin Anesth. 2004;16(3):200–6. https://doi.org/10.1016/j.jclinane.2003.08.004.
37. Herbst MO, Price MD, Soto RG. Pain related readmissions/revisits following same-day surgery: have they decreased over a decade? J Clin Anesth. 2017;42:15. https://doi.org/10.1016/j.jclinane.2017.06.009.
38. Pavlin DJ, Rapp SE, Polissar NL, Malmgren JA, Koerschgen M, Keyes H. Factors affecting discharge time in adult outpatients. Anesth Analg. 1998;87(4):816–26. https://doi.org/10.1097/00000539-199810000-00014.
39. Eskandr A, Mahmoud K, Kasemy Z, Mohamed K, Elhennawy T. A comparative study between ultrasound-guided thoracic paravertebral block, pectoral nerves block, and erector spinae block for pain management in cancer breast surgeries. A randomized controlled study. Rev Esp Anestesiol Reanim (Engl Ed). 2022;69(10):617–24. https://doi.org/10.1016/j.redare.2022.02.004.
40. Bijkerk E, Cornelissen AJM, Sommer M, Van Der Hulst RRWJ, Lataster A, Tuinder SMH. Intercostal nerve block of the anterior cutaneous branches and the sensibility of the female breast. Clin Anat. 2020;33(7):1025–32. https://doi.org/10.1002/ca.23532.
41. Walian A, Magoon R, Shri I, Kashav RC. Transversus thoracic muscle plane block for attenuating the haemodynamic response to median sternotomy: a case series. Turk J Anaesthesiol Reanim. 2022;50(6):449–53. https://doi.org/10.5152/TJAR.2022.21196.
42. Abi-Rafeh J, Safran T, Abi-Jaoude J, Kazan R, Alabdulkarim A, Davison PG. Nerve blocks in breast plastic surgery: outcomes, complications, and comparative efficacy. Plast Reconstr Surg. 2022;150(1):1e–12e. https://doi.org/10.1097/PRS.0000000000009253.
43. Boughey JC, Goravanchi F, Parris RN, Kee SS, Kowalski AM, Frenzel JC, et al. Prospective randomized trial of paravertebral block for patients undergoing breast cancer surgery. Am J Surg. 2009;198(5):720–5. https://doi.org/10.1016/j.amjsurg.2008.11.043.
44. ElHawary H, Joshi GP, Janis JE. Practical review of abdominal and breast regional analgesia for plastic surgeons: evidence and techniques. Plast Reconstr Surg Glob Open. 2020;8(12):e3224. https://doi.org/10.1097/GOX.0000000000003224.
45. Blanco R. The 'pecs block': a novel technique for providing analgesia after breast surgery. Anaesthesia. 2011;66(9):847–8. https://doi.org/10.1111/j.1365-2044.2011.06838.x.
46. Blanco R, Fajardo M, Parras MT. Ultrasound description of pecs II (modified pecs I): a novel approach to breast surgery. Rev Esp Anestesiol Reanim. 2012;59(9):470–5. https://doi.org/10.1016/j.redar.2012.07.003.
47. Aksu C, Kuş A, Yörükoğlu HU, Tor Kılıç C, Gürkan Y. Analgesic effect of the bi-level injection erector spinae plane block after breast surgery: a randomized controlled trial. Agri. 2019;31(3):132–7. https://doi.org/10.14744/agri.2019.61687.
48. Forero M, Adhikary SD, Lopez H, Tsui C, Chin KJ. The erector spinae plane block: a novel analgesic technique in thoracic neuropathic pain. Reg Anesth Pain Med. 2016;41(5):621–7. https://doi.org/10.1097/AAP.0000000000000451.
49. Hivelin M, Wyniecki A, Plaud B, Marty J, Lantieri L. Ultrasound-guided bilateral transversus abdominis plane block for postoperative analgesia after breast reconstruction by DIEP flap. Plast Reconstr Surg. 2011;128(1):44–55. https://doi.org/10.1097/PRS.0b013e3182174090.
50. Hebbard P, Fujiwara Y, Shibata Y, Royse C. Ultrasound-guided transversus abdominis plane (TAP) block. Anaesth Intensive Care. 2007;35(4):616–7.
51. Suljević I, Suljević O, Turan M, Grbo A, Šurković I. Comparison of plexus brachial blockade effect by supraclavicular and axillary approach—our experience. Acta Clin Croat. 2019;58(Suppl 1):18–22. https://doi.org/10.20471/acc.2019.58.s1.02.
52. Soberón JR Jr, Crookshank JW 3rd, Nossaman BD, Elliott CE, Sisco-Wise LE, Duncan SF. Distal peripheral nerve blocks in the forearm as an alternative to proximal brachial plexus blockade in patients undergoing hand surgery: a prospective and randomized pilot study. J Hand Surg Am. 2016;41(10):969–77. https://doi.org/10.1016/j.jhsa.2016.07.092.
53. Maxwell BG, Hansen JA, Talley J, Curtin CM, Mariano ER. Ultrasound-guided continuous median nerve block to facilitate intensive hand rehabilitation. Clin J Pain. 2013;29(1):86–8. https://doi.org/10.1097/AJP.0b013e318246d1ca.
54. Winter J, McLeod G, Quaife T, Petropolis C. Surgeon-administered ultrasound-guided peripheral nerve blocks in outpatient procedures of the upper extremity. Plast Reconstr Surg Glob Open. 2020;8(11):e3227. https://doi.org/10.1097/GOX.0000000000003227.

55. Pester JM, Varacallo M. Ulnar nerve block techniques. In: StatPearls. 2022. https://www-ncbi-nlm-nih-gov.ezproxy.bu.edu/books/NBK459208/.
56. Sehmbi H, Madjdpour C, Shah UJ, Chin KJ. Ultrasound guided distal peripheral nerve block of the upper limb: a technical review. J Anaesthesiol Clin Pharmacol. 2015;31(3):296–307. https://doi.org/10.4103/0970-9185.161654.
57. Ruan QZ, Diamond S, Zimmer S, Iorio ML. Assessing the safety and efficacy of regional anesthesia for lower extremity microvascular reconstruction: enhancing recovery. J Reconstr Microsurg. 2018;34(4):293–9. https://doi.org/10.1055/s-0037-1621726.
58. Tran DQ, Salinas FV, Benzon HT, Neal JM. Lower extremity regional anesthesia: essentials of our current understanding. Reg Anesth Pain Med. 2019:rapm-2018-000019. https://doi.org/10.1136/rapm-2018-000019.
59. Casati A, Baciarello M, Di Cianni S, Danelli G, De Marco G, Leone S, et al. Effects of ultrasound guidance on the minimum effective anaesthetic volume required to block the femoral nerve. Br J Anaesth. 2007;98(6):823–7. https://doi.org/10.1093/bja/aem100.
60. Jablonka EM, Lamelas AM, Kim JN, Molina B, Molina N, Okwali M, et al. Transversus abdominis plane blocks with single-dose liposomal bupivacaine in conjunction with a nonnarcotic pain regimen help reduce length of stay following abdominally based microsurgical breast reconstruction. Plast Reconstr Surg. 2017;140(2):240–51. https://doi.org/10.1097/PRS.0000000000003508.
61. Mavarez AC, Ahmed AA. Transabdominal plane block. In: StatPearls. 2022. https://www-ncbi-nlm-nih-gov.ezproxy.bu.edu/books/NBK560527/.
62. Rafi AN. Abdominal field block: a new approach via the lumbar triangle. Anaesthesia. 2001;56(10):1024–6. https://doi.org/10.1046/j.1365-2044.2001.02279-40.x.
63. Hebbard P. Subcostal transversus abdominis plane block under ultrasound guidance. Anesth Analg. 2008;106(2):674–5. https://doi.org/10.1213/ane.0b013e318161a88f.
64. Charlton S, Cyna AM, Middleton P, Griffiths JD. Perioperative transversus abdominis plane (TAP) blocks for analgesia after abdominal surgery. Cochrane Database Syst Rev. 2010;(12):CD007705. https://doi.org/10.1002/14651858.CD007705.pub2.
65. Wheble GA, Tan EK, Turner M, Durrant CA, Heppell S. Surgeon-administered, intra-operative transversus abdominis plane block in autologous breast reconstruction: a UK hospital experience. J Plast Reconstr Aesthet Surg. 2013;66(12):1665–70. https://doi.org/10.1016/j.bjps.2013.07.017.
66. Chin KJ, Chan V. Ultrasound-guided peripheral nerve blockade. Curr Opin Anaesthesiol. 2008;21(5):624–31. https://doi.org/10.1097/ACO.0b013e32830815d1.
67. El-Dawlatly AA, Turkistani A, Kettner SC, Machata AM, Delvi MB, Thallaj A, et al. Ultrasound-guided transversus abdominis plane block: description of a new technique and comparison with conventional systemic analgesia during laparoscopic cholecystectomy. Br J Anaesth. 2009;102(6):763–7. https://doi.org/10.1093/bja/aep067.
68. Guirguis MS, Adrada B, Santiago L, Candelaria R, Arribas E. Mimickers of breast malignancy: imaging findings, pathologic concordance and clinical management. Insights Imaging. 2021;12(1):53. https://doi.org/10.1186/s13244-021-00991-x.
69. Fracol M, Allison S, Chu Y, Yan Y, Sood R, Feld LN, et al. The palpable nodule after autologous fat grafting: distinguishing benign versus malignant lesions in breast reconstruction. Plast Reconstr Surg. 2022;150:20S–9S. https://doi.org/10.1097/PRS.0000000000009496.
70. Atasoy MM, Oren NC, Ilica AT, Güvenç İ, Günal A, Mossa-Basha M. Sonography of fat necrosis of the breast: correlation with mammography and MR imaging. J Clin Ultrasound. 2013;41(7):415–23. https://doi.org/10.1002/jcu.22061.
71. Soo MS, Kornguth PJ, Hertzberg BS. Fat necrosis in the breast: sonographic features. Radiology. 1998;206(1):261–9. https://doi.org/10.1148/radiology.206.1.9423681.
72. Genova R, Garza RF. Breast fat necrosis. In: StatPearls. 2022. https://www-ncbi-nlm-nih-gov.ezproxy.bu.edu/books/NBK542191/.
73. Kearon C. Natural history of venous thromboembolism. Circulation. 2003;107(23 Suppl 1):I22–30. https://doi.org/10.1161/01.CIR.0000078464.82671.78.
74. Needleman L, Cronan JJ, Lilly MP, Merli GJ, Adhikari S, Hertzberg BS, et al. Ultrasound for lower extremity deep venous thrombosis: multidisciplinary recommendations from the Society of Radiologists in Ultrasound Consensus Conference. Circulation. 2018;137(14):1505–15. https://doi.org/10.1161/CIRCULATIONAHA.117.030687.
75. Bates SM, Jaeschke R, Stevens SM, Goodacre S, Wells PS, Stevenson MD, et al. Diagnosis of DVT: antithrombotic therapy and prevention of thrombosis, 9th ed: American College of Chest Physicians evidence-based clinical practice guidelines. Chest. 2012;141(2 Suppl):e351S–418S. https://doi.org/10.1378/chest.11-2299.
76. Swanson E. Doppler ultrasound imaging for detection of deep vein thrombosis in plastic surgery outpatients: a prospective controlled study. Aesthet Surg J. 2015;35(2):204–14. https://doi.org/10.1093/asj/sju052.
77. Swanson E. Prospective study of Doppler ultrasound surveillance for deep venous thromboses in 1000 plastic surgery outpatients. Plast Reconstr Surg. 2020;145(1):85–96. https://doi.org/10.1097/PRS.0000000000006343.
78. Wilkins EG, Pannucci CJ. Commentary on: Doppler ultrasound imaging of plastic surgery patients for deep venous thrombosis detection: a prospective controlled

study. Aesthet Surg J. 2015;35(2):215–7. https://doi.org/10.1093/asj/sju005.
79. Horta R, Nascimento R, Valença-Filipe R, Melão L, Costa F, Esteves C, et al. The ultrasound-guided fat transplantation. Surg Innov. 2015;22(3):318–9. https://doi.org/10.1177/1553350615579731.
80. Oni G, Chow W, Ramakrishnan V, Griffiths M. Plastic surgeon-led ultrasound. Plast Reconstr Surg. 2018;141(2):300e–9e. https://doi.org/10.1097/PRS.0000000000004071.
81. Meyer A, Roof S, Gray ML, Fan CJ, Barber B, Miles BA, et al. Thermal imaging for microvascular free tissue transfer monitoring: feasibility study using a low cost, commercially available mobile phone imaging system. Head Neck. 2020;42(10):2941–7. https://doi.org/10.1002/hed.26350.
82. Xie R, Liu Q, Zhang Y, Guo C, Huang X, Liu M. A wireless infrared thermometry device for postoperative flap monitoring: proof of concept in a porcine flap model. Int Wound J. 2023;20:1839. https://doi.org/10.1111/iwj.14034.
83. Just M, Chalopin C, Unger M, Halama D, Neumuth T, Dietz A, et al. Monitoring of microvascular free flaps following oropharyngeal reconstruction using infrared thermography: first clinical experiences. Eur Arch Otorrinolaringol. 2016;273(9):2659–67. https://doi.org/10.1007/s00405-015-3780-9.
84. Obinah MPB, Nielsen M, Hölmich LR. High-end versus low-end thermal imaging for detection of arterial perforators. Plast Reconstr Surg Glob Open. 2020;8(10):e3175. https://doi.org/10.1097/GOX.0000000000003175.
85. Thiem DGE, Römer P, Blatt S, Al-Nawas B, Kämmerer PW. New approach to the old challenge of free flap monitoring-hyperspectral imaging outperforms clinical assessment by earlier detection of perfusion failure. J Pers Med. 2021;11(11):1101. https://doi.org/10.3390/jpm11111101.
86. Kohler LH, Köhler H, Kohler S, Langer S, Nuwayhid R, Gockel I, et al. Hyperspectral imaging (HSI) as a new diagnostic tool in free flap monitoring for soft tissue reconstruction: a proof of concept study. BMC Surg. 2021;21(1):222. https://doi.org/10.1186/s12893-021-01232-0.
87. Schiltz D, Taeger CD, Biermann N, Ranieri M, Klein S, Prantl L, et al. Transcutaneous oxygen measurement using ratiometric fluorescence imaging as a valid method for monitoring free flap transplants. Clin Hemorheol Microcirc. 2019;73(1):113–23. https://doi.org/10.3233/CH-199225.
88. Thiem DGE, Frick RW, Goetze E, Gielisch M, Al-Nawas B, Kämmerer PW. Hyperspectral analysis for perioperative perfusion monitoring-a clinical feasibility study on free and pedicled flaps. Clin Oral Investig. 2021;25(3):933–45. https://doi.org/10.1007/s00784-020-03382-6.
89. Landsman AS, Barnhart D, Sowa M. Near-infrared spectroscopy imaging for assessing skin and wound oxygen perfusion. Clin Podiatr Med Surg. 2018;35(3):343–55. https://doi.org/10.1016/j.cpm.2018.02.005.

Part IV

Section D. Designing Perforator flaps

15 The Ultrasound Evolution of Perforator Flaps from Lateral Thoracic Area

Giuseppe Visconti

15.1 Introduction

The lateral thoracic region is a watershed area for perforator flaps from the lateral intercostal, lateral thoracic, and subscapular systems which allows plenty of option for harvesting both free and local perforator flaps [1–7].

All potential perforator flaps from lateral thoracic area have been described for autologous breast reconstruction, both in immediate and delayed reconstruction, especially for partial breast defects after breast-conserving surgery. Based on patients' features, such flaps can be successfully used also for total breast reconstruction.

In the last decade, the approach to flap harvesting has been revolutionized by the use of ultrasound (US) technology that allows an accurate perforators' evaluation and thus a precise flap planning. US allows to define in detail the microvascular anatomy, to select the best perforator vessel closest to the defect, and finally to actualize the surgery [8–16].

In this chapter, the author describes the US-based planning of the lateral thoracic wall perforator adipocutaneous flaps, including the study of each perforator's features in terms of fascial emergence site (position), diameter of the arterial and venous component, vessel route and direction (axiality), and subcutaneous branching with particular insights on the use of such flaps for immediate and delayed, partial and total breast reconstruction.

US planning of perforator flaps from lateral thoracic area led to a technical modification of harvesting and flap transposition for partial and total breast reconstruction leading to the introduction of the "propuller" flap concept, which is the ultrasound evolution of propeller flaps [16].

Propeller perforator flap concept has been introduced by Teo TC, and it is based on a precise design where the flap width is similar to that of the defect and flap length is the sum of the defect length (for defect coverage) plus the distance between the located perforator and the defect (flap bridge) [17–21]. This design is justified because the flap is pivoted based on the perforator, which preserves its original position. To avoid perforator's twisting and kinking, the perforator should be dissected for around 3 cm to favor its gentle torsion without compromising blood flow and flap viability.

The "propuller" flap combines the propeller rotation of the skin-soft tissue paddle plus the advancement of the flap achieved by pulling the perforator flap toward the defect. This design allows to reduce the length of the flap and to use the entire flap for the reconstructive needs, rather than sacrifice part of the skin paddle as a bridge.

G. Visconti (✉)
UO Chirurgia Plastica, Dipartimento Scienze Salute della Donna, del Bambino e Sanità Pubblica—Fondazione Policlinico Gemelli IRCCS, largo Agostino Gemelli, Rome, Italy

J. P. Hong et al. (eds.), *Imaging for Reconstructive Microsurgery*,
https://doi.org/10.1007/978-981-97-7278-0_15

Moreover, without full perforator skeletonization, it increases safety and reduces morbidity related to the torsion of perforator such as twisting and/or kinking [16].

15.2 Color-Coded Duplex Sonography (CCDS)

CCDS using high-resolution ultrasound allows to have detailed information on microvascular and soft tissue anatomy of any donor site [10, 22–25]. In plastic surgery field, linear probes from 4 to 19 MhZ are the most indicated. High-frequency ultrasound (>15 MhZ) allows to expand knowledge on more superficial plane, thus allowing a further analysis of the perforator vessels and superficial microanatomy.

The anatomical details can be studied using B-mode, and information on microvascular network is better studied using color Doppler and power Doppler (Figs. 15.1 and 15.2).

In literature, different studies have demonstrated a high sensitivity of color-coded ultrasound in preoperative perforator evaluation [10, 22–25].

Compared to other imaging technology, such as multidetector CT scan angiography (MDCT) and magnetic resonance angiography (MRA)

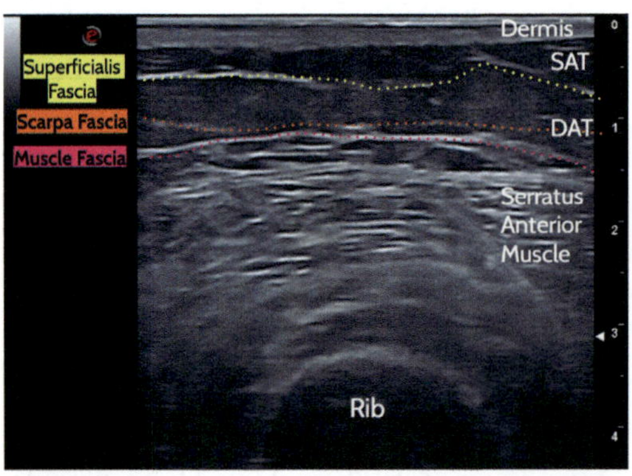

Fig. 15.1 High-frequency ultrasound B-mode visualization of the lateral thoracic area. Anatomical structures are outlined. *SAT* superficial adipose tissue, *DAT* deep adipose tissue

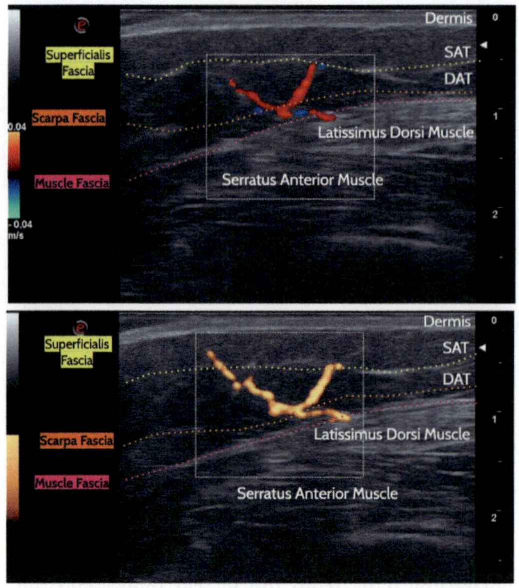

Fig. 15.2 (Above) High-frequency ultrasound color-coded visualization of a type 2 thoracodorsal artery perforator (TDAP). (Below) Same image acquired with high-frequency ultrasound power Doppler visualization that allows to clearly delineate the entire microvascular tree. *SAT* superficial adipose tissue, *DAT* deep adipose tissue

[26], US allows a live evaluation of the perforators which give the possibility to mark their location precisely on the skin. Moreover, high-frequency probes allow a resolution up to 100 μm with the possibility to visualize microvessels up to 0.2 mm in caliber, which goes beyond the ability of other imaging modalities.

Moreover, a dynamic evaluation of flow and velocity can be performed along with measuring its caliber, which helps in selecting the perforator preoperatively. The precise subfascial course of the perforator is evaluable (septal/intramuscular/mixed course) up to the source vessel, thus precisely delineating the dissection route that will be performed intraoperatively.

When planning local perforator flaps, the exact axis of perforator within the subcutaneous tissue can be delineated, which helps to precisely include the perforator tree within flap design [27].

In LVA surgery, high-frequency ultrasound is useful in preoperative evaluation of recipient venules, whereas it gives limited information on lymphatic channels compared to ultrahigh frequency [28].

15.2.1 Preoperative Color-Coded Duplex Sonography (CCDS) Study

The preoperative study is performed using high-frequency ultrasound machine with linear probes of 12 and 18 MhZ (Esaote MyLab X6, Esaote Inc., Genova, Italy).

The gross anatomy is first delineated using the 12 MhZ probe in B-mode. The rib cage, ribs, and lateral thoracic muscles are visualized (Fig. 15.1).

After having visualized the gross anatomy, the 18 MhZ probe in CCDS mode is used for mapping perforators focusing on the muscular fascia (Fig. 15.2). The entire lateral thoracic area on the side of the breast to reconstruct is scanned craniocaudal from the axilla down to the seventh rib and medial to lateral from the lateral breast margin to the posterior axillary line. When a CCDS perforator signal is found, a slower motion is used to better identify the perforator and measure its flow and its caliber. A power Doppler mode can be implemented for better visualization of subcutaneous course of the perforator.

Then the perforator is followed from the muscular fascia down to the main pedicle to determine its source vessel and to verify that perforator course is continuous. This is especially true in delayed reconstruction where previous surgery may have ligated perforators. Ligated vessels do still preserve vascular signal because of collateral branching although the perforator is not anymore connected to the source vessel below muscular fascia.

The lateral thoracic area is a watershed area for three different types of perforator flaps: thoracodorsal artery perforator (TDAP), lateral intercostal artery perforator (LICAP), and lateral thoracic artery perforator (LTAP) (Fig. 15.3).

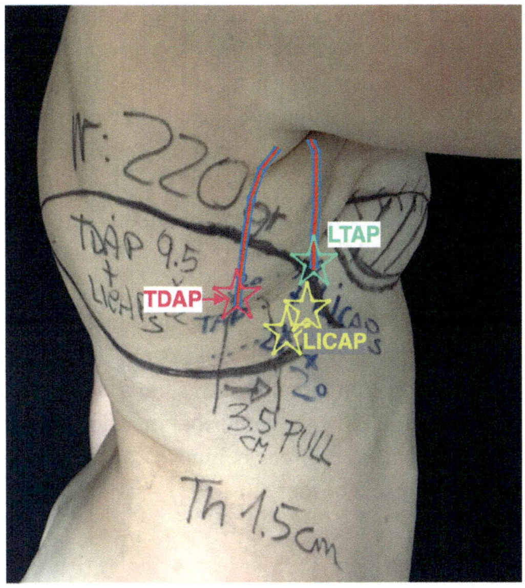

Fig. 15.3 Lateral thoracic perforator flap design based on preoperative planning with high-frequency ultrasound. Schematic design of the three sources for perforators of the lateral thoracic area is provided with pedicles (blue and red lines) and perforators' emergence (stars). *TDAP* thoracodorsal artery perforator, *LICAP* lateral intercostal artery perforator, *LTAP* lateral thoracic artery perforator

15.3 Thoracodorsal Artery Perforators (TDAP)

Thoracodorsal artery perforators are perforators branching off the thoracodorsal artery, which is the main source vessel of the latissimus dorsi muscle. Thoracodorsal artery is the other main branch coming off the subscapular artery, major branch of the axillary artery. The thoracodorsal artery continues its course downward in the axillary region reaching the undersurface of the latissimus dorsi muscle. It gives off at least one serratus branch which supplies the serratus anterior muscle before entering the latissimus dorsi muscle at around 6–8 cm from the axillary fold. The intramuscular thoracodorsal artery divides into descending (db) and transverse branch (TB) which parallels the anterior and superior muscle borders, respectively. Each of this branch gives off musculocutaneous perforators that nourish the skin. Of notice, in around 50% of the cases, the thoracodorsal artery gives off a direct cutaneous branch (also known as superficial thoracic artery of Manchot) that does usually travel around the anterior border of latissimus dorsi muscle. This is clearly visible with CCDS as the perforator is seen travelling from thoracodorsal artery to the skin around the muscle border without piercing it.

The direct branch represents the anteriormost perforator of the thoracodorsal system that otherwise is located on top of the latissimus dorsi muscle, either along the anterior muscle border (usually at least 2–3 cm behind it) or along the superior muscle border.

15.4 Lateral Thoracic Artery Perforator (LTAP)

Lateral thoracic artery also known as long thoracic artery or external mammary artery originates from the medial surface of the axillary artery. It travels downward following the lateral border of pectoralis minor muscle giving off muscular branches to serratus anterior muscle and pectoralis minor and major muscles. The LTA travels below pectoralis major muscle fascia up to a transverse line traced from the nipple, where in around 85% of cases it gives off a direct cutaneous branch nourishing the skin lateral to the breast. So far the skin vessel travels as an axial vessel within the subcutaneous tissue before entering the muscle fascia at the level of the nipple. Nearby the LTA, the thoracoepigastric vein can be found as a major cutaneous vein that can empower flap perfusion by improving venous drainage [29].

15.5 Lateral Intercostal Artery Perforator (LICAP)

Intercostal artery perforators have been described in the past for harvesting myocutaneous flap, and before the perforator era, these flaps were of limited use. The intercostal arteries travel along the inferior border of each rib, and, besides the first two, they represent a truly vascular arcade connecting the aorta with the internal mammary vessels. Intercostal arteries give off three main perforators—posterior, lateral, and anterior—which can be used for designing and harvesting adipocutaneous flaps. The lateral intercostal artery perforator (LICAP) flap has been popularized mainly as an adjunctive option for partial breast reconstruction by Hamdi, who also performed an anatomical study showing that the highest concentration of perforators is between the fifth and eight intercostal spaces and that LICAP are usually found 2.5–3.5 cm medial to the anterior border of latissimus dorsi muscle [30].

By analyzing the lateral thoracic area, LICAP perforators are the anteriormost ones, although they may be confounded with LTAP. However, LTAP are less frequent and higher located compared to LICAP which are constant and usually located below the fifth rib (Fig. 15.2).

15.6 How to Choose the Perforator for Breast Reconstruction

Perforators from the lateral thoracic area (TDAP, LTAP, LICAP) share a similar area of skin perfusion, which is the axillary-back skin roll (ABSR) which is variable between patients, based on body habitus and patients' features. As a general rule, LTAP and LICAP flaps are located closer to lateral breast pole, and thus their selection should be preferred as the entire skin paddle can be easily propelled into the breast. However, LTAP and LICAP perforators do generally nourish the back roll except the last one-third (paravertebral portion) which is better perfused by the more laterally located TDAP perforators.

Being the flap design centered on the axillary back skin roll, the vascular anatomy of the redundant soft tissue area just lateral to the lateral breast crease is studied with color-coded duplex sonography (CCDS) using high-frequency ultrasound (>15 MhZ).

15.7 US-Based Flap Planning

The presence of an axillary skin roll and soft tissue laxity in the lateral thoracic area is verified. The patient is positioned in a full lateral position with the shoulder abducted, to simulate the position in the operating room. The CDUS examination should be performed by the operating surgeon in order to acquire all the information needed for surgery, and it should not be delegated to other specialists.

The area lateral to the lateral breast crease from the fifth to the seventh intercostal space is scanned in search of the LICAP perforators. Attention is paid to locate the fascial emergence point and its route in order to confirm that it is a branch of intercostal vessels. It is usually not easy to follow the perforator in its course, at it usually has a tortuous course within multiple fascial plane in the lateral thoracic region. However, a good LICAP is frequently found here. Its average diameter is 1.2 mm, and we consider it to be adequate when over 0.9 mm.

It is very important to see the perforator course under the fascia. In case the subfascial course is not seen and the fascial emergence point is not clearly established, the suspicion emerges that the vessel was ligated at the fascial level at the previous surgery. This is especially true in case of delayed breast reconstruction or previous breast surgery. In fact, this area is very close to the breast, and previous breast surgery may have damaged the perforator.

In case no LICAP are found, the US probe is moved upward in search of the LTAP perforator, which is located similarly anterior as the LICAP but more superior than LICAP. LTAP perforators show a long subcutaneous course, and they usually pierce the muscular fascia at the midbreast level. In case LTAP is not found or small, the attention is moved toward the latissimus dorsi muscle in the search of the TDAP of the descending branch along the anterior border of the muscle in order to locate musculocutaneous perforators or eventually the direct cutaneous branch at around 8 cm from the axillary crease.

In all cases, selected perforators are analyzed in their subcutaneous course as much as possible in order to establish the precise perforator axiality.

15.8 US-Based Flap Markings

The perforator emergence location on the skin is marked as well as its axiality within the subcutaneous tissue. The flap is marked with orientation along the axillary skin roll (horizontal or oblique) paralleling as much as possible perforator subcutaneous axiality and respecting the minimum tension line. In case of LICAP and LTAP, the perforator is usually very eccentric, whereas TDAP are more centrally located.

The lateral flap margin is nearby the defect or along the lateral breast crease, according to the requirements. The flap width is determined by the pinch test, according to the possibility of direct closing of the donor site. The flap length depends on the needs. If a long flap is needed (i.e., for total breast reconstruction), its length can reach 3–4 cm from the midline in case of LICAP flap or the paramedian line in case of TDAP flap. Intraoperatively, fluorescence angiography is performed to confirm the perfused area and the non-perfused part is discharged.

The expected volume needing (i.e. estimation of mastectomy or quadrantectomy volume) is performed by weighting the resected tissue in case of immediate reconstruction and by evaluating the contralateral breast weight in case of unilateral delayed reconstruction. It is possible to grossly estimate the flap volume by applying the elliptic cylinder formula = $a \times b \times h \times 3{,}14$, where "a" is the half of the minor radius, "b" is the half of the major radius, and "h" is the elliptic cylinder height, i.e., the thickness of the flap, that we can measure with the US.

We can consider the flap volume similar to its weight [16].

15.9 The "Propuller" Flap Concept (Figs. 15.4 and 15.5)

In 2021, we report the "propuller" flap concept that we are using for over 5 years [16]. The propuller flap concept is the combination of propeller rotation of the skin-soft tissue paddle plus the advancement of the flap achieved by pulling the perforator flap toward the defect. The final flap movement is propeller + pulling, named "propuller."

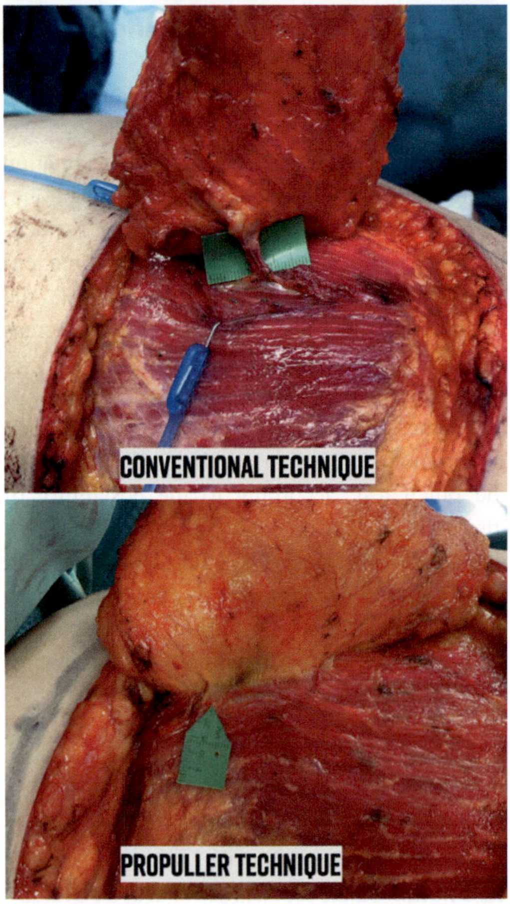

Fig. 15.4 (Above) Conventional propeller thoracodorsal artery perforator flap elevated with 3-cm perforator microdissection to favor the propeller movement without kinking and torsion. (Below) Propuller concept applied based on preoperative planning with high-frequency ultrasound. The perforator (pointed with green arrow) is only glimpsed but not fully skeletonized to favor a safe propuller movement

This design allows to reduce the length of the flap and to use the entire skin paddle for the reconstructive needs, rather than sacrificing part of the skin paddle as a bridge. Moreover, without full perforator skeletonization, it increases safety and reduces morbidity related to the torsion of perforators such as twisting and/or kinking.

The "propuller" concept is particularly interesting when applied to the lateral thoracic area. This region represents the source of several perforator flaps based on either the intercostal (ICAP), thoracodorsal (TDAP), or lateral thoracic vessel (LTAP), popularized as pedicled perforator flaps for partial breast reconstruction in the last 15 years [2].

Despite sporadic descriptions as VY advancement [31, 32] or turnover flaps [33, 34], ICAP and LTAP flaps are mostly used for breast reconstruction as propeller flaps and the TDAP as both rotation and advancement flaps to reach the breast area. As such, they all share a rotation movement to which the "propuller" concept can be applied, thus reducing the limitations in flap selection according to pedicle length, with a higher degree of freedom ruled only by the reconstructive needs. Propuller design requires the perforators is not fully skeletonized to avoid kinking/torsion during the propuller movement. For this reason, the perforator must be selected using ultrasound, and intraoperative exploration should be minimized as full perforator skeletonization will interfere with the possibility of propuller movement (Fig. 15.4).

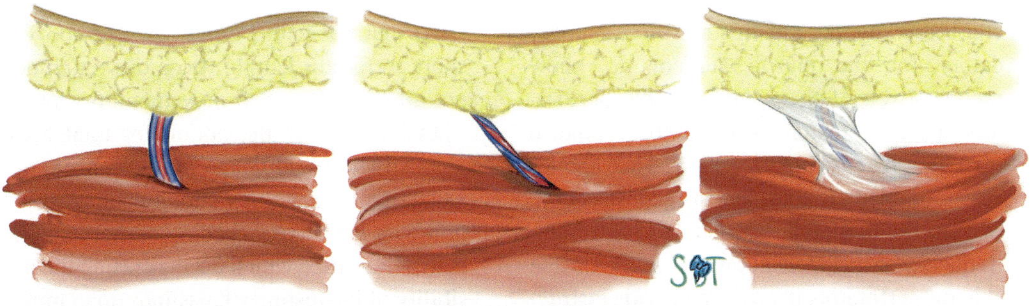

Fig. 15.5 The diagram shows the impact of traction forces on perforators in conventional and propuller perforator flaps. On the left, a conventional perforator flap with full perforator skeletonization is represented before the propeller movement, with the perforator in neutral position. The central drawing shows how skeletonized perforator flaps cannot undergo any traction, as it is entirely burdened on the perforator that represents the only attachment point of the flap. On the right, the propeller rotation and advancement is shown, the fascial cuff takes charge of the traction forces, and the perforator is not directly affected, despite the advent of the flap. This allows to propel and pull (i.e., propuller) the flap into the breast area without the risk of perforator twisting and stretching. With permission, from Visconti et al. [16]

15.10 Flap Dissection and Transfer

After local infiltration with saline solution and epinephrine 1:200.000 at the edges of the flap margins, the entire designed skin paddle is incised with beveling up to the muscle fascia. The flap is raised superficial to this fascia in the distal to proximal direction. Dissection continues along the suprafascial plane to the anterior border of the muscle and proceeds anteriorly up to the selected perforator entrance point. The other perforator vessels which are encountered along the flap dissection are observed and ligated.

The dissection proceeds until the selected perforator "is glimpsed." At this point, all the surrounding fascial adhesions that restrict the flap movement are released. The undissected perforator usually allows to retain nearby sensate nerve within the flap pedicle, sacrificing only those structures that limit the flap movement around the perforator.

Then, the best direction of flap rotation, clockwise or counterclockwise, is verified, and the flap movement is performed via propeller and advancement/pulling, meaning propuller flap movement.

Lastly, the donor site closure contributes to further push the flap lateral tissue excess at the anterior axillary line (the turning point of the pedicle) inside the breast.

In case the flap perforator is not as close to the flap edge, as it often happens in TDAP flaps, the perforator is dissected in order to allow the conventional propeller rotation, or the dissection goes along the TDA pedicle, and the flap is transposed by transposing the TDA pedicle anteriorly [7, 15, 35, 36].

15.11 Lateral Thoracic Area Perforator Flaps for Partial and Total Breast Reconstruction

Lateral thoracic area perforator flaps have been mainly described as autologous option for partial breast reconstruction, leaving the total breast reconstruction, either immediate or delayed, with indication for free perforator flap transfer such as DIEP, s-GAP, PAP, or LAP or eventually with LD myocutaneous flap. This reconstructive ladder is likely related to three main issues:

- **Perforator availability**: In delayed breast reconstruction, LTAP and LICAP may have been ligated or damaged by previous surgery because their emergence is very close to lateral breast mound. For this reason, it is mandatory for the plastic surgeon to know preoperatively if there are available perforators and their feature in order to be able to offer this reconstructive option. This applies also to immediate total breast reconstruction. In fact, the preoperative planning with high-frequency ultrasound allows to mark on the skin the perforators in order to provide instructions to the breast surgeon to be aware not to damage the perforator if oncologically possible.

- **Flap reach**: The conventional propeller design for lateral thoracic area perforator does allow a flap reach to the lateral breast pole, which makes these flaps a good indication for partial breast reconstruction. A bigger flap mobilization is possible only with TDAP and LTAP but not with LICAP which has a very short perforator length whose dissection does not allow a great flap movement. So far, the TDAP is usually the option for total breast reconstruction, although with conventional technique this requires a long pedicle dissection with very likely needing of thoracodorsal pedicle sacrifice which means erasing the possibility of harvesting a latissimus dorsi muscle flap for eventual backup reconstructive option.
- **Flap dimension and design**: For total breast reconstruction, it is very important to evaluate each patient. Skinny patients with big breast do not have enough volume to reconstruct the breast, unless a combined lateral thoracic area perforator flap and implant are considered (Fig. 15.6). Other patients may show a good

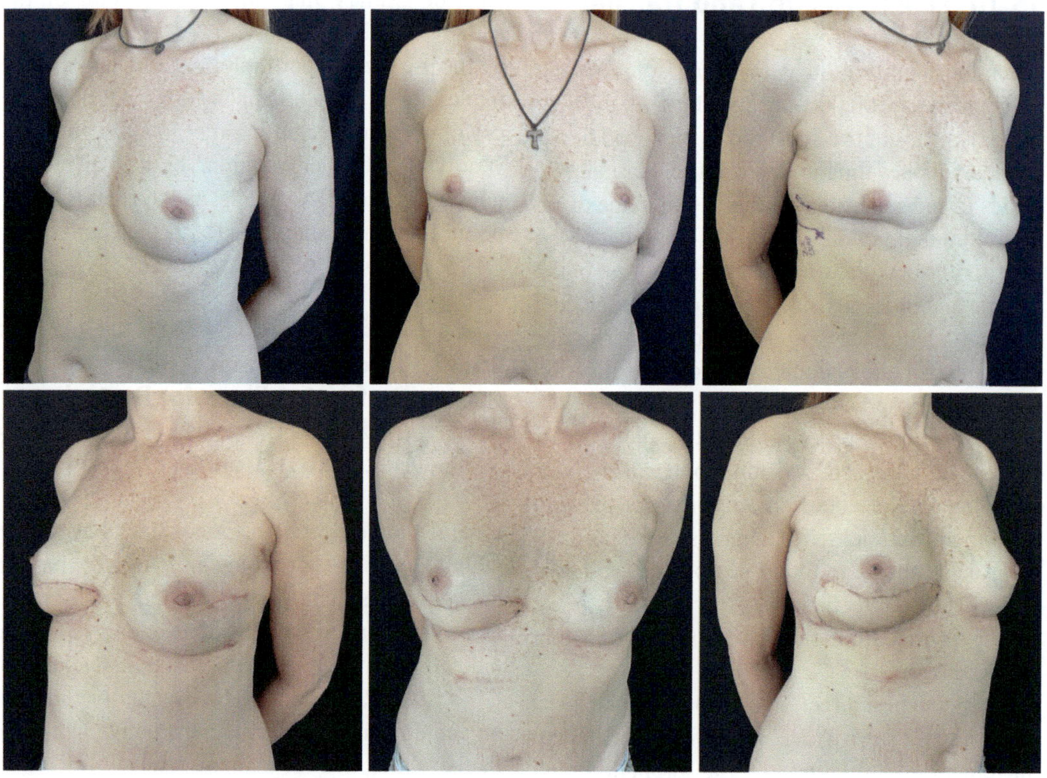

Fig. 15.6 (Above) Preoperative pictures of a 54-year-old patient with history of right quadrantectomy in the lower pole and adjuvant radiation therapy. The patient had indication for right nipple-sparing mastectomy for recurrence and contralateral prophylactic nipple-sparing mastectomy. The patient complained of breast "lower pole amputation" aspect. (Below) A 2-month postoperative picture after implant removal and breast reconstruction with LICAP propuller flap for lower pole restoration and prepectoral implant and contralateral reconstruction with prepectoral implant

representation of the ABSR, and thus they are good candidate for such reconstruction. However, preoperative ultrasound is mandatory to select the best perforator and moreover to delineate its axiality to draw the flap in the respect of angiosome.

In our experience, perforator flap from lateral thoracic area represents a precious source for partial and total breast reconstruction. The preoperative planning with ultrasound and the use of the propuller concept technique allows to expand the indication of such flaps to some cases which are alternatively considered for free perforator flap transfer.

15.12 Discussion

Pedicled perforator flaps from the lateral thoracic wall for partial and total breast reconstruction are considered a reliable surgical technique. By respecting the principle of the ideal like-for-like tissue reconstruction, the lateral thoracic wall perforator flaps represent the ideal flap for texture, color, consistency, thickness, and proximity to the defect.

In delayed total breast reconstruction, we usually can appreciate accentuation of the back skin roll as the redundant lateral thoracic tissue will further collapse laterally after the mastectomy that actually releases normal tissue adhesion. This is especially true in non-thin patients (Fig. 15.7).

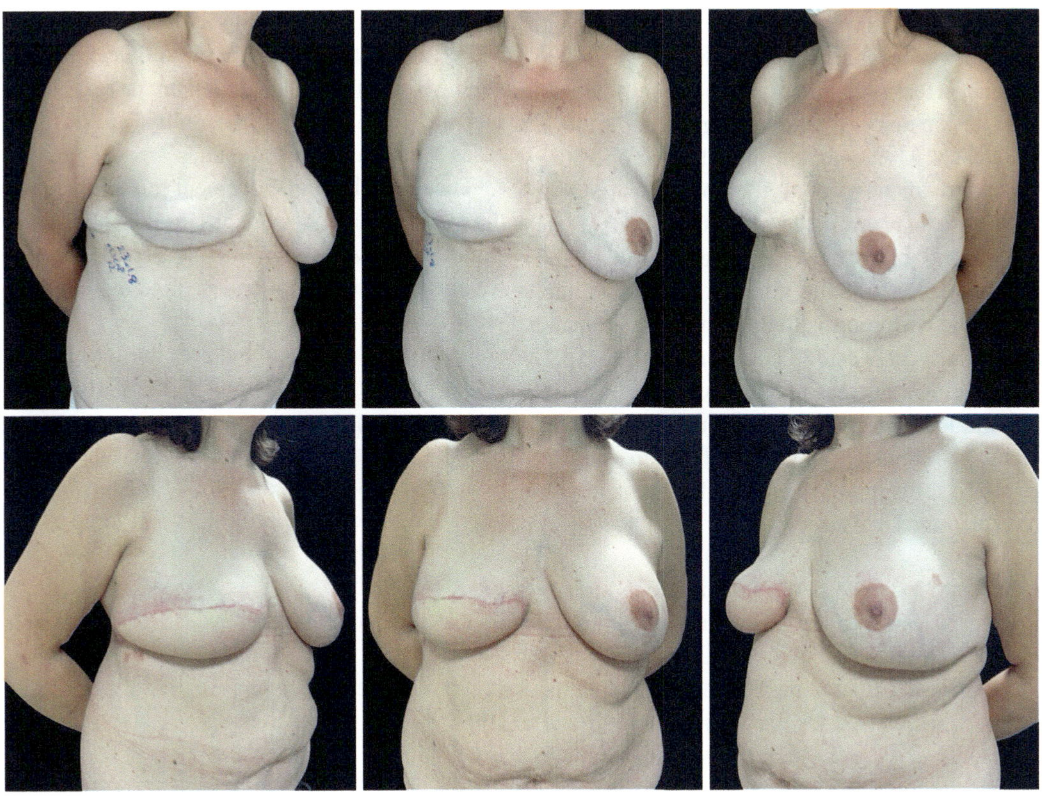

Fig. 15.7 (Above) Preoperative pictures of a 58-year-old patient with history of right skin-sparing mastectomy reconstructed with submuscular implant elsewhere 5 years before. The patient had capsular contracture Baker 3, and she was disappointed for implant shape and hardness feeling. (Below) A 5-month postoperative picture after implant removal and total breast reconstruction with TDAP propuller flap. The patient was offered but did not want revision on the contralateral side

The use of CCDS for perforator selection should be performed by the operating surgeon as lots of practical and operative information need to be acquired as described before. Such information allows the surgeon to perform a virtual "pre-surgery" during the ultrasound study that he/she will apply in the operating room. The paradigm shift in "propuller" flap concept is that perforator should be visualized and selected with ultrasound and not intraoperatively because traditional perforator skeletonization will interfere with propuller movement. To do so, the surgeon should be very confident in selecting the perforator as the other perforators encountered during surgery will be ligated. A wrong perforator selection may jeopardize the entire surgery.

The US information enables to select the best perforator in terms of caliber, position, and branching, in order to mark an elliptical flap which perforator entry point is eccentrical and close to the defect to allow a significant rotation and reach. Moreover, the detailed preoperative US-based knowledge of the local anatomy in each case may limit the skeletonization of the pedicle and improve the flap reach.

Compared to conventional perforator flap, where the perforator is traditionally skeletonized and dissected at least for 3 cm to favor the propeller movement decreasing the likelihood of twisting and kinking by distributing rotational forces along its vascular axis, in propuller flap, the perforator is only glimpsed and its skeletonization is not performed because:

- Not needed: The perforator has been already clearly seen preoperatively with ultrasound.
- Not safe in case a propuller movement is planned to be performed: The undissected tissue which surrounds the main perforator represents a security anchor, as it protects the perforator from tension and twisting and allows a more distant reach (pulling) with remarkable outcomes (Fig. 15.4).

Flap design does not change from not using ultrasound-based method; rather, what it changes is the flap dissection technique and flap movement as explained above, which is faster, safer, and in some cases more effective.

Mastering ultrasound technology in perforator detection is paramount to understand the perforator features and origin (thoracodorsal versus lateral thoracic versus intercostal) to avoid wrong flap design and eventual perforator damages.

15.13 Conclusions

Lateral thoracic flaps represent a precious source for flap harvesting for different purposes, and they can be used as local and free flaps. Ultrasound performed by the operating surgeon allows to clearly define the lateral thoracic area microvascular anatomy and thus performing a virtual surgical preoperative planning with high fidelity.

Perforator flaps from lateral thoracic area are valid option in partial and total breast reconstruction, in some cases as first option and in other cases as alternative of free flaps.

The propuller flap movement further increases the effectiveness of such flaps, as the entire tissue can be mobilized within the breast avoiding perforator skeletonization and pedicle dissection in most cases.

Propuller flap design requires mastering ultrasound preoperative planning as the perforator is selected preoperatively rather than intraoperatively. Therefore, it is reasonable that the CDUS is the operative surgeon's tool for mapping the lateral thoracic wall perforators and to appropriately plan each flap.

Conflict of Interest None.

References

1. Hamdi M, Van Landuyt K, Monstrey S, et al. Pedicled perforator flaps in breast reconstruction: a new concept. Br J Plast Surg. 2004;57(6):531–9.
2. Hamdi M, Van Landuyt K, De Frene B, Blondeel P, Monstrey S. The versatility of the inter-costal artery perforator (ICAP) flaps. J Plast Reconstr Aesthet Surg. 2006;59:644–52.
3. Hamdi M, Wolfli J, Van Landuyt K. Partial mastectomy reconstruction. Clin Plast Surg. 2007;34(1):51–62.

4. Hamdi M, Salgarello M, Barone-Adesi L, et al. Use of the thoracodorsal artery perforator (TDAP) flap with implant in breast reconstruction. Ann Plast Surg. 2008;61:143–6.
5. Angrigiani C, Grilli D, Siebert J. Latissimus dorsi musculocutaneous flap without muscle. Plast Reconstr Surg. 1995;96:1608.
6. Angrigiani C, Rancati A, Escudero E, et al. Extended thoracodorsal artery perforator flap for breast reconstruction. Gland Surg. 2015;4(6):519–27.
7. McCulley SJ, Schaverien MV, Tan VK, Macmillan RD. Lateral thoracic artery perforator (LTAP) flap in partial breast reconstruction. J Plast Reconstr Aesthet Surg. 2015;68(5):686–91.
8. Kehrer A, Sachanadani NS, da Silva NPB, et al. Step-by-step guide to ultrasound-based design of alt flaps by the microsurgeon. Basic and advanced applications and device settings. J Plast Reconstr Aesthet Surg. 2020;73(6):1081–90.
9. Visconti G, Bianchi A, Hayashi A, et al. Thin and super-thin perforator flaps elevation based on preoperative planning with ultra-high frequency ultrasound. Arch Plast Surg. 2020;47:365–70.
10. Cho MJ, Kwon JG, Pak CJ, Suh HP, Hong JP. The role of duplex ultrasound in microsurgical reconstruction: review and technical considerations. J Reconstr Microsurg. 2020;36(7):514–21.
11. Song S, Jeong HH, Lee Y, Powers H, Suh YC, Christoffi P, Suh HP, Hong JP. Direction of flap rotation in propeller flaps: does it really matter? J Reconstr Microsurg. 2019;35(8):549–56.
12. Visconti G, Bianchi A, Salgarello M, Di Leone A, Hayashi A, Masetti R, Franceschini G. Lymphatic tissue transfer: ultrasound-guided description and preoperative planning of vascularised lymph nodes, lymphatic units, and lymphatic vessels transfers. J Pers Med. 2022;12(8):1346.
13. Visconti G, Bianchi A, Hayashi A, Salgarello M. Designing an anterolateral thigh flap using ultrasound. J Reconstr Microsurg. 2022;38(3):206–16.
14. Hayashi A, Visconti G, Giacalone G, Hayashi N, Yoshimatsu H. Recent advances in ultrasound technology: ultra-high frequency ultrasound for reconstructive supermicrosurgery. J Reconstr Microsurg. 2022;38(3):193–9.
15. Salgarello M, Visconti G. Designing lateral thoracic wall perforator flaps for breast reconstruction using ultrasound. J Reconstr Microsurg. 2022;38(3):228–32.
16. Visconti G, Bianchi A, Di Leone A, Franceschini G, Masetti R, Salgarello M. The ultrasound evolution of lateral thoracic perforator flaps design and harvest for partial and total breast reconstruction. Aesthetic Plast Surg. 2024;48(5):894–904. https://doi.org/10.1007/s00266-022-03208-8. Epub 2022 Dec 14. PMID: 36517641
17. Hyakusoku H, Yamamoto T, Fumiiri M. The propeller flap method. Br J Plast Surg. 1991;44:53–4.
18. Teo TC. Reconstruccion de la extremidad inferior con colgaios de perforantes locales (Perforator local flaps in lower limb reconstruction). Cir Plas Iberolatinoam. 2006;32(4):287–292.
19. Teo TC. The propeller concept. Clin Plast Surg. 2010;37:615–25.
20. Pignatti M, Ogawa R, Hallock GG, et al. The "Tokyo" consensus on propeller flaps. Plast Reconstr Surg. 2011;127:716–22.
21. Kim JT. In: Jang BH, editor. Evolution and revolution of perforator flaps, 1st ed. 2017.
22. Thomas B, Warszawski J, Falkner F, Nagel SS, Schmidt VJ, Kneser U, Bigdeli AK. A comparative study of preoperative color-coded duplex ultrasonography versus handheld audible Dopplers in ALT flap planning. Microsurgery. 2020;40(5):561–7.
23. Kehrer A, Sachanadani NS, da Silva NPB, Lonic D, Heidekrueger P, Taeger CD, Klein S, Jung EM, Prantl L, Hong JP. Step-by-step guide to ultrasound-based design of alt flaps by the microsurgeon—basic and advanced applications and device settings. J Plast Reconstr Aesthet Surg. 2020;73(6):1081–90.
24. Feng S, Min P, Grassetti L, Lazzeri D, Sadigh P, Nicoli F, Torresetti M, Gao W, di Benedetto G, Zhang W, Zhang YX. A prospective head-to-head comparison of color Doppler ultrasound and computed tomographic angiography in the preoperative planning of lower extremity perforator flaps. Plast Reconstr Surg. 2016;137(1):335–47.
25. Cina A, Salgarello M, Barone-Adesi L, Rinaldi P, Bonomo L. Planning breast reconstruction with deep inferior epigastric artery perforating vessels: multidetector CT angiography versus color Doppler US. Radiology. 2010;255(3):979–87.
26. Cina A, Barone-Adesi L, Rinaldi P, Cipriani A, Salgarello M, Masetti R, Bonomo L. Planning deep inferior epigastric perforator flaps for breast reconstruction: a comparison between multidetector computed tomography and magnetic resonance angiography. Eur Radiol. 2013;23(8):2333–43.
27. Almadori G, De Corso E, Visconti G, Almadori A, Di Cintio G, Mele DA, Settimi S, Paludetti G, Salgarello M. Impact of internal mammary artery perforator propeller flap in neck resurfacing and fistula closure after salvage larynx cancer surgery: our experience. Head Neck. 2019;41(11):3788–97.
28. Hayashi A, Yamamoto T, Yoshimatsu H, Hayashi N, Furuya M, Harima M, Narushima M, Koshima I. Ultrasound visualization of the lymphatic vessels in the lower leg. Microsurgery. 2016;36(5):397–401.
29. Harii K, Torii S, Sekicuchi J. The free lateral thoracic flap. Plast Reconstr Surg. 1978;62(2):212–22.
30. Hamdi M, Spano A, Landuyt KV, D'Herde K, Blondeel P, Monstrey S. The lateral intercostal artery perforators: anatomical study and clinical application in breast surgery. Plast Reconstr Surg. 2008;121(2):389–96.
31. Munhoz AM, Montag E, Arruda E, Brasil JA, Aldrighi JM, Gemperli R, Filassi JR, Castro FM. Immediate conservative breast surgery reconstruction with perforator flaps: new challenges in the era of partial mastectomy reconstruction? Breast. 2011;20(3):233–40.

32. Lee JW, Kim MC, Park HY, Yang JD. Oncoplastic volume replacement techniques according to the excised volume and tumor location in small- to moderate-sized breasts. Gland Surg. 2014;3(1):14–21.
33. Kim JB, Kim DK, Lee JW, Choi KY, Chung HY, Cho BC, Park HY, Lee JY, Yang JD. The usefulness of pedicled perforator flap in partial breast reconstruction after breast conserving surgery in Korean women. Arch Plast Surg. 2018;45(1):29–36.
34. Kim JB, Eom JR, Lee JW, Lee J, Park HY, Yang JD. Utility of two surgical techniques using a lateral intercostal artery perforator flap after breast-conserving surgery: a single-center retrospective study. Plast Reconstr Surg. 2019;143(3):477e–87e.
35. Thomsen JB, Rindom MB, Rancati A, Angrigiani C. Thoracodorsal artery flaps for breast reconstruction-the variants and its approach. Arch Plast Surg. 2021;48(1):15–25.
36. Kim JT. New nomenclature concept of perforator flap. Br J Plast Surg. 2005;58:431–40.

16 Designing Perforator Flaps: Anterolateral Thigh Flaps

Min-Jeong Cho and Roman Skoracki

16.1 Introduction

With the technological advances in microsurgical instruments, microscopes, and imaging modalities, microsurgery evolved past several decades from the dawn of microsurgery to the era of supermicrosurgery and perforator flap reconstruction [1, 2]. Few advances in imaging modalities include development of multi-detector computed tomography angiography (CTA), color duplex ultrasonography (CDU), and indocyanine green (ICG) fluorescence angiography [3–5]. With these tools, microsurgeons transitioned away from relying solely on handheld Doppler ultrasound to performing a detailed preoperative planning using multiple imaging modalities that allow visualization of vascular course of pedicle, caliber of perforators, and location of perforators. With this patient-specific anatomical information, microsurgeons transitioned the goals of reconstruction from providing tissue coverage to performing anatomic and precise functional form of restoration.

Of many different flaps available, the anterolateral thigh (ALT) flap underwent the most significant changes with the evolution of microsurgery. Since its introduction in the 1980s by Song et al., the anterolateral thigh flap has served as one of workhorse flaps for various types of reconstruction [6–8]. The ALT flap became popular due to several advantages: (1) a long pedicle length, (2) ability to create chimeric flaps by including a segment of vastus lateralis muscle, (3) ability to create multi-skin island flaps based on different perforators, and (4) reliable blood supply. With increased anatomic understanding of the ALT flap, new types of flaps such as chimeric, thin, superthin, and pure skin perforator-based flaps were developed [2, 8, 9]. In contrast to the traditional method of performing flap debulking several months after the primary stage, microsurgeons are now able to customize the flap thickness and select components of flap during the initial surgery. Superthin flaps are elevated along the superficial fascia, while thin flaps are elevated along the level of the Scarpa fascia. These types of flaps allow for a greater degree of freedom when designing flaps as the composition of flaps can vary significantly based on the needs of the patient. In addition, studies have shown that a thin or superthin ALT flaps lead to decreased donor site morbidities and need for revisionary surgeries [1, 9].

Despite the versatility of these types of flaps, they are susceptible to partial and/or complete flap losses secondary to injuries to perforasomes during the suprafascial dissection. In addition, ALT perforators have a high anatomic variability,

M.-J. Cho (✉) · R. Skoracki
Department of Plastic and Reconstructive Surgery, The Ohio State University Wexner Medical Center, Columbus, OH, USA
e-mail: Min-Jeong.Cho@osumc.edu; Roman.Skoracki@osumc.edu

J. P. Hong et al. (eds.), *Imaging for Reconstructive Microsurgery*,
https://doi.org/10.1007/978-981-97-7278-0_16

and some patients do not have any ALT flap perforators [10–12]. Therefore, designing these types of ALT flaps requires precise understanding and detailed preoperative planning using imaging modalities to maximize the success of flap survival. However, most microsurgeons have limited experience with preoperative ultrasound due to the lack of access and steep-learning curve of using this technology. In this chapter, we will discuss tips and pearls of designing anterolateral thigh flap and the role of imaging in preoperative planning of the ALT flap.

16.2 Role of Imaging in Designing the Anterolateral Thigh Flap

16.2.1 Computed Tomography Angiography

Presently, there are several imaging modalities available for microsurgeons: computed tomography angiography (CTA), magnetic resonance angiography (MRA), color duplex ultrasound (CDU), and ultrahigh frequency ultrasound (UHFUS) [3, 13]. The majority of microsurgeons are familiar and comfortable with using CTA as the CTA is universally available in many centers. It provides several advantages: (1) rapid visualization of perforators and vessels as small as 0.3 mm, (2) prediction of anticipated flap volume using cross section of the CTA scan, and (3) evaluation of recipient vessels in the setting of trauma, radiation, known vessel disease, and previous surgical intervention. Given the ease of use and familiarity, CTA has become the gold standard of imaging when designing flaps, especially deep inferior epigastric perforator (DIEP) flaps [14]. However, there is limited literature on the use of CTA when designing the ALT flap.

In an anatomic study using CTA by Cohen et al., they found that ALT flap cutaneous perforator anatomy varies significantly [10]. Their study showed that ALT flap perforators were septocutaneous (34.4%), musculocutaneous (46.9%), or septomyocutaneous (18.8%). Similarly, Lakhiani et al. found in their systematic review that ALT flap perforators have high variability, and no perforators were found in 1.8% of cases [11]. These findings demonstrate the value of preoperative CTA to facilitate donor site selection and reduce operative time [12].

16.2.2 Magnetic Resonance Angiography

In contrast to computed tomography angiography, magnetic resonance angiography (MRA) offers a distinctive advantage of avoiding radiation and decreased risk against acute allergic reaction (0.07% vs. 3%) [3, 15, 16]. Studies have demonstrated that MRA has a sensitivity of 91.3–100% and a specificity of 100% in perforator mapping of DIEP flaps [17]. In addition, MRA can visualize a perforator as small as 0.8 mm, which is larger than that of CTA (0.3 mm) [18]. Presently, studies on the efficacy of MRA in designing the ALT flap are limited. Chen et al. found that MRA can be used to assess perforator course, size, and location, and their measurements are consistent with findings of CTA studies [15]. Despite the advantages, the limitations of MRAs include higher cost, longer imaging time, and lack of machine availability [18].

16.2.3 Doppler Ultrasonography

With the introduction of handheld Doppler for perforator mapping in the 1990s, it has become a popular imaging of choice to locate and evaluate vessels [3]. It typically comes as a portable unit, and the frequency of the handheld units ranges between 8 and 10 MHz. When designing the ALT flap, reconstructive surgeons use handheld Doppler to identify and confirm perforator locations. Studies have shown that handheld Doppler can detect vessels with a caliber of 0.2 mm with a sensitivity of 100% [19, 20]. However, this finding indicates that non-perforators can be identified, leading to false localization of perforators. While handheld Doppler has advantages of portability, noninvasiveness, low cost, and no radiation, few studies have shown that CTA is superior to Doppler ultrasound in decreasing the operative time [16, 18, 19, 21]. In addition, Doppler ultrasound is highly operator dependent, has a steep-learning curve, and leads to high false-positive rates.

16.2.4 Color Duplex Ultrasonography

In the era of perforator flap and supermicrosurgery, the role of ultrasound shifted from being an adjunct to a crucial tool in the setting of designing perforator flap, lymphedema surgery, and supermicrosurgery [3, 13]. In contrast to handheld Doppler, color Doppler ultrasonography (CDU) provides a real-time, surgeon-directed imaging of patient anatomy. The frequency of CDU probe for perforator mapping typically ranges from 5 to 12 MHz, and CDU offers two-dimensional color-encoded map of the blood vessels on the gray-scale tissue image [13, 22]. Typically, the blue color represents the vein, and the red color is used for the artery. In addition, an examiner can assess the velocity, caliber, direction, and course of perforators [4].

In comparison to CTA, CDU offers several advantages including increased sensitivity, accuracy, and efficiency of designing and harvesting the ALT flap [5, 23]. In a meta-analysis by Moore et al., they found that CDU has a higher perforator identification sensitivity (95.3%) than the CTA sensitivity of 90.4% [5]. However, the false-positive rate for CDU was marginally higher than that of CDU. In contrast, Kehrer et al. found that sensitivity and accuracy of CDU were 100% in their study of 18 anterolateral thigh and six superficial circumflex iliac artery flaps [23]. These findings reveal that CDU has a higher specificity and sensitivity but it is susceptible to a high interobserver variability [24]. The variability could be secondary to differences in experiences and familiarity of using CDU. However, the benefits of using CDU include significant reduction of harvest and operative times of ALT flaps by minimizing unexpected anatomic variability of perforasomes [24, 25].

16.3 Designing the Anterolateral Thigh Flap

16.3.1 Using the ABC System

The most popular and conventional method of designing the ALT flap is using the anterior superior iliac spine (ASIS) to the superolateral patella axis as a landmark. First, the extremity of choice would be placed in a neutral position without rotations to avoid incorrect placement of perforator location. The position of the leg should be carefully monitored during prepping and draping to prevent any rotation. Once the leg is in a neutral position and it is draped, then the ASIS and the superolateral corner of the patella are palpated. A line is drawn connecting the two landmarks, and the midpoint of the line is marked. As described by Yu et al., this point serves as the location of perforator B. Then, a point located approximately 5 cm proximal to perforator B is designated as perforator B. Similarly, perforator C is 5 cm distal to perforator B (Fig. 16.1). Yu et al. found that the ABC system is more accurate than a handheld Doppler examination in identifying perforators [26]. Once the potential location of perforators has been identified, multiple tissue components can be harvested using various types of combinations based on the need of the patient.

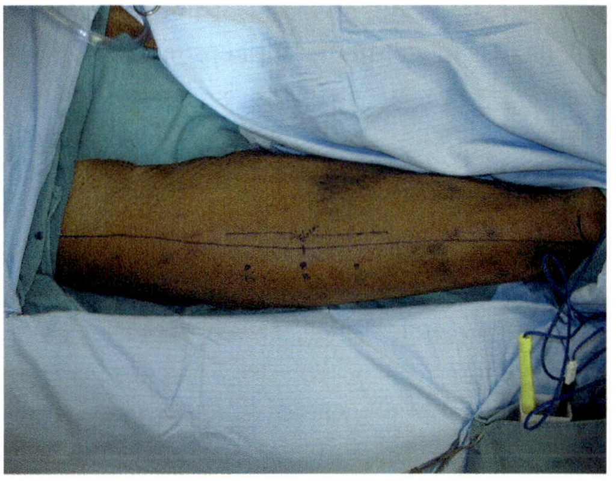

Fig. 16.1 Designing of the anterolateral thigh flap using the ABC system

16.3.2 Using Color Duplex Ultrasonography

Due to the recent popularity of the CDU, there are various types of CDU available for reconstructive surgeons. Historically, CDUs came with a bulky and heavy base, which significantly limited its portability [3]. With technological advances, portable CDUs that can be accessed through smartphone applications became available. Its ultrasound probe is connected to smartphone or tablets, and the application is used to select different presets [27]. In addition, it provides several modes including B-mode, M-mode, color Doppler, power Doppler, and pulsed wave Doppler. In contrast to traditional CDUs, these portable CDUs use a lower frequency probe, which provides increased depth but with low resolution. However, portable CDUs can visualize perforators as small as 0.85 mm and are effective devices when designing the ALT flap [4, 22, 27]. In our center, we use the Butterfly IQ+ probe (Burlington, MA) connected to any smartphone or tablet via an application (Fig. 16.2). The frequency of this ultrasound probe ranges from 1 to 10 MHz.

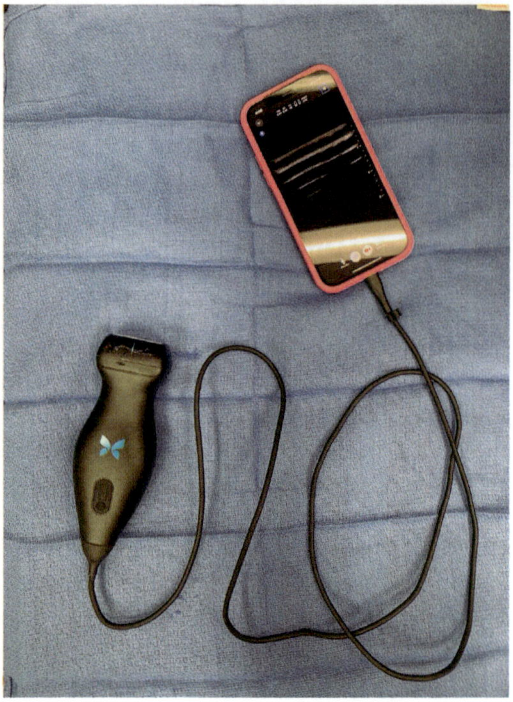

Fig. 16.2 A portable color duplex ultrasound connected to a smartphone

Similar to the conventional method of designing the ALT flap, the axis between the ASIS and the lateral patella is marked. We then identify the potential location of perforators A, B, and C as described above. Then, a musculoskeletal preset is selected, and an ultrasound probe is positioned transversally to the midpoint of the ASIS-lateral patella axis to identify quadriceps muscle bellies. First, skin (hyperechoic), subcutaneous (hypoechoic), fascia (hyperechoic), and muscle (hypoechoic) are identified (Fig. 16.3). While the subcutaneous tissue is hypoechoic, it can be mildly more hyperechoic than the skeletal muscle. The superficial fascia is typically identified as a hyperechoic line between superficial and deep adipose tissues. The deep fascia is characterized as a hyperechoic band located above hypoechoic muscle bellies. Once the examiner has become familiar with distinctive tissue characteristics on ultrasound, the septum between muscle bellies of vastus lateralis and rectus femoris is identified. First, the depth of the ultrasound probe is increased to identify the patient's femur. It can be localized to a circular, hyperechoic structure with a hypoechoic center. Hypoechoic structures above the femur are muscle bellies of quadriceps. To facilitate the identification of muscles, the examiner can ask the patient to extend his or her knee joint, which would allow visualization of the vastus lateralis and the rectus femoris gliding against each other. Typically, the vastus intermedius muscle is located superficial to the femur. Then, the rectus femoris is located superficial and medial to the vastus intermedius, while the vastus lateralis is located lateral and

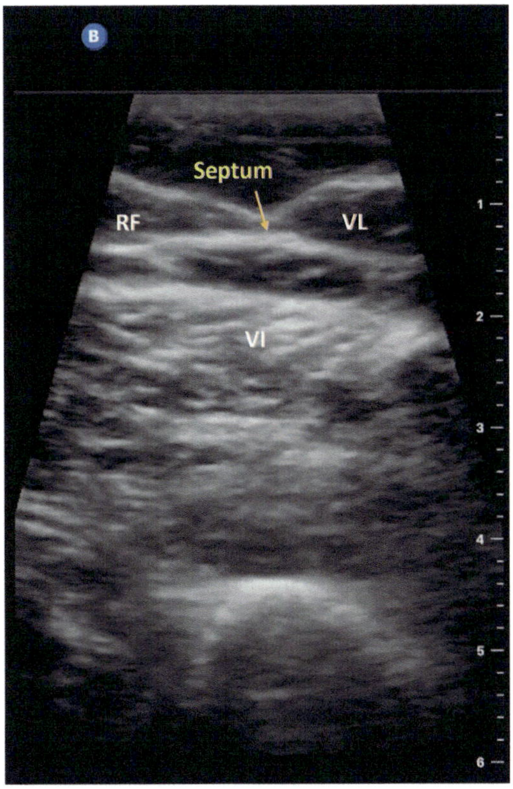

Fig. 16.3 B-mode ultrasound examination of the anterolateral thigh. The yellow arrow indicates the intermuscular septum between the rectus femoris (RF) and vastus lateralis (VL) muscle. The vastus intermedius (VI) muscle is located inferior to the septum

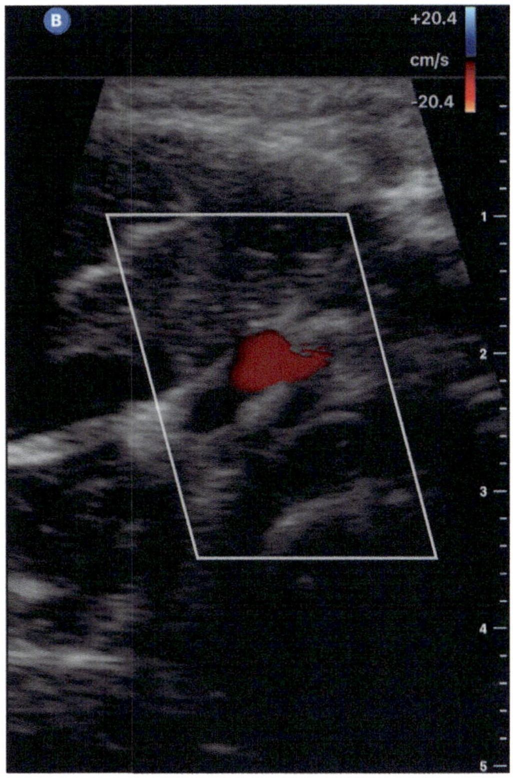

Fig. 16.4 Color duplex ultrasound examination of the anterolateral thigh flap showing a septocutaneous anterolateral thigh perforator

superficial. The septum between two muscle bellies is characterized as a hyperechoic layer.

Once the septum has been identified, then the preset of CDU is switched to vascular preset to localize perforators. Duplex mode is enabled, and the probe is gently moved proximally and distally at the perforator B location while carefully searching for perforators piercing the deep fascia (Fig. 16.4). Signs of perforators include any hint of pulsating colored structures superficial or deep to the deep fascia. Once perforators have been identified, its course, caliber, and velocity are assessed. With this detailed anatomical information, creativity and efficiency of designing the ALT flap are increased.

16.4 Technical Considerations

Case 1 Designing a Chimeric ALT Flap Using the ABC System

A patient presented with squamous cell carcinoma involving the hypopharynx and larynx after failing radiotherapy. Given the previous radiotherapy, and the extent of anticipated defect, ablative team anticipated a partial laryngopharyngectomy. As pharyngoesophageal reconstruction in the setting of a radiated field demands significant attention to detail, careful dissection, and coordinated care, detailed preoperative discussion and planning with the ablative team was performed [7]. After discussion of potential donor sites, the patient preferred thigh-based

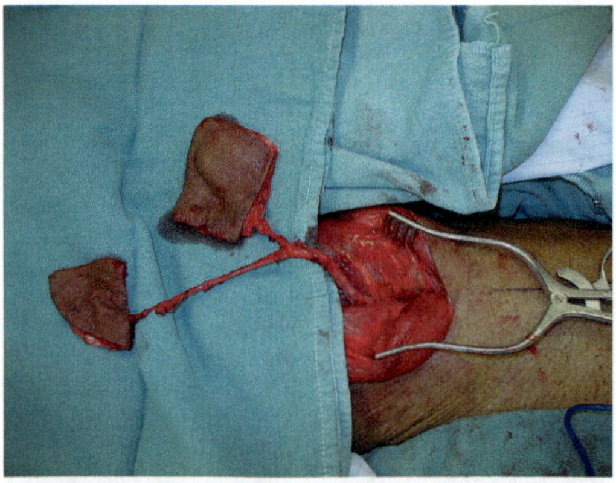

Fig. 16.5 A chimeric anterolateral thigh flap with two skin paddles for reconstruction using the B perforator and resurfacing using the C perforator in the case example 1

flaps to avoid any visible donor site scars over his forearm. As the patient had thin thighs, the decision was made to harvest a chimeric ALT flap with two skin paddles for reconstruction and resurfacing. As described above, the location of potential perforators A, B, and C were determined using the ABC system.

To reconstruct partial laryngectomy defect, a rectangular-shaped skin paddle (5 × 10 cm) was centered on the perforator B location. Then, a triangular-shaped skin paddle (5 × 7 cm) was centered on the perforator C to provide anterior neck reconstruction of radiated neck skin and to provide a flap monitoring segment (Fig. 16.5). Once the designing of a chimeric ALT flap was complete, we proceeded with flap dissection. First, a straight, anterior incision was made at the anterior midline of the thigh. The fascial incision was made 1–2 cm more medial than the skin incision to recruit additional cuff of fascia to promote additional layer of closure. Then, subfascial dissection was continued to intraoperatively identify the location of perforators. The location of perforators found by handheld Doppler coincided with the true location of perforators intraoperatively. At this time, flap design can be altered based on the true location of perforators. The proximal skin paddle can be based on perforator A or B, and the distal skin paddle is usually based on perforator C. If there are no two suitable perforators available, then the vastus lateralis muscle can be harvested with a skin graft for resurfacing of neck. Lastly, the perforators of the anteromedial thigh (AMT) flap can be examined using the same anterior skin incision if there are no suitable ALT flap perforators identified.

Case 2 Designing a Thin ALT Flap Using Color Duplex Ultrasound

A patient presented with a soft tissue defect with an exposed bone over the right lateral malleolus after motorcycle crush. Given the extent and location of defect, preoperative planning of the ALT flap using color Doppler ultrasound was performed. We determined that the patient would require a thin ALT flap with a piece of fascia to provide additional support and durable coverage over the bone. In addition, a thin ALT flap was chosen to prevent bulkiness of flap, which can prevent appropriate shoe wearing and lead to multiple revisionary surgeries. As described previously, we identified a septocutaneous B perforator and a septocutaneous C perforator using a portable CDU. We then designed an elliptical skin paddle (10 × 8 cm) with a plan to harvest a piece of the vastus lateralis fascia laterally (Fig. 16.6). Once the incision was made, we started the dissection in a sub-Scarpa fascia until we were 1 cm away from the location of the B perforator. Typically, the superficial fascia is encountered first, and the fascia can be identified

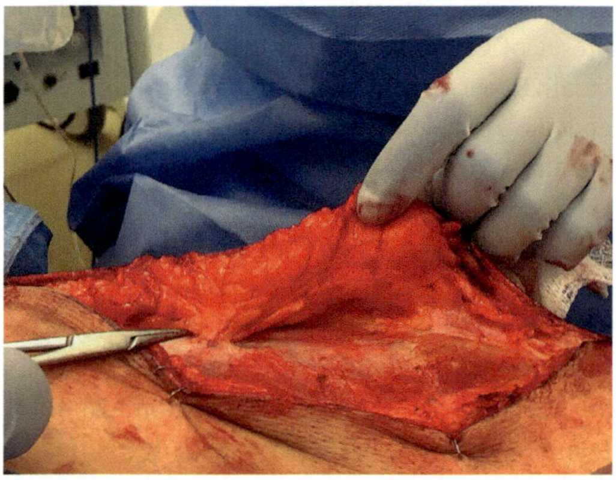

Fig. 16.6 Designing of a thin anterolateral thigh flap using preoperatively identified perforator using color duplex ultrasound in the case example 2

at the level when superficial fat (small lobules which are vertically oriented) changes to deep fat (large lobules without vertical orientation). Then, the Scarpa fascia layer is encountered after the superficial fascia, which is thinner than the Scarpa fascia. We then transitioned the dissection plan to suprafascial layer to prevent injuries to perforasomes. During the dissection, we left a cuff of loose alveolar prescarpal fat along the perforator. We then identified the C perforator, and a 5 × 8 cm vastus lateralis fascia around the C perforator was incised. We then isolated each perforator and identified the pedicle of the ALT flap.

In this case, we were able to minimize the need for a secondary revision procedure as CDU allowed us to freestyle the flap. Typically, the ALT flap is debulked at the second stage due to the concerns of potentially causing partial flap loss. However, varying degrees of flap thickness can be harvested using an ultrasound. With CDU, vascular arborization of perforators can be visualized, and suitability of perforators can be preoperatively determined [1, 28, 29]. As described by Visconti et al., there are two types of perforator arborization: In type 1, perforators course from the muscular fascia to the superficial fascia without branching, and, in type 2, perforators start branching at the level of the Scarpa fascia [29]. Type 1 perforators are typically used for designing a superthin or pure skin perforator-based flap as the perforator takes a direct course toward the superficial fascia, allowing a safe dissection of the flap. Once the superficial fascia has been identified, the dissection would continue until the perforator has been encountered. Superthin flaps are ideal for defects requiring low-profile reconstruction, such as the dorsum of the foot and hand, palate, and tongue [30]. For the pure skin perforator-based flap, the flap elevation starts at the subdermal plane. In contrast, type 2 perforators are not suitable for superthin or pure skin perforator-based flaps as these perforators branch prior to the superficial fascia. Thus, type 2 perforators cannot be easily traced as there is no direct perforator course. Therefore, type 2 perforators are suitable for a thin flap, which are elevated at the level of the Scarpa fascia. While thin and superthin ALT flaps can be designed without the aid of CDU, the flap vascularity can be compromised, leading to partial/flap failure.

16.5 Conclusion

Achieving successful reconstruction using a chimeric, thin, superthin, or perforator-based anterolateral thigh flaps is challenging due to high anatomic variability in these types of flaps. While these types of flaps allow a greater degree of freedom in designing, they are susceptible to partial and/or complete flap losses secondary to injuries to perforasomes. With the introduction of color Doppler ultrasound, microsurgeons have refined designing different types of anterolateral thigh flap by obtaining details of patient-specific anatomy. In addition, CDU allows facilitation of perforator selection, which leads to decrease in operative time and donor site morbidity. Therefore, we believe CDU is an invaluable tool for any reconstructive surgeons who are interested in performing patient-specific reconstruction.

References

1. Diamond S, Seth AK, Chattha AS, Iorio ML. Outcomes of subfascial, suprafascial, and super-thin anterolateral thigh flaps: tailoring thickness without added morbidity. J Reconstr Microsurg. 2018;34(3):176–84. https://doi.org/10.1055/s-0037-1607426.
2. Glass GE, Staruch RM, Sivakumar B, Stotland MA. Thin and superthin free flaps: an innovative approach to pediatric extremity reconstruction. J Plast Reconstr Aesthet Surg. 2022;75(11):3970–8. https://doi.org/10.1016/j.bjps.2022.06.090.
3. Cho MJ, Kwon JG, Pak CJ, Suh HP, Hong JP. The role of duplex ultrasound in microsurgical reconstruction: review and technical considerations. J Reconstr Microsurg. 2020;36(7):514–21. https://doi.org/10.1055/s-0040-1709479.
4. Kehrer A, Sachanadani NS, da Silva NPB, et al. Step-by-step guide to ultrasound-based design of alt flaps by the microsurgeon—basic and advanced applications and device settings. J Plast Reconstr Aesthet Surg. 2020;73(6):1081–90. https://doi.org/10.1016/j.bjps.2019.11.035.

5. Moore R, Mullner D, Nichols G, Scomacao I, Herrera F. Color Doppler ultrasound versus computed tomography angiography for preoperative anterolateral thigh flap perforator imaging: a systematic review and meta-analysis. J Reconstr Microsurg. 2022;38(7):563–70. https://doi.org/10.1055/s-0041-1740958.
6. Song YG, Chen GZ, Song YL. The free thigh flap: a new free flap concept based on the septocutaneous artery. Br J Plast Surg. 1984;37(2):149–59. https://doi.org/10.1016/0007-1226(84)90002-x.
7. Hanasono MM, Weinstock YE, Yu P. Reconstruction of extensive head and neck defects with multiple simultaneous free flaps. Plast Reconstr Surg. 2008;122(6):1739–46. https://doi.org/10.1097/PRS.0b013e31818a9afa.
8. Maruccia M, Fallico N, Cigna E, et al. Suprafascial versus traditional harvesting technique for free antero lateral thigh flap: a case-control study to assess the best functional and aesthetic result in extremity reconstruction. Microsurgery. 2017;37(8):851–7. https://doi.org/10.1002/micr.30248.
9. Suh YC, Kim SH, Baek WY, Hong JW, Lee WJ, Jun YJ. Super-thin ALT flap elevation using preoperative color Doppler ultrasound planning: identification of horizontally running pathway at the deep adipofascial layers. J Plast Reconstr Aesthet Surg. 2022;75(2):665–73. https://doi.org/10.1016/j.bjps.2021.09.051.
10. Cohen OD, Abdou SA, Nolan IT, Saadeh PB. Perforator variability of the anterolateral thigh flap identified on computed tomographic angiography: anatomic and clinical implications. J Reconstr Microsurg. 2020;36(8):616–24. https://doi.org/10.1055/s-0040-1713668.
11. Lakhiani C, Lee MR, Saint-Cyr M. Vascular anatomy of the anterolateral thigh flap: a systematic review. Plast Reconstr Surg. 2012;130(6):1254–68. https://doi.org/10.1097/PRS.0b013e31826d1662.
12. Smith RK, Wykes J, Martin DT, Niles N. Perforator variability in the anterolateral thigh free flap: a systematic review. Surg Radiol Anat. 2017;39(7):779–89. https://doi.org/10.1007/s00276-016-1802-y.
13. Visconti G, Hayashi A, Hong JP. The new imaging techniques in reconstructive microsurgery: a new revolution in perforator flaps and lymphatic surgery. Arch Plast Surg. 2022;49(4):471–2. https://doi.org/10.1055/s-0042-1751099.
14. Steenbeek LM, Peperkamp K, Ulrich DJO, Hummelink S. Alternative imaging technologies for perforator mapping in free flap breast reconstructive surgery—a comprehensive overview of the current literature. J Plast Reconstr Aesthet Surg. 2022;75(11):4074–84. https://doi.org/10.1016/j.bjps.2022.06.100.
15. Chen FR, Kerluku J, Mintz D, et al. Noncontrast magnetic resonance imaging of perforators for preoperative evaluation of anterolateral thigh flaps. Plast Reconstr Surg Glob Open. 2020;8(10):e3174. https://doi.org/10.1097/gox.0000000000003174.
16. Kiely J, Kumar M, Wade RG. The accuracy of different modalities of perforator mapping for unilateral DIEP flap breast reconstruction: a systematic review and meta-analysis. J Plast Reconstr Aesthet Surg. 2021;74(5):945–56. https://doi.org/10.1016/j.bjps.2020.12.005.
17. Agrawal MD, Thimmappa ND, Vasile JV, et al. Autologous breast reconstruction: preoperative magnetic resonance angiography for perforator flap vessel mapping. J Reconstr Microsurg. 2015;31(1):1–11. https://doi.org/10.1055/s-0034-1372475.
18. Wade RG, Watford J, Wormald JCR, Bramhall RJ, Figus A. Perforator mapping reduces the operative time of DIEP flap breast reconstruction: a systematic review and meta-analysis of preoperative ultrasound, computed tomography and magnetic resonance angiography. J Plast Reconstr Aesthet Surg. 2018;71(4):468–77. https://doi.org/10.1016/j.bjps.2017.12.012.
19. González Martínez J, Torres Pérez A, Gijón Vega M, Nuñez-Villaveiran T. Preoperative vascular planning of free flaps: comparative study of computed tomographic angiography, color Doppler ultrasonography, and hand-held Doppler. Plast Reconstr Surg. 2020;146(2):227–37. https://doi.org/10.1097/prs.0000000000006966.
20. Thomas B, Haug V, Falkner F, et al. A single-center retrospective comparison of Duplex ultrasonography versus audible Doppler regarding anterolateral thigh perforator flap harvest and operative times. Microsurgery. 2022;42(1):40–9. https://doi.org/10.1002/micr.30775.
21. Schneider CM, Palines PA, Womac DJ, Tuggle CT, St Hilaire H, Stalder MW. Preoperative computed tomography angiography for ALT flaps optimizes design and reduces operative time. J Reconstr Microsurg. 2022;38(6):491–8. https://doi.org/10.1055/s-0041-1740122.
22. Visconti G, Bianchi A, Hayashi A, Salgarello M. Designing an anterolateral thigh flap using ultrasound. J Reconstr Microsurg. 2022;38(3):206–16. https://doi.org/10.1055/s-0041-1740126.
23. Kehrer A, Lonic D, Heidekrueger P, et al. Feasibility study of preoperative microvessel evaluation and characterization in perforator flaps using various modes of color-coded duplex sonography (CCDS). Microsurgery. 2020;40(7):750–9. https://doi.org/10.1002/micr.30648.
24. Haribhakti VV, Thorat TS, Powle VR, Virarkar MK. Prospective study to analyse the efficiency of acoustic Doppler v/s colour duplex ultrasound in locating perforators for antero-lateral thigh flap in reconstructive head and neck surgery. J Plast Reconstr Aesthet Surg. 2021;74(9):2026–33. https://doi.org/10.1016/j.bjps.2020.12.088.
25. Kim S, Lee HR, Yun JH, et al. Preoperative perforator localization in anterolateral thigh free flap using acoustic Doppler and computed tomography angiography. Laryngoscope Investig Otolaryngol. 2022;7(6):1790–7. https://doi.org/10.1002/lio2.958.

26. Lin SJ, Rabie A, Yu P. Designing the anterolateral thigh flap without preoperative Doppler or imaging. J Reconstr Microsurg. 2010;26(1):67–72. https://doi.org/10.1055/s-0029-1234023.
27. Lindsey JT Jr, Smith C, Lee J, St Hilaire H, Lindsey JT Sr. Mapping 216 perforator flaps using highly portable tablet-based color Doppler ultrasound (PT-CDU). J Reconstr Microsurg. 2022;38(2):115–20. https://doi.org/10.1055/s-0041-1731676.
28. Seth AK, Iorio ML. Super-thin and suprafascial anterolateral thigh perforator flaps for extremity reconstruction. J Reconstr Microsurg. 2017;33(7):466–73. https://doi.org/10.1055/s-0037-1601422.
29. Visconti G, Bianchi A, Hayashi A, et al. Thin and superthin perforator flap elevation based on preoperative planning with ultrahigh-frequency ultrasound. Arch Plast Surg. 2020;47(4):365–70. https://doi.org/10.5999/aps.2019.01179.
30. Innocenti M, Calabrese S, Tanini S, Malzone G, Innocenti A. A safer way to harvest a superthin perforator flap. Plast Reconstr Surg. 2021;147(3):466–9. https://doi.org/10.1097/prs.0000000000007676.

17 Imaging for Superficial Circumflex Iliac Artery Perforator (SCIP) Flap

Hyung Hwa Jeong and Hyun Suk Peter Suh

17.1 Introduction

The groin free flap, based on the superficial circumflex iliac artery (SCIA), was first described by Taylor et al. in 1973 [1]. Later, Koshima et al. introduced a modification of the SCIA, called the superficial circumflex iliac artery perforator (SCIP), in 2004 [2]. This yields a thin and pliable flap that can be elevated in a supra-fascial dissection above the deep fascia. Although the introduction of the SCIP flap was quite long ago, its popularity has grown in the last decade. It is now considered an ideal flap option that is comparable to the anterolateral thigh (ALT) flap and the deep inferior epigastric artery perforator (DIEP) flap. The main advantage of the SCIP flap is its thin elevation, which provides good contour and conceals the donor site scar [3]. Its application in reconstruction is vast, especially in the head and neck and lower extremity region, because of its thin and pliable nature [4].

Supplementary Information The online version contains supplementary material available at https://doi.org/10.1007/978-981-97-7278-0_17.

H. H. Jeong · H. S. P. Suh (✉)
Department of Plastic and Reconstructive Surgery, Asan Medical Center, University of Ulsan College of Medicine, Seoul, South Korea

17.2 Anatomical Perspective

The vascular supply of the SCIP flap is different from other free flaps. Its perforator is a direct skin perforator that arises from a large caliber vessel, pierces the deep fascia, and directly goes to the subcutaneous layer to nourish the skin and subcutaneous tissue. The SCIA system is composed of two different branches: the superficial (medial) branch and the deep (lateral) branch. The superficial branch of the SCIA is a direct cutaneous branch with a large caliber, located relatively medially. Generally, it arises from the main trunk of SCIA at the medial border of the sartorius and then penetrates the deep fascia within an oval of 4.2 × 2 (vertical × horizontal) cm, with the center of the oval located 4.5 cm lateral and 1.5 cm superior from the lateral corner of the pubic tubercle [2, 5]. The superficial branch runs in a superolateral direction and crosses the inguinal ligament at the lateral third [6]. After the penetration of the deep fascia, it is reported that there are two types of superficial branches: direct anchoring to the dermis and axial pattern toward the anterior superior iliac spine (ASIS) [5]. There are some debates about the traveling layer of the superficial branch of SCIA. Suh et al. reported that it almost directly enters the superficial fat layer, whereas the cadaveric study by Zubler et al. reported that the superficial branch runs in the deep fat layer and then gives off several skin perforators before coming to the superficial fat layer.

J. P. Hong et al. (eds.), *Imaging for Reconstructive Microsurgery*,
https://doi.org/10.1007/978-981-97-7278-0_17

The deep branch of the SCIA is located beneath the deep fascia and penetrates the deep fascia at the lateral border of the sartorius. It nourishes the sartorius muscle, deep fascia, and iliac bone [6]. It is a true perforator that enters the subcutaneous layer after entering the sartorius muscle and penetrates the sartorius muscle fascia [7]. Some articles advocate using the deep branch as the main pedicle, which ensures a longer pedicle and wider perfusion area [6, 8]. However, tedious intramuscular dissection should be followed if the deep branch of the SCIA is used as the main pedicle of the flap. Furthermore, it is reported that the size of the superficial branch is generally larger than the deep branch: 1.55 ± 0.25 mm vs. 1.33 ± 0.26 mm, respectively [8].

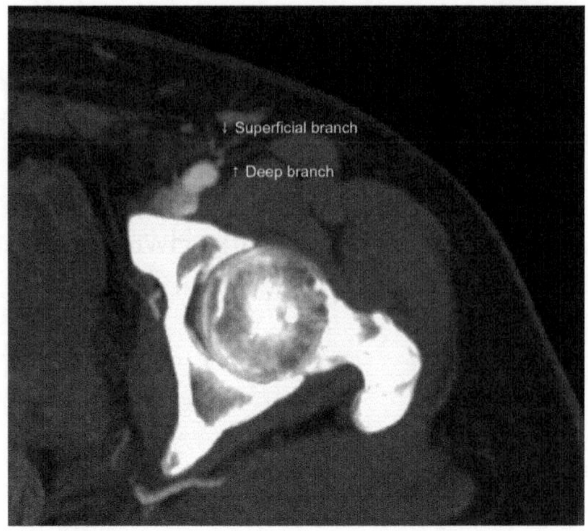

Fig. 17.1 CT angiography finding of the superficial and deep branch of SCIA

17.3 Computed Tomography (CT) Angiography

CT angiography (CTA) is a widely used imaging modality in preoperative planning for the SCIP flap. It has the advantage of providing detailed resolution and three-dimensional information with relatively low cost and complications [9]. CTA can detect vessels with small calibers, less than 0.3 mm [9], making it the gold standard modality for reconstructive operation planning. As the caliber of SCIP is less than 2 mm, it is advised to use multi-detector CT and fine-cut images less than 1 mm.

To identify the vessel, the superolateral corner of the pelvic tubercle and ASIS should be found as bony landmarks. The superficial branch of SCIA generally runs more medially and vertically and also runs in a similar course with SCIV, whereas the lateral branch goes more laterally and horizontally, and its main side branch runs in an inferior and lateral direction below the inguinal ligament [6]. Based on these characteristics, tracing the vessel in axial view is possible.

In the groin area, many vascular systems arise from the same area, such as the pudendal system and superficial inferior epigastric vessel, which makes exact tracing difficult, especially at the area where SCIA originates from the femoral artery. It is advisable to trace the vessel from the distal (around ASIS) (see Fig. 17.1).

17.4 Utilizing CTA for SCIP Flap Design

CTA is superior in providing the overall anatomical course of the target vessel, and it can be well utilized for SCIP flap planning. By using the CTA image, operators can overlook the course and the point piercing the deep fascia and superficial fascia. It is possible to mark those points by measuring the distance from the fixed (bony) landmark—ASIS and pubic tubercle. A high correlation rate with surgical findings and CTA was reported [5]. Pereira et al. introduced the planning method by using CTA to design the SCIP flap according to the known axis (ASIS-inguinal crease) and then marking the point where the superficial branch pierces the deep fascia (point D) and superficial fascia (point S) over the drawn SCIP flap design to ensure the target pedicle is included in the flap design [10, 11].

However, there are several pitfalls in utilizing CTA in planning the SCIP flap. Unlike other flaps using musculocutaneous perforator or septocutaneous perforator, the intramuscular portion of

SCIP is small as its nature of direct cutaneous perforator. Therefore, it is relatively hard to identify the source vessel and the point perforating the deep fascia in axial image, whereas the perpendicular penetration point of musculocutaneous or septocutaneous perforator is well visualized in axial view. Furthermore, the SCIP area generally has a small amount of subcutaneous fatty tissue compared with DIEP, especially in thin patients with low BMI. Therefore, it is relatively hard to identify the perforator in the CTA axial image compared to other flaps.

17.5 Handheld Acoustic Doppler

The handheld acoustic Doppler has its advantages due to the thin nature of the superficial circumflex iliac artery perforators (SCIP). The mean flap thickness of SCIP is reported to be 2–22 mm [4, 6, 12], making the handheld Doppler optimal in finding the pedicle of SCIP, which lies relatively shallow. Several articles have reported its effectiveness in finding the pedicle of SCIP [11, 13]. However, its high false-positive value and lack of visualized information have also been reported [9, 14]. Despite these limitations, the handheld Doppler can still be used as a supportive tool in preoperative mapping due to its light, mobile nature. It can also be utilized intraoperatively to find the real-time location of the target vessel.

17.6 Color Doppler Ultrasound

Color Doppler ultrasound (CDU) can overcome the limitations of CTA and the handheld Doppler. CDU can provide real-time anatomical information, including the size and depth of the vessel [14], as well as physiologic information such as flow velocity and volume of the vessel. Although CDU has a steep learning curve, it is becoming increasingly popular as an essential tool for reconstructive surgeons.

CDU is an ideal imaging modality for SCIP as it can provide real-time information about the highly variable vessel anatomy that can be confusing in CTA. Additionally, CDU can distinguish between veins and arteries, which is difficult in CTA. Furthermore, CDU can be used relatively unhindered by tissue thickness. With a high-frequency probe (more than 20 MHz), less than 1 cm depth can be scanned with high resolution.

17.7 Settings

The frequency of the probe does not have to be high. Typically, a 5–13 MHz linear probe is enough to find the perforators. B-mode is ideal for visualizing general tissue morphology and localizing large vessels and measuring their size. Skilled individuals can also detect small branches such as the middle trunk of the superficial branch in B-mode by adjusting the gain and focus depth. Utilizing the preset "thyroid mode" is advisable [15].

In color Doppler mode, the pulse of the vessel can be visualized in a color signal, making it easier to distinguish the vessel from surrounding structures. However, image delay can occur if the region of interest increases, and the Doppler signal can hide or exaggerate the vessel structure. Operators can adjust the gain and PRS scale, but this can also induce delay and false signal detection. For beginners, localizing the vessel by color Doppler mode and then visualizing and measuring the exact appearance of the vessel are advised (Figs. 17.2 and 17.3).

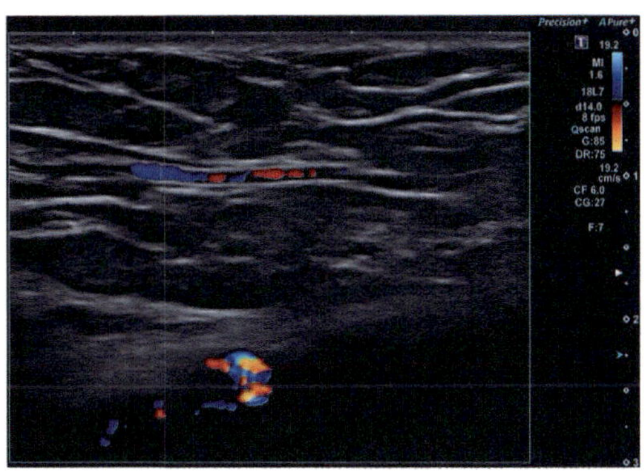

Fig. 17.2 Axial view of superficial branch and visualized flow in color Doppler mode

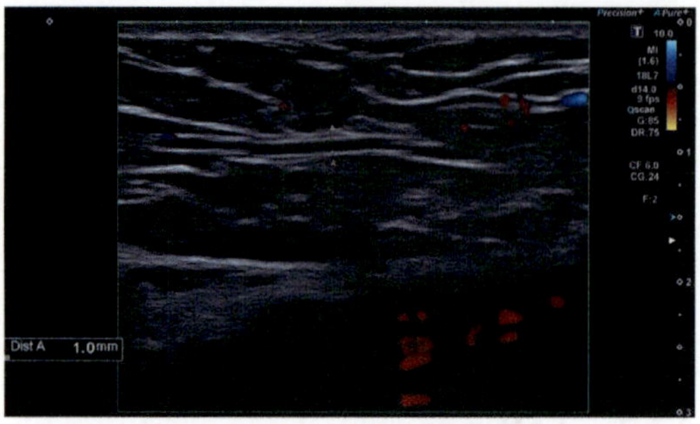

Fig. 17.3 Measuring the size of the branch

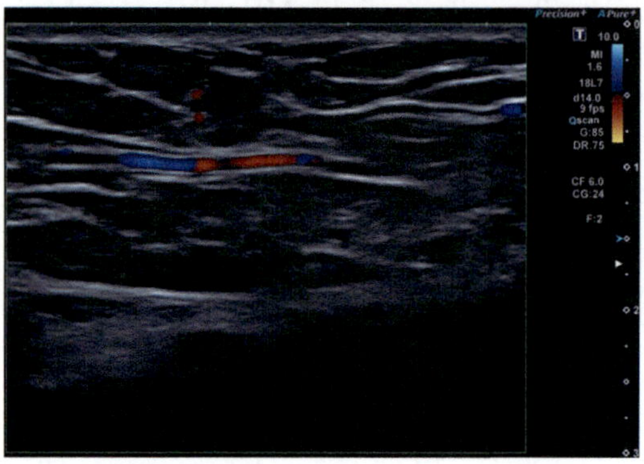

Fig. 17.4 Power Doppler mode

Table 17.1 Recommended setting for CDU

	B-mode	Color Doppler
Probe	Linear ~15 MHz	
Frequency	14 MHz	7–14 MHz
Gain	25–35 dB	15–30 dB
Depth/focus	1–3 cm[a]	
PRS scale	na	14.4 cm/s
Wall filter	na	Minimal

[a] Examiner can adjust according to the actual depth

Power Doppler mode is also effective in visualizing small vessels. It is an optimized setting for low-flow and small vessels by encoding the power of blood flow and tissue motion (clutter). It has been reported to have superior sensitivity in the depiction of vessel morphology and tissue perfusion [16], making it useful in finding the SCIA branches with small caliber (Fig. 17.4). Optimal settings for each mode are documented in Table 17.1.

17.8 Tips for Transducer Placement

To locate the perforators easily, draw a reference line starting from the line between the lateral border of the pubic tubercle and the ASIS, based on the surface anatomy of SCIP [11]. Since the superficial and deep branches of SCIA generally run almost parallel to the reference line, placing the transducer vertically to the reference line has an advantage. This enables the easy visualization of the lumen of the perforator (Fig. 17.5). Placing the probe parallel to the reference line has an advantage in visualizing the overall axis of the perforator (Fig. 17.6). For those who are not

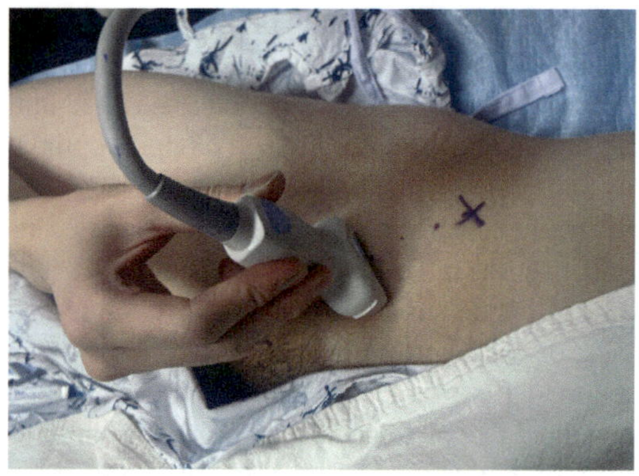

Fig. 17.5 Transverse placement of transducer to the reference line

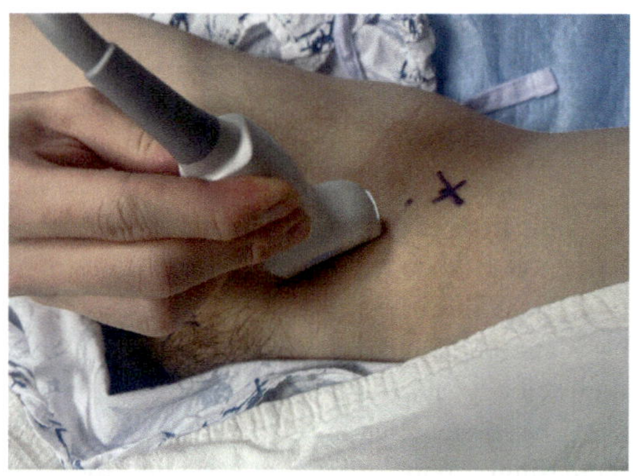

Fig. 17.6 Longitudinal placement of transducer to the reference line

familiar with ultrasound, it is helpful to use the vertical placement of the transducer first to locate the lumen of the target perforator. Then, by placing the lumen at the center of the monitor and rotating the transducer by 90°, the overall axis of the vessel can be visualized.

17.9 Comprehensive Use of Imaging Modality

CT angiography has the advantage of providing comprehensive imaging, including the surrounding tissue. Utilize CTA to get an overall view of both branches and mark the point of piercing the deep fascia and superficial fascia. Then, use ultrasound to find the exact course of the vessel. By placing the transducer over the marked points, prompt mapping of the vessel is possible. CDU has a superior advantage in tracing the vessel, especially for thin patients, compared to CTA, as mentioned above. If the power Doppler mode is used, smaller caliber perforators can be visualized even at the most distal part of the superficial branch.

References

1. Daniel RK, Taylor GI. Distant transfer of an island flap by microvascular anastomoses. A clinical technique. Plast Reconstr Surg. 1973;52(2):111–7.
2. Koshima I, Nanba Y, Tsutsui T, Takahashi Y, Urushibara K, Inagawa K, et al. Superficial circumflex iliac artery perforator flap for reconstruction of limb defects. Plast Reconstr Surg. 2004;113(1):233–40.
3. Narushima M, Iida T, Kaji N, Yamamoto T, Yoshimatsu H, Hara H, et al. Superficial circumflex iliac artery pure skin perforator-based superthin flap for hand and finger reconstruction. J Plast Reconstr Aesthet Surg. 2016;69(6):827–34.
4. Altiparmak M, Cha HG, Hong JP, Suh HP. Superficial circumflex iliac artery perforator flap as a workhorse flap: systematic review and meta-analysis. J Reconstr Microsurg. 2020;36(8):600–5.
5. Suh HSP, Jeong HH, Choi DH, Hong J. Study of the medial superficial perforator of the superficial circumflex iliac artery perforator flap using computed tomographic angiography and surgical anatomy in 142 patients. Plast Reconstr Surg. 2017;139(3):738–48.
6. Zubler C, Haberthür D, Hlushchuk R, Djonov V, Constantinescu MA, Olariu R. The anatomical reliability of the superficial circumflex iliac artery perforator (SCIP) flap. Ann Anat. 2021;234:151624.
7. Gentileschi S, Servillo M, Garganese G, Fragomeni S, De Bonis F, Cina A, et al. The lymphatic superficial circumflex iliac vessels deep branch perforator flap: a new preventive approach to lower limb lymphedema after groin dissection-preliminary evidence. Microsurgery. 2017;37(6):564–73.
8. Gentileschi S, Servillo M, De Bonis F, Albanese R, Pino V, Mangialardi ML, et al. Radioanatomical study of the pedicle of the superficial circumflex iliac perforator flap. J Reconstr Microsurg. 2019;35(9):669–76.
9. Nassar AH, Maselli AM, Manstein S, Shiah E, Slatnick BL, Dowlatshahi AS, et al. Comparison of various modalities utilized for preoperative planning in microsurgical reconstructive surgery. J Reconstr Microsurg. 2022;38(3):170–80.
10. Pereira N, Parada L, Kufeke M, Troncoso E, Roa R. A new planning method to easily harvest the superficial circumflex iliac artery perforator flap. J Reconstr Microsurg. 2020;36(3):165–70.
11. Goh TLH, Park SW, Cho JY, Choi JW, Hong JP. The search for the ideal thin skin flap: superficial circumflex iliac artery perforator flap—a review of 210 cases. Plast Reconstr Surg. 2015;135(2):592–601.
12. Kueckelhaus M, Gebur N, Kampshoff D, Hiort M, Varnava C, Harati K, et al. Initial experience with the superficial circumflex iliac artery perforator (SCIP) flap for extremity reconstruction in Caucasians. J Plast Reconstr Aesthet Surg. 2022;75(1):118–24.
13. He Y, Jin S, Tian Z, Fang Z, Ma C, Tao X, et al. Superficial circumflex iliac artery perforator flap's imaging, anatomy and clinical applications in oral maxillofacial reconstruction. J Craniomaxillofac Surg. 2016;44(3):242–8.
14. Cho MJ, Kwon JG, Pak CJ, Suh HP, Hong JP. The role of duplex ultrasound in microsurgical reconstruction: review and technical considerations. J Reconstr Microsurg. 2020;36(7):514–21.
15. Schiltz D, Lenhard J, Klein S, Anker A, Lonic D, Heidekrueger PI, et al. Do-it-yourself preoperative high-resolution ultrasound-guided flap design of the superficial circumflex iliac artery perforator flap (SCIP). J Clin Med. 2021;10(11):2427.
16. Martinoli C, Pretolesi F, Crespi G, Bianchi S, Gandolfo N, Valle M, et al. Power Doppler sonography: clinical applications. Eur J Radiol. 1998;27(Suppl 2):S133–40.

18 Usability of Imaging Modalities for DIEP/SIEA Flap Design and Planning

Tomoyuki Yano

18.1 Introduction

Nowadays, the DIEP flap has become the gold standard for free flap breast reconstruction. The DIEP flap can provide a large amount of adipose tissue with a wide skin paddle for any kind of shape and size of the breast. Its vascular pedicle is anatomically stable and provides multiple perforators for flap harvesting. When the DIEP flap is used for breast reconstruction by experienced surgeons, the surgical result is promising, and there is only a small risk for postoperative flap problems, such as fat necrosis and flap loss.

Therefore, patients have rather high expectations for success in breast reconstruction using the DIEP flap. Moreover, as the risks for BIA-ALCL after implant breast reconstruction have been reported, there has been more and more demand for free flap breast reconstruction. In addition, some patients want breast reconstruction with the SIEA flap, which entails less donor site morbidity than the DIEP flap.

To meet your patients' needs and satisfaction for free flap breast reconstruction, surgeons should conduct full planning before the reconstructive surgery to reduce the risk of intraoperative trouble and the whole surgical time. Reconstructive microsurgery is not an easy or fast surgical procedure. Lie [1] reported complete DIEP flap failure occurred on average in 1.12% of cases, and partial fat necrosis, which needs surgical intervention, ranged from 0 to 11% of cases based on the review of 693 DIEP flap breast reconstruction articles with 17,096 patients. Therefore, surgeons always keep several backup plans for unexpected intraoperative problems to avoid these complications.

Sufficient preoperative evaluation of perforator vessels and the flap pedicle might avoid unnecessary and unfavorable sacrifice and dissection in the donor site, which reduces donor site morbidity of your patient. Mennie [2] reported that the incidence rate for postoperative abdominal hernia was 2.45% in their cohort study of 7929 patients.

In the past, the technique of reconstructive microsurgery was thought to be a kind of art, and surgeons performed the procedures based on their surgical sensibilities, personal experience, and subjective observations. Lately, the usability of imaging devices such as duplex ultrasound, CT angiography, and ICG has been re-evaluated, and new findings using these devices have been reported [3–7].

In this chapter, I would like to introduce the usability of CT angiography, MR angiography, duplex ultrasound, and ICG for DIEP/SIEA flap planning and harvesting.

T. Yano (✉)
Department of Plastic Surgery, Cancer Institute Hospital, Tokyo, Japan
e-mail: yanoaprs@icloud.com

J. P. Hong et al. (eds.), *Imaging for Reconstructive Microsurgery*,
https://doi.org/10.1007/978-981-97-7278-0_18

18.2 Perforator and Pedicle Vessel Evaluation with CT Angiography and MR Angiography

A handheld Doppler is a small and simple device for detecting the approximate location of perforator vessels in the whole body. Because this device is available in most hospitals and is easy to use even for beginners, some surgeons may say a handheld Doppler is enough for preoperative marking for perforator vessels before harvesting abdominal flaps. On the other hand, CT angiography has an obvious advantage over a handheld Doppler. CT angiography can give information about the whole images of perforator vessels and flap pedicle course in the abdomen. Surgeons can understand the intramuscular course of the flap pedicle and the distribution of its peripheral branch in the adipose tissue before surgery. When there are several sizable perforators in the right and left sides of the abdomen, it is recommended to avoid the perforator that has a long intramuscular course (Fig. 18.1). During intramuscular dissection, surgeons perform meticulous dissection around the pedicle and ligation of small side branches. The more you do dissection and ligation around the flap pedicle, the more you will have a chance of damaging perforator vessels and the rectus muscle. CT angiography will tell you not only the size and distribution of the candidate perforators but also which side of the pedicle is easiest and simplest to dissect. When you find a robust perforator with a short intramuscular course on both sides of the abdomen, it might be a good opportunity for your residents or less experienced surgeons to take on the challenge of harvesting DIEP flaps.

In addition, CT angiography will give you extra information about superficial abdominal vessels such as the SIEA and SIEV. When you recognize a certain size of the SIEA branching from the femoral artery (Fig. 18.2a, b), it might be a possible candidate for SIEA flap breast

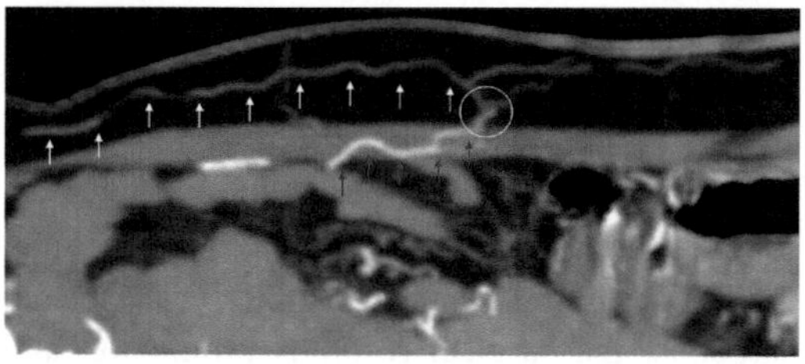

Fig. 18.1 The preferred large perforator (yellow circle) which has a good connection with the SIEV (white arrow) but has a long intramuscular course (red arrow)

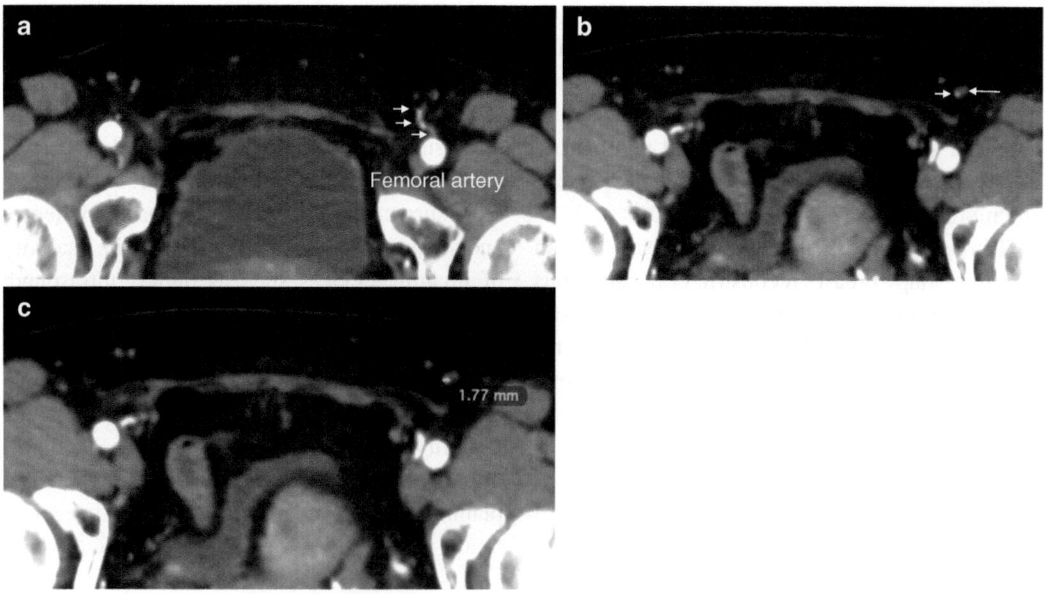

Fig. 18.2 (a) Upper left: white arrows show the SIEA branching from the femoral artery. (b) Upper right: white short and long arrows indicate the SIEA and SIEV, respectively. (c) Lower left: the SIEA showed 1.77 mm in its diameter

reconstruction. Spiegel [8] reported that a patient with a SIEA greater than 1.5 mm would be an appropriate candidate for a safe SIEA flap harvesting (Fig. 18.2c).

Also, you can check the size and approximate location of the SIEV (Fig. 18.2b) as a lifeboat for flap congestion.

When you consider performing a CT angiography examination of your patient, you should check whether your patient has a history of asthma, severe thyroid disease, or allergy to a contrast agent. A patient with these medical histories might have a risk for adverse reactions to contrast agents. In such cases, MR angiography will be an alternative option to evaluate donor site perforators and pedicle vessels. When you try to assess perforator and pedicle vessels with MR angiography, some adjustments and changes in MR angiography settings are needed to obtain satisfactory images of these vessels. It is important to discuss what you want to see and focus on MR angiography images with a radiologist before performing MR angiography on your patients.

Moreover, it is recommended to use scopolamine butylbromide to reduce intestine vermiculation, which can cause artifacts in abdominal wall images with MR angiography. If these images are taken properly, MR angiography will give you almost the same information about the perforator and pedicle vessels (Fig. 18.3). Unfortunately, MR angiography cannot be applied to a patient if the patient has a certain tissue expander in the breast because the device has metal parts.

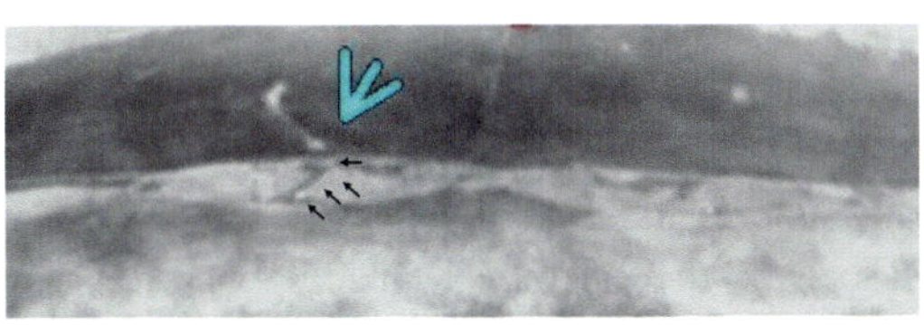

Fig. 18.3 Perforator and its pedicle evaluation with MR angiography. The large blue arrow shows the perforator arising from the rectus muscle, and the black arrows indicate the intramuscular course of the flap pedicle

18.3 Perforator and Pedicle Vessel Evaluation with Duplex Ultrasound

The usage of duplex ultrasound in the DIEP or SIEA flap harvesting was not common in the past. Recently, Cho and Hong [9] reported on the practicality of using duplex ultrasound in microsurgical reconstruction. Duplex ultrasound will give you extra information for flap harvesting, which enables you to perform the procedure safely.

A handheld Doppler and CT angiography will give you the approximate location and size of perforator vessels arising from the rectus muscle. Still, they do not provide you with the quality and exact location of perforator vessels. Sometimes you can find several good perforator vessels with CT angiography, but finding too many candidates might confuse beginners on which one to choose and include in the flap. In that situation, a duplex ultrasound can provide information about the quality, size, and velocity of perforator vessels (Fig. 18.4a, b). With this information, you can choose and include the largest perforator with reasonable velocity for your flap and mark the second largest perforator in the contralateral side as a backup perforator in case there is unexpected damage to the initially planned perforator or a need for a bi-pedicled flap harvesting.

Another important point is to find and mark alternative drainage systems other than the DIEV, i.e., the SIEV and SCIV. If surgeons experience many DIEP flap breast reconstructions, they probably realize the importance of preparing a second drainage system as a lifeboat when they have drainage trouble or flap congestion. Shen [10] reported that the takeback rate due to flap compromise was 5.8%, according to their review of 40,431 cases. Of flap trouble, 59.5% was caused by veinous anastomotic failure, 27.9% was arterial, and 2.3% was a combination of both. Since 2017, we have had 727 cases of free flap breast reconstruction, and the flap compromise rate was 3.6%. Of these, 38.5% was due to veinous trouble, and 19.2% was a combination of

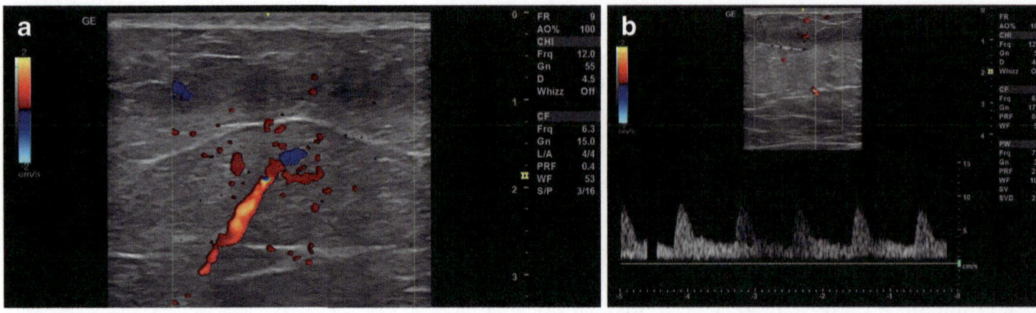

Fig. 18.4 (**a**) Left: a large perforator arising from the rectus muscle. (**b**) Right: perforator velocity was evaluated with a pulse-wave mode of ultrasound

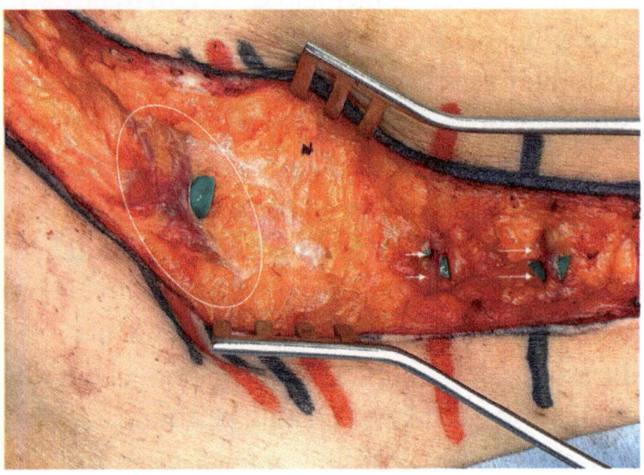

Fig. 18.5 White long and short arrows indicate the SIEV and SIEA, respectively, just under the preoperative marking with duplex ultrasound. The white circle shows a set of SICA and its concomitant veins just below the marking

artery and vein trouble. According to Shen's report and our data, around 50% or more flap compromise is caused by veinous-related problems. In addition, Shen [10] reported that the success rate for flap takeback surgery was 64.8%, and our data shows a rate of 69.2%. Regarding veinous thrombosis, we had a 71.4% success rate for salvage surgery with reanastomosis or creating extra drainage using a vein graft.

For this reason, it is important to find and mark superficial veins as backup drainage systems in case of flap congestion. In clinical settings, you can find these veins in exactly the same place under the markings (Fig. 18.5). And also the marking of superficial vessels will help you find an interposition graft vein if you need it for vein grafting.

In addition, there is an increasing demand for less invasive surgery, especially less donor site morbidity, in patients. The SIEA flap has an apparent advantage concerning this point. Patients do not need to worry about postoperative abdominal bulging. They can reconstruct breasts without damaging the rectus muscles or sacrificing the major artery and vein. Moreover, an idea has been suggested by Yano [11] of a combined SIEA- and SCIP-based double-pedicled abdominal flap for breast reconstruction, a revised technique to augment arterial blood flow and increase the drainage channel by including two separate flap pedicles. A duplex ultrasound will help surgeons to decide how to draw a design for these flaps.

As superficial vessels exist in superficial subdermal tissues, it is recommended to use a high-frequency ultrasound device that has a 48 MHz linear probe. However, a high-frequency ultrasound is still not common in general clinical practice. An 8–10 MHz probe will be an alternative option to scan subdermal structures. When you trace superficial vessels, the color Doppler mode is unnecessary, and the B mode is enough to detect vessels. You can scan and find superficial vessels in the lower abdomen around the lower incision line of the DIEP or SIEA design. Usually, these vessels exist between the dermis and superficial fascia or just below the superficial fascia in the abdomen (Fig. 18.6). You can distinguish superficial arteries and veins with their characteristic features. The superficial artery shows a pulsation movement under B mode scanning (Fig. 18.6). The superficial vein will show its mosaic pattern in its lumen (Fig. 18.7), and superficial veins can easily collapse by pressure through the skin surface (Fig. 18.8a, b).

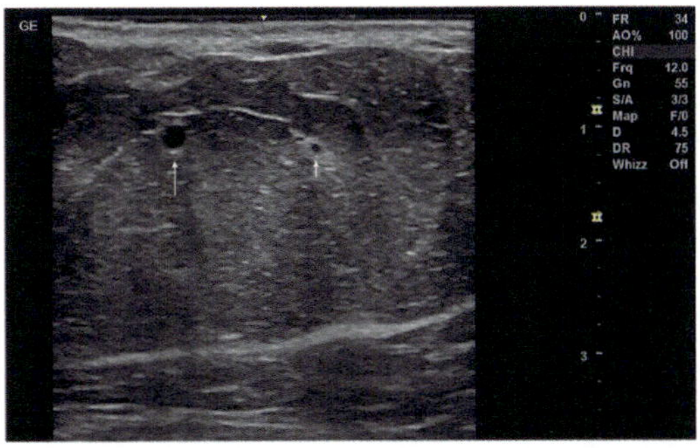

Fig. 18.6 Pedicle vessel evaluation with a 12 MHz probe of duplex ultrasound. White long and short arrows indicate the SIEV and SIEA, respectively. The SIEA shows a thicker vascular wall compared to the SIEV. Usually, the SIEA is smaller than the SIEV in size as well. The SIEA shows apparent pulsation, and the SIEV can easily collapse with pressure through the skin during ultrasound observation

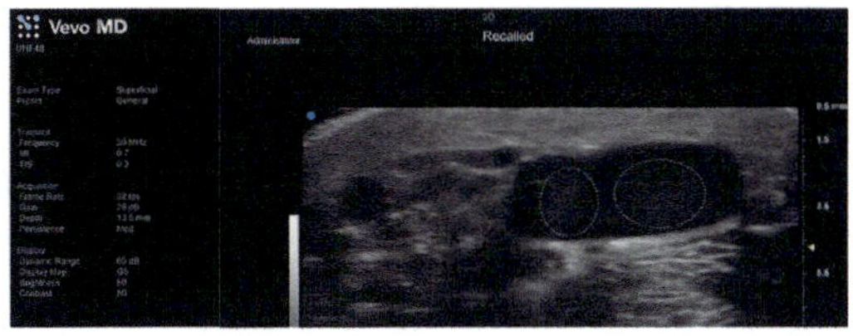

Fig. 18.7 Evaluated with a 48 MHz probe, the white dotted circle shows a mosaic pattern inside the SIEV

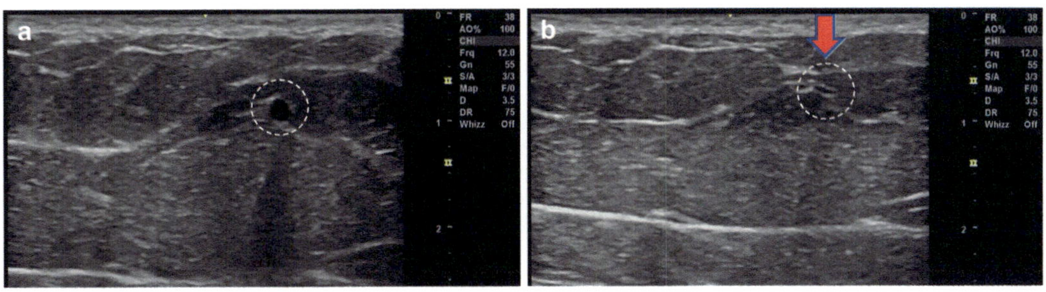

Fig. 18.8 (**a**) Left: the white dotted circle indicates the SIEV. (**b**) Right: the large red arrow represents pressure through the skin surface, and the white dotted circle shows a collapsed SIEV with an external force

After finding this artery and vein, these vessels can be traced back to their origin, and their course can be marked on the skin surface. Sometimes, the SIEV and SCIV will join together at the proximal side. You can measure the exact location and depth of these vessels. Surgeons can avoid damaging these vascular pedicles accidentally. Sometimes, these superficial pedicle vessels run under the dermis, contrary to the surgeon's predictions and experiences. Therefore, using a duplex ultrasound for preoperative examination and flap design is very worthwhile.

18.4 Harvested Flap Evaluation with an ICG Device

After finishing dissection of the abdominal flap, it is strongly recommended to evaluate flap viability and viable area mapping with an ICG device. Usually, fluorescence shows three transitions, a strong fluorescence area (green zone), a weak fluorescence area (yellow zone), and a no signal area (red zone). In our experience, it is safe to use an area where there is strong fluorescence with ICG (green zone), and surgeons should ignore areas that have only weak fluorescence

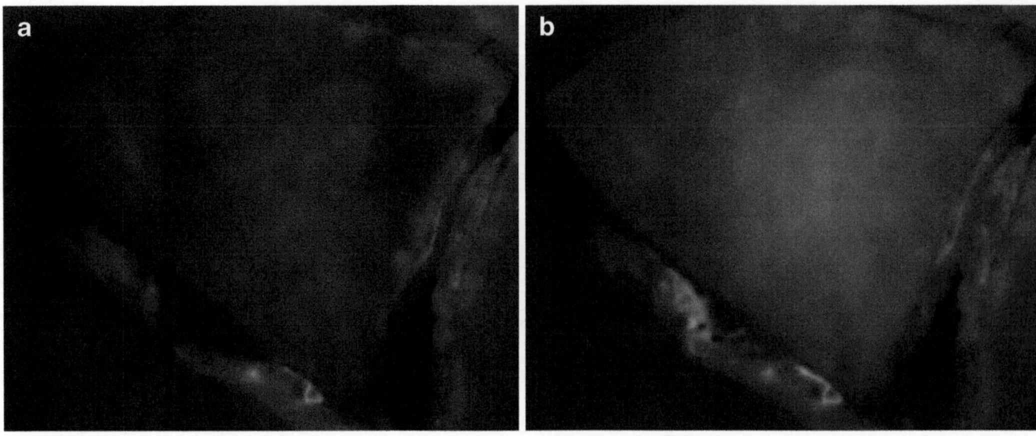

Fig. 18.9 (**a**) Left: flap congestion with ICG evaluation. The split DIEP flap was harvested with DIEA and DIEV flap pedicle, and ICG fluorescence showed a particular pattern. ICG fluorescence appeared only around the flap perforator and the peripheral margin of the flap. (**b**) Right: after releasing the SIEV to have extra venous drainage, the ICG fluorescence area extended to the whole area of the flap. These findings implied the SIEV was the dominant drainage system in this flap, or DIEV pedicle might have unexpected damage

(yellow zone) or no signal areas (red zone). If you use abdominal flaps for extremity defects or chronic ulcers, a yellow zone of the flap can be considered. On the other hand, yellow zone should be discarded for breast reconstruction because such areas have a risk for postoperative fat necrosis and may cause your patient to complain about a hard mass or an unexpected partial atrophy in the reconstructed breast due to deficient blood flow. In this case, surgeons should consider using a bi-pedicled flap to have extra blood flow to satisfy the original flap design.

Recently, Yoshimatsu reported [7] that ICG evaluation can detect flap drainage insufficiency, i.e., flap congestion. In Fig. 18.9, the flap showed slight redness after flap dissection, and ICG showed a characteristic low fluorescence pattern in the whole part of the flap with the deep inferior epigastric vessels (Fig. 18.9a). The flap showed remarkable improvement in its ICG fluorescence area after releasing the SIEV (Fig. 18.9b). In this case, the flap design changed to include SIEV, and SIEV anastomosed to the internal mammary vein in a retrograde fashion.

18.5 Flap Design: Step-By-Step Guidance

Step 1: Initial perforator marking (Fig. 18.10).

Start by marking approximate candidate perforators, with one to three points on each side of the abdomen according to the CT angiography and handheld Doppler findings.

Step 2: Find and mark superficial arteries and veins (Fig. 18.11a–c).

You can find and mark the superficial artery, SIEA (Fig. 18.11a), and superficial veins, SIEV (Fig. 18.11b), in the lower abdomen (Fig. 18.11c) using duplex ultrasound. You can harvest the SIEA flap or combine the SIEA and SCIP flap for breast reconstruction when you can find sizable superficial systems after starting dissection. Alternatively, you can preserve or include superficial veins to your flap as a lifeboat vessel when you face flap congestion.

Step 3: Choose preferred perforators (Fig. 18.12a–d).

Evaluate the intramuscular course of the perforator pedicle with CT angiography, and you

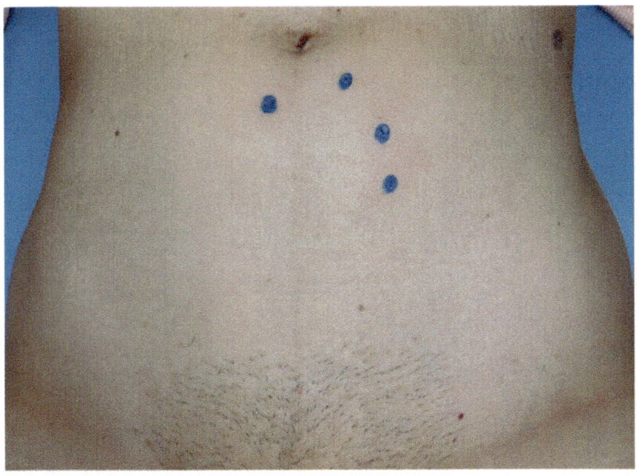

Fig. 18.10 Initial marking of candidate perforators according to CT angiography and handheld Doppler evaluation

should decide which side of the pedicle to use. It is always recommended to choose the side that has a robust perforator with a good connection to the superficial vessel system (Fig. 18.12a) and a perforator pedicle with a short intramuscular course (Fig. 18.12a).

Using a duplex ultrasound to confirm the dominant perforators of both the right and the left side of the abdomen. Select perforating branches that have a significant diameter and spread toward the superficial layers (Fig. 18.12b). Additionally, it is advisable to measure the blood flow velocity, as we believe having a higher peak velocity results in a wider blood flow spread into your flap

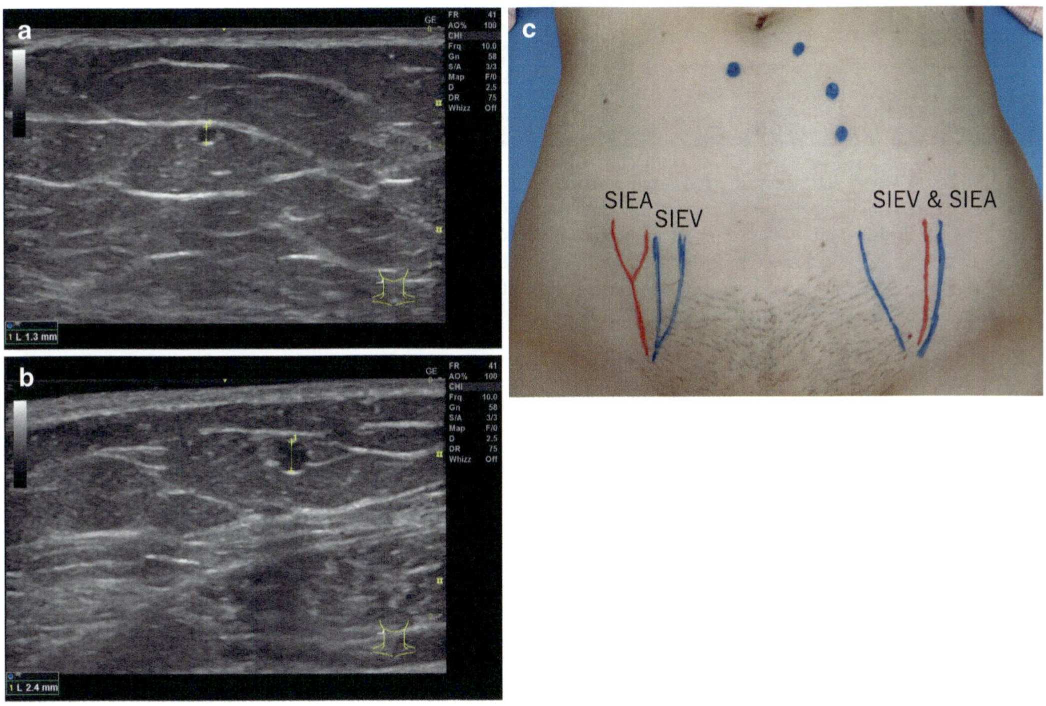

Fig. 18.11 (**a**) Upper left: the SIEA with the size of 1.3 mm with 8–10 MHz probe B mode ultrasound evaluation. (**b**) Lower left: the SIEV with the size of 2.4 mm with B mode 8–10 MHz probe ultrasound evaluation. (**c**) Right: markings of the SIEA and SIEV running course according to the 8–10 MHz probe ultrasound evaluation onto the patient abdomen

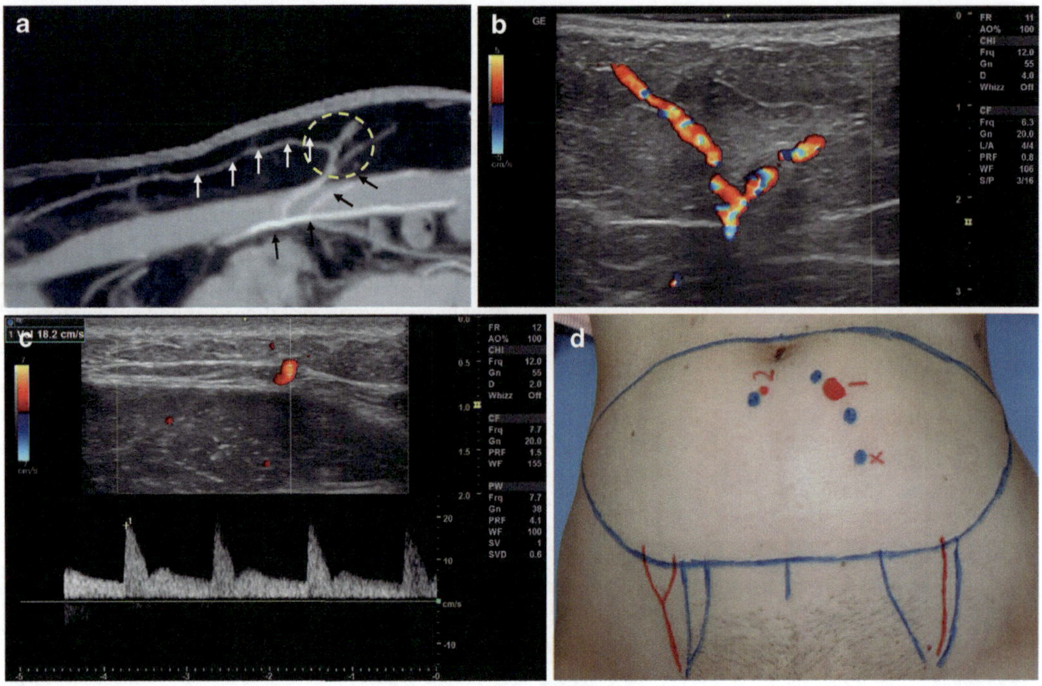

Fig. 18.12 (a) Upper left: the preferred large perforator (yellow circle) which has a good connection with the SIEV (white arrow) and it has a short intramuscular course (black arrow). (**b**) Lower left: the preferred large and widespread perforator was observed with 8–10 MHz probe ultrasound. (**c**) Upper right: the first choice perforator has an adequate velocity with ultrasound evaluation. (**d**) Lower right: Based on the findings of these ultrasound evaluations, prioritize the selection of perforators, mark the orientation of superficial blood vessels, and conclude the final flap design

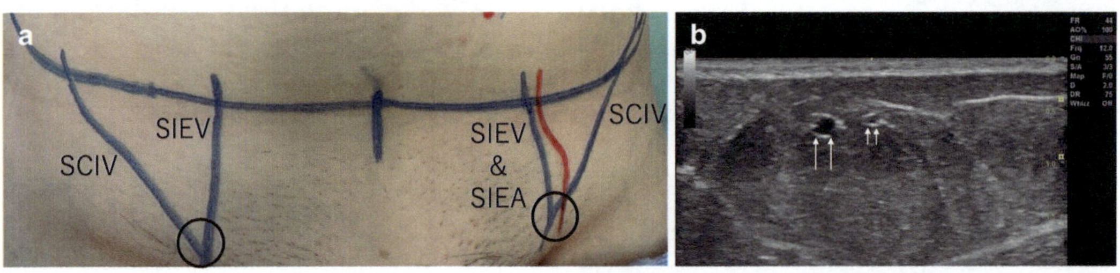

Fig. 18.13 (**a**) Markings and relations between the SIEV and SCIV. (**b**) Both veins came closer and joined together at its proximal side with an ultrasound evaluation

(Fig. 18.12c). After a duplex ultrasound examination, you can mark the dominant perforator on one side of the abdomen and the second candidate on the other side of the abdomen (Fig. 18.12d). You can switch to the other side in case you have trouble during perforator or pedicle dissection.

Step 4: Mark additional drainage veins (Fig. 18.13a, b)**.**

Use a duplex ultrasound to mark extra drainage veins, the SIEV and SCIV, on your flap design (Fig. 18.13a, b). Usually, the SIEV will be included in your flap with a length of 2–3 cm. If you mark the SCIV, you can find it easily and fast when you need an interposition vein graft.

Step 5: Use an ICG device to evaluate flap perfusion (Fig. 18.14)**.**

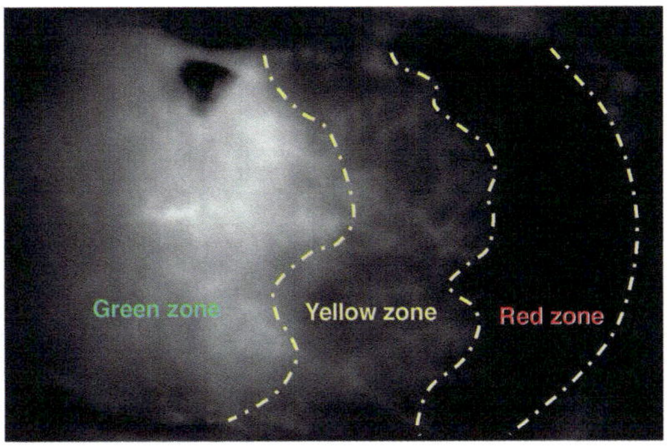

Fig. 18.14 ICG evaluation after the flap harvesting. You can classify into three categories, green zone, yellow zone, and red zone, according to the fluorescence intensity of ICG

Evaluate viable areas of the flap and divide it into three zones, green, yellow, and red zones, to finalize flap design. To obtain satisfactory results, yellow and red zones should be discarded. When you need to use yellow and red zones to add extra volume to reconstruct large breast, additional intra-flap anastomosis or using extra drainage vessels is needed to improve the vascularity of the flap.

18.6 Tips and Pearls

- When drawing the flap design line of the caudal side of the abdominal flap, it is recommended to mark the line as low as possible while still allowing closure of the primary donor site to be performed. With a lower abdominal flap design, it is easier to find and dissect a SIEV and SCIV of sufficient size.
- When evaluating the size and velocity of perforators in the abdomen, it is better to use the color flow mode of the duplex ultrasound. On the other hand, normal B mode with a probe of more than 8–10 MHz is enough for finding a superficial venous system. Due to slight discrepancies in the position of perforators indicated by a handheld Doppler and ultrasound, it is advisable, especially for beginners, to perform image assessment using ultrasound when you make a flap design.
- The ICG fluorescence result gives you better objective flap perfusion information than the pinprick test and capillary refill.

References

1. Lie KH, Barker AS, Ashton MW. A classification system for partial and complete DIEP flap necrosis based on a review of 17,096 DIEP flaps in 693 articles including analysis of 152 total flap failures. Plast Reconstr Surg. 2013;132:1401–8.
2. Mennie JC, Mohanna PN, O'Donoghue JM, Rainsbury R, Cromwell DA. Donor-site hernia repair in abdominal flap breast reconstruction: a population-based cohort study of 7929 patients. Plast Reconstr Surg. 2015;136:1–9.
3. Perez-Iglesias CT, Laikhter E, Kang CO, Nassar AH, Maselli AM, Cauley R, Lee BT. Current applications of ultrasound imaging in the preoperative planning of DIEP flaps. J Reconstr Microsurg. 2022;38:221–7.
4. Teunis T, Voss MRH, Kon M, Maurik JFMM. CT-angiography prior to DIEP flap breast reconstruction: a systematic review and meta-analysis. Microsurgery. 2013;33:496–502.
5. Mijuskovic B, Tremp M, Heimer MM, Boll D, Aschwanden M, Zeindler J, Kurzeder C, Schaefer DJ, Haug MD, Kappos EA. Color Doppler ultrasound and computed tomographic angiography for perforator mapping in DIEP flap breast reconstruction revisited: a cohort study. J Plast Reconstr Aesthet Surg. 2019;72:1632–9.
6. Wade RG, Watford J, Wormald JCR, Bramhall RJ, Figus A. Perforator mapping reduces the operative time of DIEP flap breast reconstruction: a systematic review and meta-analysis of preoperative ultrasound, computed tomography and magnetic resonance angiography. J Plast Reconstr Aesthet Surg. 2018;71:468–77.
7. Yoshimatsu H, Karakawa R, Scaglioni MF, Fuse Y, Tanakura K, Yano T. Application of intraoperative indocyanine green angiography for detecting flap congestion in the use of free deep inferior epigastric perforator flaps for breast reconstruction. Microsurgery. 2021;41:522–6.
8. Spiegel A, Khan FN. An intraoperative algorithm for use of the SIEA flap for breast reconstruction. Plast Reconstr Surg. 2007;120:1450–9.
9. Cho MJ, Kwon JG, Pak CJ, Suh HP, Hong JP. The role of duplex ultrasound in microsurgical reconstruction: review and technical considerations. J Reconstr Microsurg. 2020;36:514–21.
10. Shen AY, Lonie S, Lim K, Farthing H, Hunter-Smith DJ, Rozen WM. Free flap monitoring, salvage, and failure timing: a systematic review. J Reconstr Microsurg. 2021;37:300–8.
11. Yano T, Yoshimatsu H, Karakawa R, Fuse Y, Kuramoto Y, Shibata T, Suesada N, Miyashita H. Use of a combined SIEA and SCIP based double pedicled abdominal flap for breast reconstruction. Microsurgery. 2021;41:319–26.

Medial Sural Perforator Free Flap for Head and Neck Reconstructions

19

Jong-Woo (JW) Choi and Young-Chul Kim

19.1 Introduction

The head and neck reconstructions could be categorized into three major areas. The one is the facial surface reconstruction including all facial subunits such as forehead, nose, eyelid, lip, and cheek. The other is facial skeletal and muscular reconstruction such as the facial muscles and nerves. The last one is the intraoral and pharyngeal reconstructions. In narrower sense of head and neck reconstructions, this type of reconstruction is regarded as the head and neck reconstruction especially for the head and neck cancer management.

There are some unique features in the clinical application of the perforator free flaps for head and neck reconstructions in the management of head and neck cancer. Firstly, if the intraoral reconstruction or pharyngeal reconstruction fails, the other conservative alternative usually does not work. Therefore, flaps for head and neck reconstruction in narrow sense should be a success without even local flap compromise which will lead to fistula formation. Secondly, the flaps insetted intraorally or in pharyngeal area tend to be inevitably located three-dimensionally while being folded or being curved. These features might endanger the kinking of the small perforators used for head and neck reconstructions. Finally, in order to minimize the longer operation time, two-team approach would be ideal. For this purpose, free flap harvest from lower extremities is preferred in many institutions.

In head and neck reconstructions for intraoral cancer managements, ALT free flap would be the most popular choice although the partial tongue defects could be reconstructed with traditional radial forearm free flap. Of course, any perforator free flaps could be used for intraoral reconstructions. Among the various options, medial sural perforator free flap could be an option. Considering the bulk and thickness of the original donor site for the perforator free flap, medial sural perforator free flap could be adequate for intraoral reconstruction. In addition, it allows us to perform the two-team approach without discomfort.

The functional oropharyngeal reconstruction requires various flaps according to the size and location of the defect. The fasciocutaneous free flap such as radial forearm flap, anterolateral thigh perforator flap, and thoracodorsal perforator flap would be the most common in choice for oropharyngeal reconstruction. But, in terms of volume or thickness of the flaps for anatomical reconstructions, radial forearm free flap is sometimes too thin, and anterolateral thigh free flap is often too thick depending on each patient's characteristics. When we encounter these situations, the application of the medial sural perforator free

J.-W. (JW). Choi (✉) · Y.-C. Kim
Department of Plastic and Reconstructive Surgery, Asan Medical Center, Seoul, South Korea

J. P. Hong et al. (eds.), *Imaging for Reconstructive Microsurgery*,
https://doi.org/10.1007/978-981-97-7278-0_19

flaps for oropharyngeal reconstructions seems to be very beneficial.

The insufficient volume of the reconstructed flap may result in functional deficit like swallowing or speaking difficulty. Likewise, the overcorrected volume of the reconstructed flap may cause similar functional problems postoperatively that need the secondary debulking procedures.

In order to overcome these limitations, we felt the need of intermediate flap which has the medium thickness or volume for anatomical reconstruction as possible. Based on my experiences with application of the medial sural perforator free flap to oropharyngeal reconstructions, the indications and limitations of this flap to help other surgeons to understand the advantages and disadvantages of the medial sural perforator free flap for oropharyngeal reconstruction will be described.

19.2 Anatomy

The locations of the medial sural perforators somewhat remain controversial (Fig. 19.1). According to the anatomical study by Thione et al. in 2004, all perforators gathered between 7 and 18 cm from the popliteal crease; 34.2% of perforators arose on the midline of the medial head of gastrocnemius muscle; before entering the fascia, the perforator artery diameter was on average 0.5 mm. Two configurations of the intramuscular course of perforators were found. On average, length of flaps was 12.9 cm, and width was 7.9 cm; all 38 perforators were musculocutaneous: one perforator was always found (on average, 1.9 per flap). Sixty-six percent of perforators originated from the lateral branch of the medial sural artery and 34% from the medial one [3].

Similarly, Kim et al. in Korea reported the anatomical and clinical investigation based on dissections performed on 40 legs from 20 cadavers; the authors identified the location of the first and second perforators of the medial sural artery. The authors found that the main perforators of the medial sural artery were located on a line drawn from the midpoint of the popliteal crease to the midpoint of the medial malleolus. The hip joint was flexed in supine position, and the knee joint was flexed into a 90-degree angle, thus making it possible to observe the first perforator, which was approximately 8 cm from the midpoint of the popliteal crease, and the second perforator, which was approximately 15 cm from the popliteal crease. A series of 21 clinical cases with soft tissue defects were successfully treated using the medial sural artery perforator flap, including 18 free flaps and three pedicled flaps. There were seven cases of hand recon-

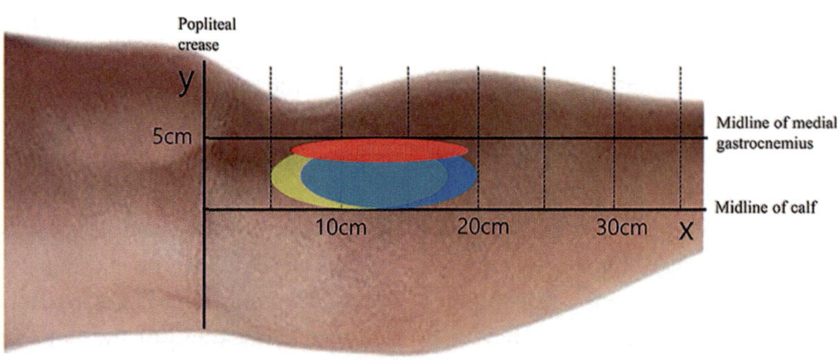

Fig. 19.1 Location of perforators based on Cartesian coordinate system. The midline of the calf is determined as x axis, while the popliteal crease is set as y axis. Okamoto et al. found the perforators (yellow-colored area) 5.5–17.2 cm (mean 11.6) from the popliteal crease and 0.5–4.5 cm from the calf midline [1]. Cavadas et al. found the perforators (blue-colored area) 8.5–19 cm (mean 14.2) from the popliteal crease [2]. Thione et al. found them (red-colored area) between 7 and 18 cm from the popliteal crease, and 34.2% of perforators arose 1 cm medially from the midline of the medial head of gastrocnemius muscle [3]

struction and 14 cases of lower extremity reconstruction [4].

Recently, Fu Chan Wei et al. showed the clinical application of the medial sural perforator free flap for the head and neck reconstructions. This study revealed that flap sizes ranged from 8 × 4 to 12 × 14 cm. The mean pedicle length was 12.7 cm, the mean flap thickness was 4.8 mm, the mean number of total perforators was 2.7 ± 1.5 (range, 1–5), and the mean number of sizable perforators was 1.6 ± 0.7 (range, 1–3). The mean distance from the perforator perpendicular to the popliteal crease was 11.4 ± 2.7 cm. No perforators were found less than 6 cm or more than 18 cm from the popliteal crease. Most sizable perforators (85.4%) entered the medial gastrocnemius muscle at a relative distance of one-fifth to one-third of the lower leg length measured from the popliteal crease [5].

According to my personal experiences regarding the applications of the medial sural perforator free flaps to the head and neck reconstructions, the vertical location for the major sizable medial sural perforators ranges from 6 to 15 cm (average = 9.1 cm) from the popliteal crease. The transverse distances from the midlines which connect the midpoint of the popliteal fossa and Achilles tendon ranged from 1.0 to 5 cm (average = 2.7 cm). Most of the sizable medial sural perforators were found within the triangle which consists of the line from the midpoint of the popliteal crease to medial calcaneus and the line from the midpoint of the popliteal crease to Achilles tendon. When it comes to the thickness of the medial sural perforator free flaps, the thickness of the flap ranged from 4 to 10 mm (average: 5.9 mm). The average vertical dimension of the flaps was 10.6 cm (4.5–15 cm). The average transverse dimension of the flaps was 5.8 cm (4–7 cm). The average length of the pedicles was 10.7 cm. The length of pedicles ranged from 8 to 15 cm. In addition to this, the dominant venae comitantes were evident in 15 cases. One vena comitans was much bigger in diameter than the others. No cases required additional debulking surgery owing to bulk of the flaps or the deficient volume of the flap.

19.3 Flap Design

Flap design for head and neck reconstruction is an important issue. Because the restoration of the original anatomic structures is essential for functional head and neck reconstruction, sophisticated design of flap is crucial in addition to the success of the microsurgical anastomosis and elevation of the perforator flaps.

As the chemoradiation evolves, the pattern of the intraoral defects is changing as well in some parts. For the tonsil cancer, the chemoradiation already becomes the first option. If the chemoradiation fails, the salvage surgery and reconstruction could be chosen. Although the recent trends in the management of the head and neck cancer emphasize the efficacy of the chemoradiation therapy, the surgical resection remains as the one of the most important roles in the treatment of the head and neck cancer yet [6]. During the past decades, the treatment of the head and neck cancer has strikingly evolved as the reconstruction method with the free flap transfer using the microsurgical techniques developed. As a result, more aggressive surgical resection and radiation therapy became possible [7–9]. Presently, the main goals of the head and neck reconstruction following the oral cancer ablation surgery have been focused on the anatomical and functional reconstruction. In order to minimize the functional deficit after the surgical resections, it is necessary to restore the three-dimensional anatomical structures of the oral and oropharyngeal area as possible.

The design of the flap begins with the identification of suitable perforator. Various ways of schematic mapping have been suggested to facilitate preoperative identification of the most common location of the perforator (Fig. 19.2). Most frequently used method, suggested by Kim et al., indicates a hemi-circle with a radius of 2 cm, drawn 8 cm distally from the midpoint of popliteal crease to the prominence of medial malleolus [4]. Later, this line was frequently used as landmark by other authors. Choi et al. reported that the most sizable perforator was located within a triangle formed by the line from the midpoint of

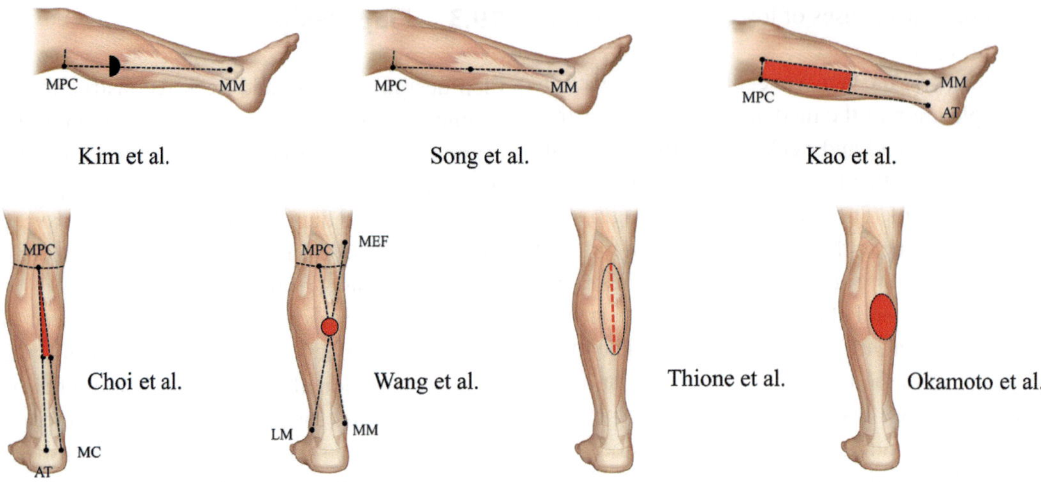

Fig. 19.2 Schematic mapping of medial sural artery perforator. (**a**) Kim et al. indicate a hemi-circle with a radius of 2 cm, drawn 8 cm distally from the midpoint of popliteal crease (MPC) to the prominence of medial malleolus (MM). (**b**) Song et al. searched the perforator around the single point located at the midpoint between Kim's lines. (**c**) Kao et al. used multiple landmarks, which consists of four lines including popliteal crease, line between the MPC and the Achilles tendon (AT), line along the distal border of medial gastrocnemius muscle, and the line from the medial tibial condyle to the prominence of the MM. (**d**) Choi et al. emphasized the closer location of perforator to the midline. They drew a triangle formed by the line from the midpoint of the popliteal crease to the medial calcaneus (MC) and the line from the MPC to the AT. (**e**) Wang et al. drew a circle with a radius of 4 cm centered at the intersection of the line connecting the medial epicondyle of the femur (MEF) and the prominence of the lateral malleolus (LM) and Kim's line. (**f**) Thione et al. suggested that perforators are located within the midline of the medial gastrocnemius muscle. (**g**) Okamoto et al. found the perforators in the distal half of the medial gastrocnemius muscle

the popliteal crease to the medial calcaneus and the line from the midpoint of popliteal crease to the Achilles tendon [10]. In their findings, the sizable perforators were located closer to the midline. Song et al. searched the perforator around the single point located at the midpoint between Kim's lines [11]. Wang et al. drew a circle with a radius of 4 cm centered at the intersection of the line connecting the medial epicondyle of the femur and the prominence of the lateral malleolus and Kim's line [12]. Thione et al. reported that most perforators were located within the midline of the medial gastrocnemius muscle, drawn vertically along the midline of the muscle, while Okamoto et al. reported that most perforators were found in the distal half of the medial gastrocnemius muscle, which showed interracial variance between Asians and Caucasians [1]. Similarly, Pease et al. implied that the location of the popliteal crease might vary among individuals and recommended the use of fibular head and intermuscular septum as fixed landmarks [13]. Kao et al. proposed the use of multiple landmarks to increase the reliability of perforator mapping. The intersection consists of four lines including popliteal crease, line between the midpoint of the popliteal crease and the Achilles tendon, line along the distal border of medial gastrocnemius muscle, and the line from the medial tibial condyle to the prominence of the medial malleolus [5].

19.4 Ultrasound Assessment and Surgical Technique

Preoperatively, the locations of the medial sural perforator flap are marked using handheld Doppler and color duplex ultrasonography. Color duplex ultrasonography is employed to provide localization of the perforators, determine the main course of the pedicle vessel, and assess the surrounding anatomy. In addition, the portable handheld Doppler is used to double-check the location of the perforator immediately before surgery. Both calves are thoroughly evaluated to identify perforators with suitable diameter and flow and to assess the intramuscular course, which facilitates easier dissection with a shorter intramuscular course.

To locate the medial sural artery perforator using duplex ultrasound, the procedure begins with B-mode ultrasound to gain a comprehensive understanding of the anatomy in the medial calf region. The primary focus is on marking the medial border of the gastrocnemius muscle, serving as the initial reference point for the perforator search. Transitioning to the color Doppler setting on the ultrasound machine follows. Fine-tuning the imaging parameters, including depth, gain, and color gain, is essential to achieve optimal visualization of blood flow. The scanning process commences by moving the transducer horizontally along the medial border of the gastrocnemius muscle, progressing from the proximal end, closer to the knee, to the distal end near the ankle. Throughout this process, vigilance is maintained to identify the distinctive appearance of the medial sural artery perforator, typically recognized as a small artery displaying color flow signals that emerge from the deeper tissue layers and extend toward the skin's surface (Fig. 19.3).

One-fourth of the cases are done with two-team approach to avoid unnecessary incision on medial calf area. Getting the lower leg abducted and knee flexed, the elevation of the medial sural flap is undertaken on supine position. After making incision on one side, the perforators are looked for to determine whether it could be used for pedicle or not. And then the other incisions are done to harvest the flap. Subfascial elevations are done. Being cautious not to injure the perforators, the medial sural artery and veins are dissected according to its route. Afterward, the dissection is quite straightforward because the location of the medial sural artery is quite shallow compared to the other perforator flaps. But numerous muscular branches may be encountered. These are ligated with micro-hemoclips or bipolar cauterizations. After getting enough length of pedicle, the flap is completely elevated.

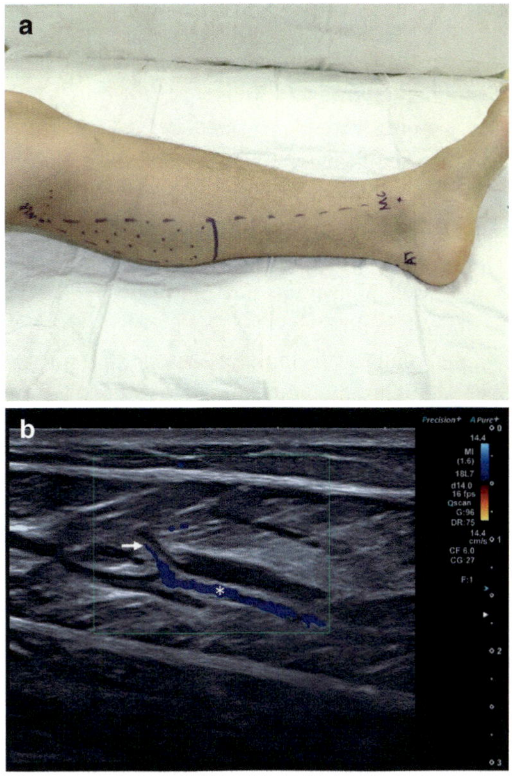

Fig. 19.3 Preoperative ultrasonographic marking. (**a**) Perforators are found in the triangle formed by the line from the midpoint of the popliteal crease to the medial calcaneus and the line from the midpoint of popliteal crease to the Achilles tendon. (**b**) Note the medial sural artery perforator (arrow) arising from the intramuscular course of the medial sural artery

19.5 Case Example

Case 1

One first case was for the reconstruction of the base of the tongue. The first perforator located 6 cm from the popliteal crease along the imaginary line to medial calcaneus was used. The second and third perforators could not be found. The diameter of the perforator was very small, but pulsation was confirmed. The dissection of the medial sural pedicle was done up to the medial popliteal artery. Thus, the end point of the pedicle showed the right-angled shape. Although the vascular flow was a little concerned because of this tortuous route, the circulation of the flap had looked like good after the microanastomosis.

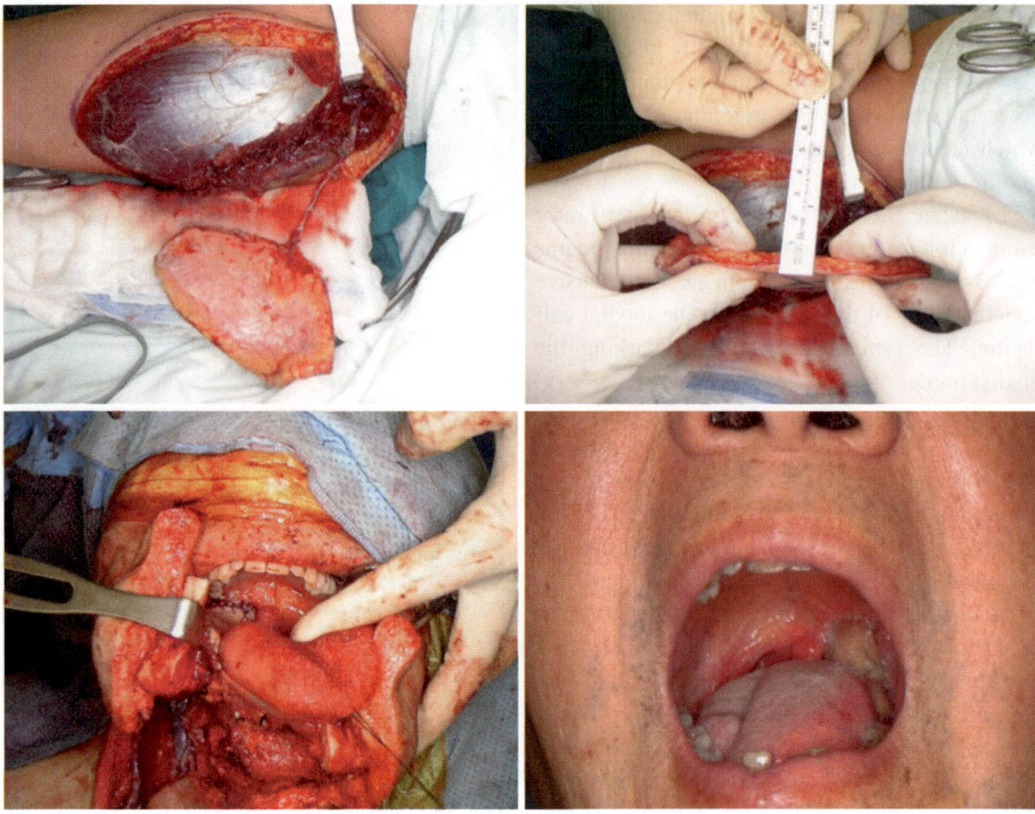

Fig. 19.4 Case 1: Tongue base reconstruction. A perforator located 6 cm from the popliteal crease was used for this case. The flap showed venous congestion at 24 h post-operatively, but salvage operation failed. The flap was taken down and replaced by forearm free flap

But, 24 h after the surgery, the flap became purple abruptly, and the salvage procedure was done but failed. Immediate mouth floor reconstruction was done again with radial forearm free flap. The forearm flap worked very well afterward without any complication or functional deficit (Fig. 19.4).

Case 2

After previous failure, medial sural perforators with less than 1 mm were no more used in my cases, even when the pulsation of the perforators was confirmed. However, if multiple sizable perforators were identified, this could be another indication for successful survival. When a single perforator was used, the diameter of the perforator should be greater than 2 mm. Afterward, no cases failed using medial sural perforator free flaps for the oropharyngeal reconstruction.

This case was done with multiple perforators arising from the first and second perforators located 8 cm and 12 cm from the popliteal crease along the imaginary line to medial calcaneus. A 14-cm-length pedicle was harvested for the reconstruction of the tonsil and soft palate defect (Fig. 19.5).

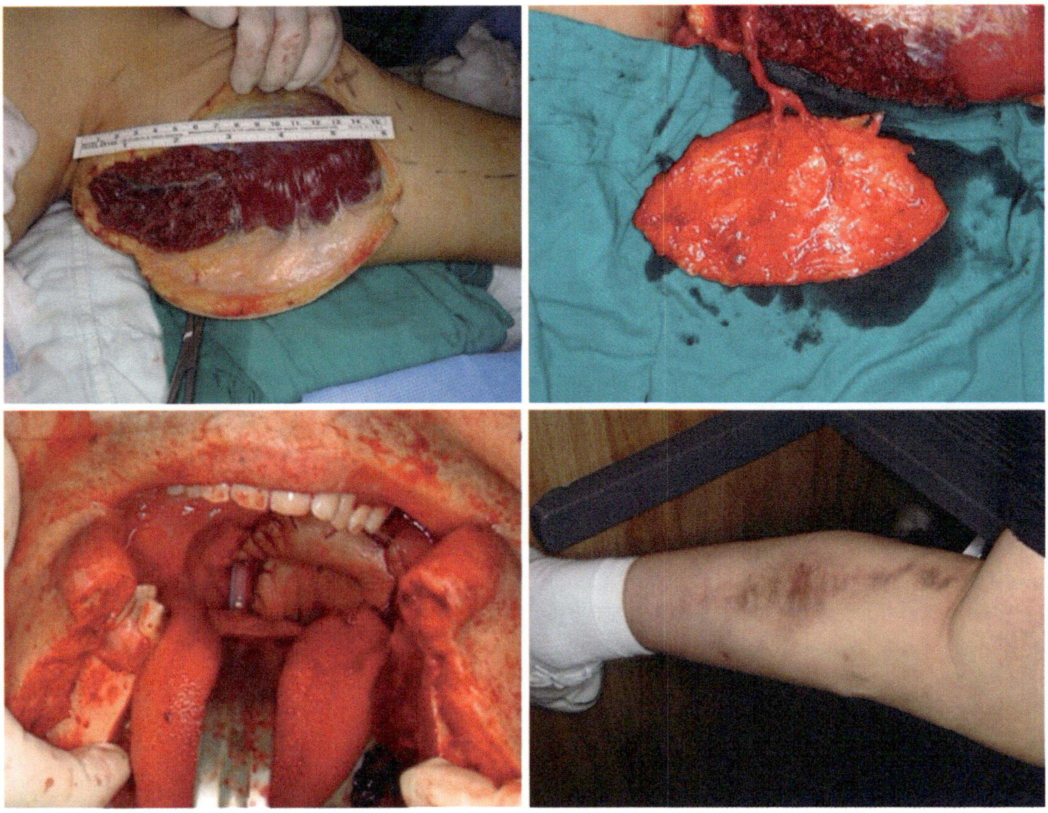

Fig. 19.5 Case 2: Soft palate and tonsil reconstruction. In this case, multiple perforators located 8 and 12 cm from the popliteal crease were used. Obtaining multiple sizable perforators or single large perforator at least 2 mm in diameter allows successful flap survival in head and neck reconstruction. Appearance of donor site scar is acceptable

19.6 Modification

The medial sural artery is known to have two branches, medial and lateral branches. I prefer the medial branch of medial sural perforators for my series. Although sometimes the lateral branch of the medial sural vessels could provide excellent perforators, the medial branch of medial sural vessels seems to provide better sizable perforators in my understanding. Moreover, the proximity to the sural nerve and vein made us to use the simultaneous harvesting of the additional vein source and nerve for venous drainage and sensate or functional flap. In addition, I have tried to dissect as many perforators as possible in order to ensure the flap survival in cases of head and neck reconstructions because the vascular setting around neck area might cause the rotations or kinking of the vessels. And the wound problems due to the flap failure for head and neck reconstructions could delay the postoperative radiotherapy or chemotherapy, which might result in failure of whole management of head and neck cancer.

19.7 Pitfalls

Because the technique using the perforator free flaps has evolved quite enormously recently, various new perforator flaps have been introduced [2, 14–17]. Therefore, the microsurgeons tend to try the new perforator flap more frequently than before. Although the freestyle perforator-based free flaps are getting popularity, it must be true that the surgeon should know the characteristic trait in vascular anatomy according to the variety of the legions. As the freestyle perforator-based free flaps have been emphasized too much, the specific information regarding the anatomic locations or vascular territories tends to be easily ignored in recent era. But, without the basic knowledge of these, there seems to exist the possibility to get in trouble for successful applications of the newly introduced perforator flaps [18–20].

The failed two cases of the medial sural perforator free flaps for oropharyngeal reconstructions seem like related to these pitfalls. Regarding the first failed case, we found the first and second perforators on the medial aspect of the calf. The diameter of the first perforator was larger than that of the second perforator. Thus, we chose the first perforator for pedicle. But the first perforator was too short for mouth floor reconstruction. In our experience, first perforators were useful for tonsil reconstruction where direct route exists from the recipient vessel to the tonsillar area. On the contrary, the perforator flaps for hemitongue defect or mouth floor defect seem to need the second or third perforator in terms of the length of the total pedicle because the route to the perforator flaps from the recipient vessel should follow the neck, tongue base, and finally tongue and mouth floor. A length of 5–6 cm is often too short to be used for mouth floor reconstruction close to the symphysis area. Because the perforator vessel should route in tortuous course in the head and neck area, the shortage of the length in the pedicle would contain the higher risk for failure. We seemed to ignore this fact. In addition to this, we had tried to get more length of pedicle through the dissection up to the dividing ends of the medial and lateral branch of the medial sural arteries as possible. But this might endanger the perforator flap because of the turbulent flow on the ligated dividing vessel branches.

The failure of the second case would be owing to the selection of the non-sizable perforator. In this case, when first and third perforators were not found, we have better stop the elevation and try other options instead. We overestimated the meaning of the pulsation of the perforator than the diameter at that time. That seems to be the reason why we failed the application of the medial sural perforator free flap for oropharyngeal reconstruction.

Medial sural perforator free flaps could be one more alternative in case of medium-sized defects in which radial forearm or ALT perforator free flaps would not be adequate in point of flap volumes.

19.8 Further Readings

Further discussions can be made regarding the versatile use of this flap with chimeric design. Recently, several studies have reported the chimeric concept of supplying different perforators to the skin paddles and gastrocnemius muscle in different types of head and neck region [21, 22]. Versatile application of chimeric design has been made for reconstruction of tongue, pharyngoesophageal, and oropharyngeal defects. The chimeric design allows for reconstruction of the three-dimensional structures and prevention of the fistula formation and provides inner resurfacing for frozen neck and mobile units for functional reconstruction.

Basically, this chimeric flap includes skin paddle and muscle part. The concept of chimeric flap can be also used to create two skin paddles based on distinct skin perforator. Furthermore, surrounding tissue can be used as composite flaps, such as plantaris tendon for sling structure, sural nerves for cutaneous innervation, and saphenous vein for vein graft. The muscle itself can be used to obliterate dead space or can be used as functional component by motor nerve innervation.

The application of chimeric medial sural perforator flap is based on predictable and reliable anatomy of the flap. The medial sural artery originates directly from the popliteal artery or common sural artery and descends to the medial head of the gastrocnemius muscle. Along the course of medial sural artery, it has usually two opposite branches, the medial and lateral branches. The medial branch of medial sural artery which supplies the medial gastrocnemius muscle part can be used as muscle part of the flap, while the perforators from opposite lateral branch are used for supplying the skin paddle. To do this, maximal length of pedicle should be dissected beyond the dividing ends of the medial and lateral branch of the medial sural artery. When sufficient length of the pedicle is not assured, the pedicle may be kinked or twisted during inset of the chimeric components, jeopardizing the flap survival.

The chimeric flap allows the best restoration of oral and pharyngeal functions, such as swallowing, speech, and tongue mobility [11, 23]. Speech and swallowing functions are highly related with thickness and extensibility of the flap. The speech intelligibility and articulation require fine control of tongue movement, thus requiring pliable and easily stretched tissues, while swallowing function is related with adequate bulk in tongue base reconstruction. Thin to moderate thickness of the skin paddle allows best restoration of oropharyngeal and pharyngo-esophageal defect, where too bulky tissue can be a disadvantage, restricting tongue and pharyngeal movement. The chimeric medial sural perforator flap meets these requirements. The thickness and volume of the skin paddle can be adjusted according to the extent of the defect. When tissue bulk is required or dead space occurs, such as in tongue base and mouth floor, muscle flaps can be added in the internal aspect of the flap. When the oral commissure is involved, the plantaris tendon can be easily harvested between the gastrocnemius and the soleus muscle and used for static suspension of the lip against the gravity.

Related with donor site functions, this flap is often compared with conventional fasciocutaneous flap, the radial forearm flap. The donor site morbidity of the medial sural perforator flap includes sensory disturbance and muscular weakness. This may occur when skin graft coverage is required for larger flap coverage or when the gastrocnemius muscle has been damaged. Mostly, overall donor site morbidities were higher in the traditional option [24, 25]. The radial forearm free flap always requires skin graft and is often related with conspicuous scar in the forearm, with temporary weakness. Sometimes, tendon exposure and sensory deficits, or numbness, may be problematic. Compared with the radial forearm, the donor site scar of the medial sural perforator flap is located in the posterior aspect of the lower leg, and sometimes primary closure can be achieved if the skin is lax.

19.9 Conclusion

The medial sural perforator flap is a good alternative for small- to medium-sized defect in head and neck reconstruction. This flap allows three-dimensional reconstruction of intraoral and pharyngeal structure, owing to its pliable nature to be easily folded and curved, and functional restoration of the oropharyngeal region, with adequate bulkiness to facilitate swallowing and speaking. Comprehensive understanding of the pedicle anatomy and mapping the sizable perforator can ensure the success of the flap survival. Furthermore, chimeric medial sural artery perforator flap can be used for complex head and neck defects to provide adequate tissue bulk and functional restoration.

References

1. Okamoto H, Sekiya I, Mizutani J, Otsuka T. Anatomical basis of the medial sural artery perforator flap in Asians. Scand J Plast Reconstr Surg Hand Surg. 2007;41(3):125–9.
2. Cavadas PC, Sanz-Giménez-Rico JR, Gutierrez-de la Cámara A, Navarro-Monzonís A, Soler-Nomdedeu S, Martínez-Soriano F. The medial sural artery perforator free flap. Plast Reconstr Surg. 2001;108(6):1609–15; discussion 16–7.
3. Thione A, Valdatta L, Buoro M, Tuinder S, Mortarino C, Putz R. The medial sural artery perforators: anatomic basis for a surgical plan. Ann Plast Surg. 2004;53(3):250–5.
4. Kim HH, Jeong JH, Seul JH, Cho BC. New design and identification of the medial sural perforator flap: an anatomical study and its clinical applications. Plast Reconstr Surg. 2006;117(5):1609–18.
5. Kao HK, Chang KP, Chen YA, Wei FC, Cheng MH. Anatomical basis and versatile application of the free medial sural artery perforator flap for head and neck reconstruction. Plast Reconstr Surg. 2010;125(4):1135–45.

6. Scher RL, Esclamado RM. Organ and function preservation: the role of surgery as the optimal primary modality or as salvage after chemoradiation failure. Semin Radiat Oncol. 2009;19(1):17–23.
7. Mowry SE, Ho A, Lotempio MM, Sadeghi A, Blackwell KE, Wang MB. Quality of life in advanced oropharyngeal carcinoma after chemoradiation versus surgery and radiation. Laryngoscope. 2006;116(9):1589–93.
8. Arce K, Bell RB, Potter JK, Buehler MJ, Potter BE, Dierks EJ. Vascularized free tissue transfer for reconstruction of ablative defects in oral and oropharyngeal cancer patients undergoing salvage surgery following concomitant chemoradiation. Int J Oral Maxillofac Surg. 2012;41(6):733–8.
9. Sewnaik A, Keereweer S, Al-Mamgani A, Baatenburg de Jong RJ, Wieringa MH, Meeuwis CA, et al. High complication risk of salvage surgery after chemoradiation failures. Acta Otolaryngol. 2012;132(1):96–100.
10. Choi JW, Nam SY, Choi SH, Roh JL, Kim SY, Hong JP. Applications of medial sural perforator free flap for head and neck reconstructions. J Reconstr Microsurg. 2013;29(7):437–42.
11. Song X, Wu H, Zhang W, Chen J, Ding X, Ye J, et al. Medial sural artery perforator flap for postsurgical reconstruction of head and neck cancer. J Reconstr Microsurg. 2015;31(4):319–26.
12. Wang X, Mei J, Pan J, Chen H, Zhang W, Tang M. Reconstruction of distal limb defects with the free medial sural artery perforator flap. Plast Reconstr Surg. 2013;131(1):95–105.
13. Pease NL, Ong J, Townley WA. Fixed reference points in mapping medial sural artery perforator location. J Plast Reconstr Aesthet Surg. 2015;68(4):589–90.
14. Hallock GG. Anatomic basis of the gastrocnemius perforator-based flap. Ann Plast Surg. 2001;47(5):517–22.
15. Hallock GG. The medial sural (medial gastrocnemius) perforator local flap. Ann Plast Surg. 2004;53(5):501–5.
16. Sano K, Hallock GG, Hamazaki M, Daicyo Y. The perforator-based conjoint (chimeric) medial sural (medial gastrocnemius) free flap. Ann Plast Surg. 2004;53(6):588–92.
17. Chen SL, Yu CC, Chang MC, Deng SC, Wu YS, Chen TM. Medial sural artery perforator flap for intraoral reconstruction following cancer ablation. Ann Plast Surg. 2008;61(3):274–9.
18. Lin CH, Lin YT, Hsu CC, Ng TW, Wei FC. The medial sural artery perforator flap: a versatile donor site for hand reconstruction. J Trauma. 2011;70(3):736–43.
19. Mao C, Zhang L, Cui QJ, Peng X, Wang Y, Yu GY. [A preliminary study on free medial sural artery perforator flap for head and neck reconstruction following tumor ablation]. Zhonghua Kou Qiang Yi Xue Za Zhi. 2011;46(12):742–746.
20. Xie XT, Chai YM. Medial sural artery perforator flap. Ann Plast Surg. 2012;68(1):105–10.
21. Lee CH, Chang NT, Hsiao JC, Chu YY, Lin CH, Kao HK, et al. Extended use of chimeric medial sural artery perforator flap for 3-dimensional defect reconstruction. Ann Plast Surg. 2019;82(1S Suppl 1):S86–94.
22. Ooi ASH, Ng MJM, Sudirman SRB, Chang D. The chimeric medial sural artery perforator flap as the ideal for partial tongue reconstruction: a case series and technical refinements. J Plast Reconstr Aesthet Surg. 2021;74(10):2613–21.
23. Mughal M, Gabuniya N, Zoccali G, Roblin P, Townley W. Functional outcomes of the medial sural artery perforator flap in oral cavity reconstruction. Ann Plast Surg. 2020;85(3):256–9.
24. Kao HK, Chang KP, Wei FC, Cheng MH. Comparison of the medial sural artery perforator flap with the radial forearm flap for head and neck reconstructions. Plast Reconstr Surg. 2009;124(4):1125–32.
25. Ng MJM, Goh CSL, Tan NC, Song DH, Ooi ASH. A head-to-head comparison of the medial sural artery perforator versus radial forearm flap for tongue reconstruction. J Reconstr Microsurg. 2021;37(5):445–52.

Part V

Section E. application for lymphedema surgery - *will review all applicable modalities for these approaches, which is the most valuable modality?. It is talking about the algorithm of application imaging*

Finding Functional Lymphatic Vessels

20

Alessandro Bianchi and Giuseppe Visconti

20.1 Introduction

Imaging techniques for visualisation of the lymphatic system are less developed than those for imaging of the vascular system for two main reasons. First, the lymphatic system is more difficult to "make visible". It is not apparent to the naked eye, even under the microscope, and its organisation as a one-way transport network makes the entire system impossible to enhance with a single injection. Thus, the imaging of the lymphatic system is traditionally performed after interstitial (e.g. intradermal, subcutaneous, intramuscular) injections of tracers, and several factors must be taken into account to enable efficient uptake by the lymphatics of that specific tissue. Second, the importance of the lymphatic system in health and disease has been historically underappreciated [1].

Lymphatic vessels were among the latest macroscopical structures to become visible to anatomists, and while the lymph nodes have been dissected and mapped since the ancient times [2, 3], even nowadays the identification of these tiny, colourless and impalpable structures represents the key point of lymphatic surgery [4].

The advances in lymphatic imaging have represented the driving force for the improvement in lymphatic surgery, as well as for the comprehension of the lymphedema itself. As the physiopathology of lymphedema was progressively understood, it became clear that the key to success in physiologic surgery was not merely the localisation of lymphatic vessels to perform LVA [5] but the identification of functional lymphatics and even more of the appropriate collectors among the functional ones [6].

This concept applies also to the transfer of lymphatic tissues, as all the hypothesis about the mechanisms of action shares a common point: vial and active lymphatics must be included in the transplant to make it effective [7–20].

The recent trend to localise functional lymphatics to maximise the efficacy of LVA surgery leads to enormous changes in LVA indications, preoperative planning and execution, and the present classifications and staging systems of lymphedema are losing their clinical significance.

As such, this chapter will leave out scores and stages, as every lymphedema patient needs a customised treatment planning, and focus on the only question still important nowadays: can you find functional, overloaded, propulsive lymphatic that can be used for LVA?

A. Bianchi · G. Visconti (✉)
UO Chirurgia Plastica, Dipartimento Scienze Salute della Donna, del Bambino e Sanità Pubblica—Fondazione Policlinico Gemelli IRCCS—Largo Agostino Gemelli, Rome, Italy

J. P. Hong et al. (eds.), *Imaging for Reconstructive Microsurgery*,
https://doi.org/10.1007/978-981-97-7278-0_20

20.2 Imaging of Functional Lymphatic Vessels for Lymphedema Evaluation and Surgical Planning

The identification of functional lymphatic vessels has its role in the evaluation of lymphedema, in deciding the appropriate treatment path and in the preoperative planning for LVA to select the lymphatic vessels suitable for anastomosis.

Traditionally, patients who demonstrate pitting oedema and responsiveness to nonsurgical therapy are favourable candidates for physiologic procedures. This is because these clinical findings correspond to a disease stage characterised by the accumulation of lymphatic fluid caused by structural lymphatic defects that can be corrected through LVA or lymphatic tissue transfer. On the other hand, in more advanced lymphedema, the main feature is an increased adiposity and ablative surgery is indicated [20]. While this concept may be true in some cases, the clinical expression of lymphedema is strongly related to the lifestyle of each patient, the adaptive response of the lymphatic system to injury/malformation and the efficacy of the decongestive therapy, so the clinical features may not always be an accurate indicator of the disease progression phase [17].

Lymphatic vessels are becoming more and more visible nowadays, so the indirect signs of their presence cannot be considered anymore the criterion to offer patients the big chance of undergoing physiologic surgery.

Traditionally, LVA was considered indicated in early to moderate lymphedema cases, while the advanced diseases were candidates for lymphatic tissue transfer. Nowadays, the lymphatic imaging showed how lymphatic vessels can be detected also in advanced lymphedema that can hide the presence of large functional collectors, suitable for LVA. Advanced lymphedema cases were not devoid of lymphatic vessels, it was the imaging technology inapt to find them; thus, the present contrast-based staging systems cannot be employed anymore in deciding the treatment plan of each patient [6].

The lymphatic system of each patient must nowadays be "seen" and understood, and the treatment plan customised to its features. The imaging modalities that are presently employed for this purpose are lymphoscintigraphy, near-infrared fluorescence lymphangiography, magnetic resonance lymphangiography, ultrasound imaging and photoacoustic imaging.

The technical details and the interpretation methods of these modalities have been treated elsewhere in this book, so this chapter will focus on their applicability to the identification of functional lymphatics.

The ideal imaging modality should offer a comprehensive evaluation of the lymphatic function of the affected area, give an in-depth visualisation of lymphatic vessel anatomy and detect lymphatic functionality, show the course in three dimensions and together display the venous network that will function as an anastomotic acceptor site [21]. None of the imaging modalities encompasses all the need for the evaluation and treatment of lymphedema, so they have to be combined to obtain the appropriate answers to the questions that each lymphedema case may pose.

20.3 Lymphoscintigraphy

Of all the imaging modalities for lymphedema, lymphoscintigraphy has been used for the longest period of time. Every patient with clinical suspect of lymphedema should undergo lymphoscintigraphy, which is nowadays considered the gold standard for functional evaluation of the lymphatic system and has characteristics that make it an ideal first-level examination [1, 22].

With a gamma camera, whole-body images are obtained to get a gross overview of the lymphatic uptake of a 99m-technetium-labeled contrast agent.

The standard lymphoscintigraphy method is represented by the rest subcutaneous lymphoscintigraphy (SubQ-RL). After colloid injection, two imagings are usually acquired: early and late scans. Early scans may take up to 30–60 min, whereas late scans are acquired from 3 to 6 h from injection [23]. Several qualitative and quantitative parameters may categorise patients into severity types. The qualitative information contributes to adequate diagnosis and staging including the visualisation of the inguinal or axially lymph nodes, the lymphatic vessels, the lymphatic leakage into the subcutaneous tissue and the uptake in popliteal or antecubital nodes [22]. Although the acquired images are typically low resolution, their qualitative analysis provides descriptive information about the symmetry of the tracer uptake in the lymphatics and lymph nodes of the healthy and lymphedematous limb, as well as the presence of dermal backflow [24, 25]. Quantitative parameters reflect the overall functionality of the lymphatic system by assessing the lymph transport and are derived primarily from the arrival time in the proximal lymph nodes (transit time TT or tracer appearance time) or clearance rate from the injection site. The transport index is a scoring of several subjective observations indicating the normal or abnormal lymphatics [23].

Although SubQ-RL is the most diffuse method, it shows several limitations, as it is a time-consuming exam, with poor imaging resolution due to high background activity from injection sites, and makes very difficult also an interpretation of results and transport index (TI) evaluation. The more recent intradermal rest-stress lymphoscintigraphy (ID-RSL) is able to overcome some limitations of standard RSL. Diluted 99mTC-nanocolloids in neutral pH solution are intradermally injected into the first digital space of hand and/or foot for limbs evaluations. The acquisition protocol takes less than 1 h only, and it is differentiated in rest scan (within the first 10 min), stress scan (after 2 min of exercise) and late scan (30–60 min after injection). This acquisition protocol is based on the evidence that a healthy limb shows symmetric visualisation of locoregional nodes (axillary or inguinal) with stress scan (within 10–12 min after injection) compared to a lymphedematous limb where the trace appearance time (TAT) is delayed or absent. Moreover, ID-RSL provides higher resolution images with minimal background activity, qualitative data such as stagnation points, more precise visualisation of dermal backflow areas, compensation phenomena as well as dynamic data such as intrinsic lymphatic pump (rest), combined intrinsic and extrinsic function (stress) and lymphedema diffusion (late) [23]. The main limitations of ID-RSL are bidimensional and gross imaging, but it still allows the instrumental diagnosis of lymphedema and the evaluation of lymphatic system impairment and residual function (Figs. 20.1 and 20.2).

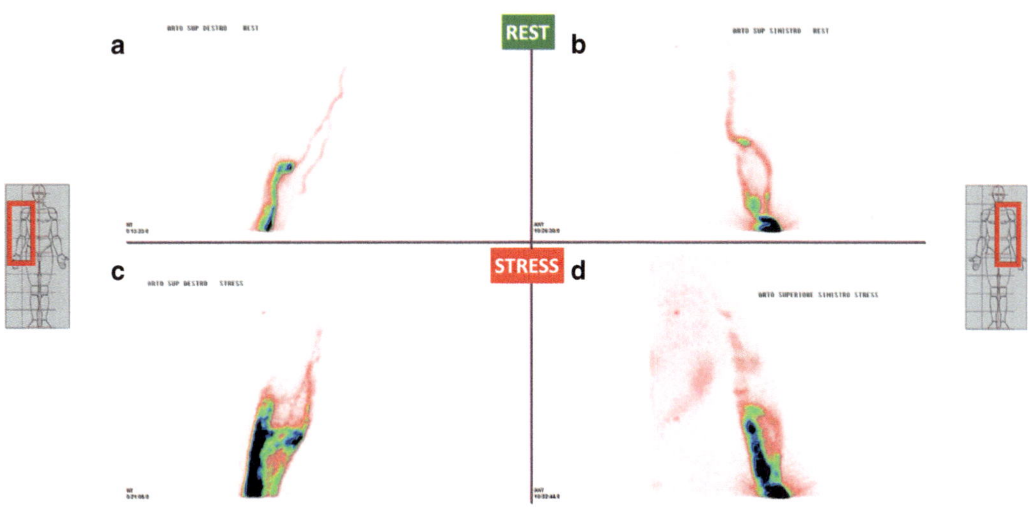

Fig. 20.1 Upper limbs. Rest scans (**a**, right; **b**, left); stress scans (**c**, right; **d**, left). Female, 74-year-old, BMI = 23. Bilateral BCRL (clinical stage 2), right ALND 0/33, left ALND 0/17, CH, RT. Rest scan shows the lymphatic collector along right cephalic vein (**a**) and a collateral in the left forearm (**b**). Stress scans show a dermal backflow of right forearm (**c**) and a tracer stagnation in the left forearm in basilic region. (With permission, From Hayashi and Visconti [4])

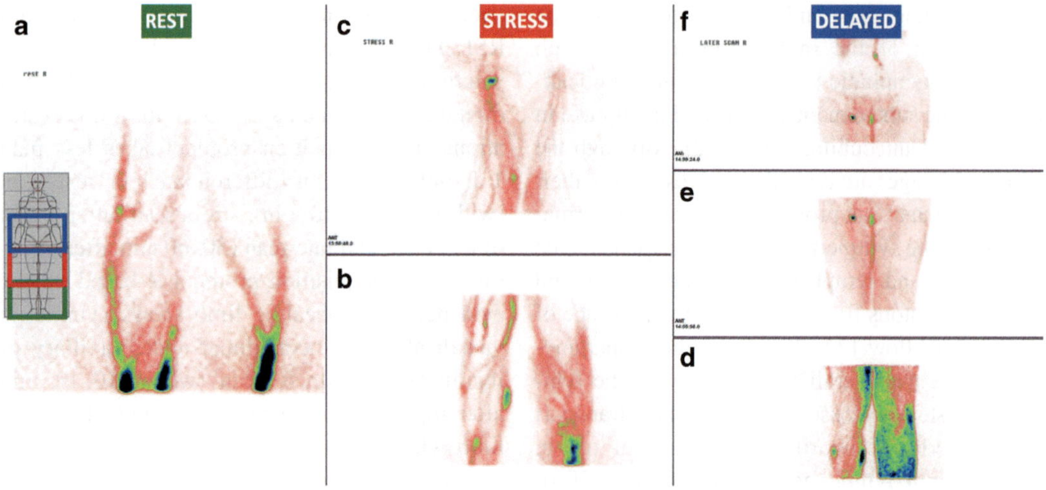

Fig. 20.2 Lower limbs. Rest scan (**a**, legs); stress scans (**b**, legs; **c**, thighs); delayed scans (**d**, legs; **e**, thighs; **c**, iliac region). Female, 48-year-old, BMI = 24. Endometrial cancer, PLND 2/26, CH, RT. Rest scan shows a tract of lymphatic collector along small saphena. Stress scans show the presence of collaterals. Delayed scans show dermal backflow of left leg and uptake of superior iliac nodes. (With permission, From Hayashi and Visconti [4])

For the purpose of finding functional lymphatics, lymphoscintigraphy has to be intended as a first-level screening examination. The exam is not time-consuming for the surgeon, so it can be requested to all patients with clinical suspect of lymphedema. If dilated lymphatic collectors can be visualised at this examination, the patient can be candidate to LVA and will undergo further examinations at the moment of the surgical planning. In case of primary lymphedema, it can show if the impairment is assimilable to an obstructive pattern and thus is eligible for LVA without other investigations. It can also highlight compensation pathways, like the Mascagni path for upper limb lymphedema, that can be not equally clear with the other imaging modalities, thus indicating what not to touch during LVA.

20.4 Near-Infrared Fluorescence Lymphography

Near-infrared fluorescence lymphography (NIRF-L), most commonly named indocyanine green lymphography (ICG-L), uses the fluorescence properties of indocyanine green for real-time visualisation of the lymphatic vessels and to assess the global function of the lymphatic system of the investigated area. This noninvasive and radiation-free tool is an effective modality for the evaluation of lymph circulation and the diagnosis of lymphedema and provides useful information for LVA, as it allows a live visualisation of superficial lymphatic channels before dermal backflow takes space. This is especially true in patients with early to mild lymphedema. The possibility to mark lymphatic channels on the skin allows to optimise skin incision locations and may aid the surgeon during the procedure [26]..

ICG is an optical tracer agent (water-soluble tricarbocyanine dye with around 5% of sodium iodide), and the fluorescent images are digitalised by infrared camera devices. ICG imaging can detect lymphatic channels located up to 2 cm deep from the skin surface if there is no fascia, muscle or bone above the channels. So normal ICG-L shows superficial lymphatic channels (collectors, precollectors and capillaries) [27]. ICG-L findings are classified into two patterns: linear and dermal backflow (DB) patterns, the latter one including the splash, stardust and diffuse patterns. Linear pattern is more frequently observed in normal limbs and mild lymphedema cases [27]. Nevertheless, linear patterns can be transitorily observed also in moderate and severe cases in thinner areas and before DB takes space. DB patterns represent the pathologic sign of lymphedema; it can both arise from linear patterns and be the only progression modality of the tracer, in case no functional collectors are still visible with this imaging modality. The splash pattern consists of scattered dye twinkling in thin lines and tortuous lymphatic channels [27]. It expresses an early stage of lymphedema in which valves between lymphatic collectors and precollectors collapse and reverse flow from the collectors to the precollectors occurs [27]. The stardust pattern demonstrates dimly luminous, spotted fluorescent signals. It occurs with progression of lymphedema, the reverse flow through the efferent precollectors generates the typical spotted image. In diffuse pattern, the dye is widely distributed, without twinkling or identifiable spots. The number of spots visualised on ICG-L increases to the point that they merge and cannot be distinguished from each other [27].

The severity staging based on the proximal to distal extension of different DB correlates with the clinical classifications of lymphedema and has been used to select the appropriate treatment option.

LVA was considered not as effective as in earlier stages because the function of the lymphatic channels is already lost. Actually, nowadays, even patients with diffuse pattern can undergo tremendous improvements if overloaded, yet functional collectors can be identified with other imaging modalities [6].

ICG-L has nowadays a worldwide diffusion and is the most used tool per LVA preoperative planning. This is comprehensive, as it is real time, easy to use, directly performed by the operating surgeon and safe, and it can detect lymphatic channels as linear patterns that can be marked directly on patient's skin. But even if identification of lymphatic vessels as fluorescent linear patterns is possible in most cases of mild to moderate lymphedema, ICG lymphography cannot show lymphatic flow in deep layers or if masked beneath dermal backflow pattern, and it is contraindicated in iodine-allergic patients. It has been also reported the possibility of functional lymphatic evaluation by visualising the pulsatile behaviour of lymphatics, but this is true in an even minor subset of early lymphedema patients [21].

So behind a linear pattern, many questions stay unsolved, including how deep is the lymphatic channel, where exactly in relation with other structures, how many lymphatics do actually correspond to a single fluorescent line, how ectatic and how propulsive they are. Moreover, there is a total absence of information about the tissues.

Still, this is the era of the direct visualisation of functional lymphatics, and ICG-L, despite it being of great value as the only option for preoperative LVA planning for a decade, has the limits of being an indirect enhancement of the lymphatic channels.

On the other hand, this exam is a fundamental first approach for the location of functional lymphatics, as it keeps a comprehensive overview of the limb whole system function, giving information about the affected area (extension and origin of DB) and the selected channels, whether they have been selected by ICG-L itself or by more recent methodologies.

20.5 Magnetic Resonance Lymphangiography

Magnetic resonance lymphangiography (MRL) imaging is performed after the interstitial injection of gadolinium-based contrast agents that create a positive enhancement signal. Owing to the high imaging depth of MRI, 3D volumetric images of the lymphatic vasculature can be obtained, and the images obtained from MRL depict lymphatic anatomy with a high spatial and temporal resolution without radiation exposure [21]. Compared to ICG-L, also MRL provides data regarding location and transport capacity of lymphatic channels and the presence and extension of dermal backflow, but in adjunct to ICG-L MRL gives an image of the entire limb, quantity and quality of the superficial and deep lymphatics and a three-dimensional image that can be critically reviewed by the surgeon in the preoperative evaluation [28].

MRL is a direct visualisation tool and, as such, gives information not only on the lymphatic vessels but also on the limb tissues, in terms of liquid versus fatty and fibrotic accumulation [29].

The functional lymphatics are identified as the structures that take and transport the contrast agent, the calibre can be calculated and they can be simultaneously highlighted from the origin to the lymph nodes or the most proximal point before their closure [28].

The reproducibility of the images and their translation to clinical use depend on the standardised placement of the patient into the MR machine, and to create a system of coordinates (generally the position in relation to palpable bony structures), that may vary from one centre to another, so that the surgeon can transpose the radiological information on patients' skin. In this planar coordinate system, the depth is added, thanks to the 3D images [1].

The literature showed that in the same patient MRL is able to identify more lymphatics, and this is comprehensible considering the depth possibility of this tool. The decision about the point where to interrupt the lymphatic vessels can take into account the relationship with a fluid oedematous area, the most proximal point before its interruption, and there is the possibility to spare the healthy lymphatics by considering that they are the ones that go from the origin to the lymph nodes with no interruptions [28].

MRL can be used also to localise the recipient venule, with the same coordinate system. According to different centres, this may be performed by a double contrast injection or with a single injection and an appropriate processing of the acquired images [4].

Also some morphological features may help the radiologist in discerning the lymphatic vessels from the vascular structures.

Non-contrast MRI lymphography has been used for imaging of the lymphatic system. The use of heavily T2-wighted sequences for the imaging allows for highlighting the signal from the stagnant fluid in the tissues and in the lymphatics while depressing the signs from the tissue itself, so giving information about the localisation of the oedema or the leak in the lymphatics. However, non-contrast MRI is able to make the lymphatic vessels visible only when they become dilated and filled with stagnant fluid [21].

MRI lymphangiography is a useful adjunct to ICG-L, allowing the identification of lymphatics that are invisible to ICG, and adds information about the whole lymphatic system and the tissues, and the tridimensional mapping allows for the localisation of recipient venules as well.

On the other hand, this exam is not directly performed by the surgeon, requires a strong radiologic collaboration and above all is not a live examination.

The application to venule mapping has many limitations, as magnetic resonance is not the exam of choice for the venous system, the study of venous dynamics cannot be performed and this is a fundamental part of LVA surgery.

20.6 Ultrahigh-Frequency Ultrasound

The idea of applying the ultrasound (US) to the lymphatic system derives from its usage in the venous preoperative mapping for LVA, as ultrasound examination is the gold standard to study the venous dynamics. The superiority of US for venule selection compared to all the other available tools is clear, and this is a critical aspect as the venules are as important as lymphatics for the efficacy of LVA [30].

The introduction of conventional high-frequency ultrasound (CHFUS) first and ultrahigh-frequency ultrasound (UHFUS) later revealed a powerful tool for the identification of functional lymphatic vessels, as it is a direct visualisation method, performed by the operating surgeon, that is radiation-free and real time, with an in-depth analysis of lymphatic vessel anatomy and dynamic function. Moreover, it is the only non-contrast-based tool, so it does not depend on the choice of injection sites and on the characteristics of the selected contrast agent [31–34].

The adjunct of CHFUS to ICG-L allowed to overcome the limitations of ICG lymphography as it detects lymphatic vessels masked by dermal backflow patterns or located in deeper layers and can be performed in iodine-allergic patients. Furthermore, CHFUS added new information, as it clarifies relationship with the skin and surrounding tissues and structures, and this is very useful for lymphatic surgeons. However, CHFUS may be very difficult and, above all, still lacked an in-depth evaluation of lymphatic functionality [32].

The introduction of ultrahigh-frequency ultrasound (UHFUS), with frequencies as high as 70 MHz and resolution as fine as 30 μm, permits more precise detection of small-sized anatomical structures. UHFUS provides unprecedented clear images of the lymphatic vessels along with valuable dynamic information. The resolution is that high that evaluation of wall thickness compared to the lumen diameter is possible, and lymphatic fluids moving inside the lumen and functioning valve can be visualised in some cases [19, 31].

Lymphatic channels show as intermittent homogeneous, hypoechoic and specular misshapen images in sagittal B-mode with no colour seen with colour Doppler mode. Lymphatic vessels show no convergence seen with arteries, venules and nerves and are less likely to collapse when pressure is applied to the skin with the transducer, and the expansion of functional lymphatic vessels can be observed with the same manoeuvre.

The accuracy of UHFUS in detecting the lymphatic vessels preoperatively and the anatomic characteristic showed to be comparable to direct histologic evaluation [35].

The whole limb can be scanned, for how long and all the times that the surgeon needs, and the real-time evaluation allows to observe a lymphatic channel from different perspectives, as well as directly observe the spontaneous contractions and dilations of propulsive lymphatics. The channels can be followed from the origin to their end point in the lymph nodes, or it is possible to observe the course up to the calibre restriction and closure of the lumens when they are blocked [4] (Figs. 20.3, 20.4 and 20.5).

Instead of generating a standard staging system, US has been used to classify the lymphatic collectors in lymphedema into two types, based on the functionality of the lymphatic collectors.

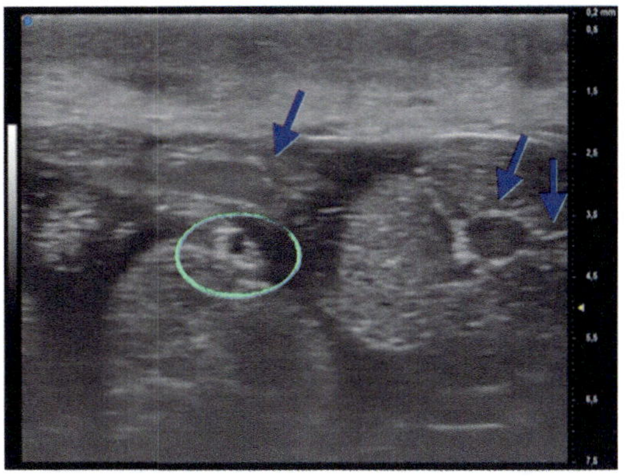

Fig. 20.3 The lymphatic channel found on ulnar side of forearm is circled in green. Notice the severe swelling. A suitable recipient venule with two branches (blue arrows) has been found nearby the lymphatic channel. Notice also the precious anatomic preoperative information get. One of the vein branches is passing above the lymphatic channel. So we already know how to proceed with dissection before opening the wound. (With permission, From Hayashi and Visconti [4])

Type 1 (or functional) lymphatics include the ectatic channels and dilated propulsive channels with high lymph flux, and type 2 lymphatics refer to lymphatics with an advanced degeneration status that show a thick wall compared to the lumen, not expandable even under stimuli [35].

The application of UHFUS to advanced lymphedema cases revealed the ability to detect functional lymphatics also in patients with a total absence of lymphatics at lymphoscintigraphy and no linear pattern at ICG-L. [6]

The reported limitations of UHFUS are the in-depth penetration and the operator dependency [21].

The 70 MHz probe has a penetration of 1 cm, and the 48 MHz probe of 2,5 cm. But as the examination is real time and dynamic, the probe can be pushed against the tissues reducing the thickness and at the same time expanding the functional channels while causing the collapse of the vascular structures. So the 70 MHz probe can be used distally also in advanced cases, and the 48 MHz probe also in the most proximal areas.

US has a demanding learning curve compared to the other modalities and is obviously operator-dependent.

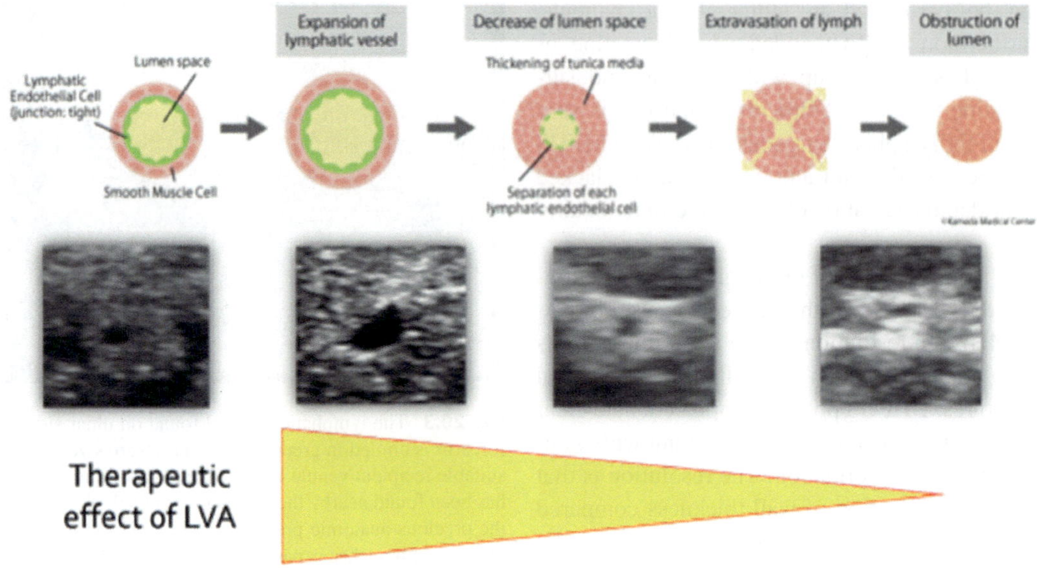

Fig. 20.4 Evaluation of degenerative status in the lymphatic vessels using UHFUS. High echoic region around the low echoic region shows degenerative status of smooth muscle cells and hyperplasia of collagenous fibres in the lymphatic vessels. (With permission, From Hayashi and Visconti [4])

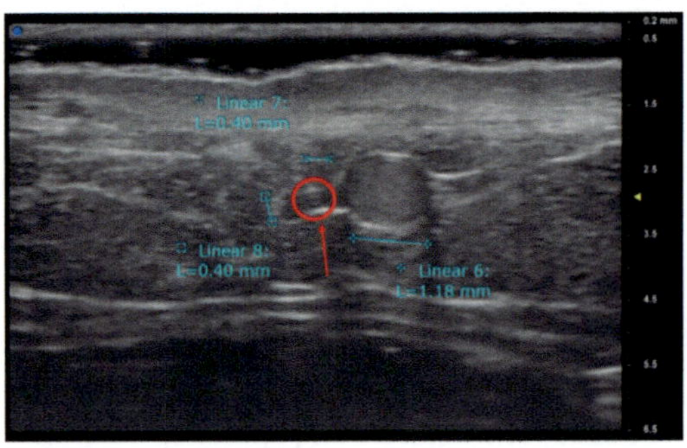

Fig. 20.5 Selection of the appropriate vein for LVA using UHFUS. Appropriate vein which is the branch of main trunk and has valve for LVA (red circle) can be selected using UHFUS preoperatively

20.7 Conclusions

The actual trend in lymphedema surgery is toward a personalised surgery, featured on each patient's characteristics, with incision sites unique for each individual and established on the base of the preoperative selection of propulsive lymphatics and reflux-free venules.

Lymphoscintigraphy is a useful first-level examination, in most cases sufficient to select the patient candidate to LVA, and provides a useful global system assessment. ICG-L represents a second-level examination in cases where the scintigraphic examination is not diriment and is the first important step in the preoperative planning. It combines a real-time whole-system assessment and the anatomical localisation of lymphatic channels, but its limitations make it reductive to stand alone in the preoperative planning of LVA.

The direct visualisation tools, including the contrast-based MRI-L and the non-contrast-based US, allow to add the anatomical and functional details that are necessary to maximise the efficacy of LVA. MRI-I gives a whole comprehensive representation of the lymphatic system but is a static examination, and the evaluation of lymphatic functionality relies on their dimension and tracer uptake. US offers the value of a real-time and dynamic evaluation in the hands of the operating surgeons, with anatomical and functional details impossible to obtain in a state manner, at the cost of a harder learning curve.

References

1. Polomska AK, Proulx ST. Imaging technology of the lymphatic system. Adv Drug Deliv Rev. 2021;170:294–311. https://doi.org/10.1016/j.addr.2020.08.013. Epub 2020 Sep 3. PMID: 32891679.
2. Natale G, Bocci G, Ribatti D. Scholars and scientists in the history of the lymphatic system. J Anat. 2017;231(3):417–29.
3. Irschick R, Siemon C, Brenner E. The history of anatomical research of lymphatics—From the ancient times to the end of the European renaissance. Ann Anat. 2019;233:49–69.
4. Hayashi A, Visconti G. Supermicrosurgical lymphaticovenular anastomosis: a practical textbook. HV Projects; 2020.
5. Yamamoto T, Yamamoto N, Yoshimatsu H, et al. Factors associated with lymphosclerosis: an analysis on 962 lymphatic vessels. Plast Reconstr Surg. 2017;140:734–41.
6. Visconti G, Hayashi A, Bianchi A, Tartaglione G, Bartoletti R, Salgarello M. Lymphaticovenular anastomosis for advanced-stage peripheral lymphedema: expanding indication and introducing the hand/foot sign. J Plast Reconstr Aesthet Surg. 2022;75(7):2153–63. https://doi.org/10.1016/j.bjps.2022.02.012. Epub 2022 Feb 20. PMID: 35367158.
7. Visconti G, Bianchi A, Salgarello M, Di Leone A, Hayashi A, Masetti R, Franceschini G. Lymphatic tissue transfer: ultrasound-guided description and preoperative planning of vascularised lymph nodes, lymphatic units, and lymphatic vessels transfers. J Pers Med. 2022;12(8):1346. https://doi.org/10.3390/jpm12081346. PMID: 36013294; PMCID: PMC9410514.
8. Scallan JP, Zawieja SD, Castorena-Gonzales JA, et al. Lymphatic pumping: mechanics, mechanisms and malfunction. J Physiol. 2016;594(20):5749–68.
9. Suami H, Scaglioni MF. Anatomy of the lymphatic system and the lymphosome concept with reference to lymphedema. Semin Plast Surg. 2018;32:5–11.
10. Standring S. Gray's anatomy. The anatomical basis of clinical practice. Elsevier Limited; 2008.
11. Szube A, Rockson SG. Lymphedema: anatomy, physiology and pathogenesis. Vasc Med. 1997;2:321–6.
12. Von der Weid PY. Lymphatic vessel pumping. Adv Exp Med Biol. 2019;1124:357–77.
13. Conti F. Medical physiology. Physiology of organs and systems. Edi-Ermes s.r.l.; 2010.
14. Mihara M, Hara H, Hayashi Y, et al. Pathological steps of cancer-related lymphedema: histological changes in the collecting lymphatic vessels after lymphadenectomy. PLoS One. 2012;7(7):e41126.
15. Visconti G, Salgarello M, Hayashi A. The recipient venule in supermicrosurgical lymphaticovenular anastomosis: flow dynamic classification and correlation with surgical outcomes. J Reconstr Microsurg. 2018;34(8):581–9. https://doi.org/10.1055/s--0038-1649518. Epub 2018 May 12. PMID: 29753301.
16. Suami H, Koelmeyer L, Mackie H, et al. Patterns of lymphatic drainage after axillary node dissection impact arm lymphedema severity: a review of animal and clinical imaging studies. Surg Oncol. 2018;27:743–50.
17. Liu N, Wang B. Functional lymphatic collectors in breast cancer-related lymphedema arm. Lymphat Res Biol. 2014;12(4):232–7.
18. Schaverien MV, Coroneos CJ. Surgical treatment of lymphedema. Plast Reconstr Surg. 2019;144(3):738–58.
19. Hayashi A, Visconti G, Yamamoto T, et al. Intraoperative imaging of lymphatic vessels using ultra high-frequency ultrasound. J Plast Reconstr Aesthet Surg. 2018;71(5):778–80.
20. Kung TA, Champaneria MC, Maki JH, Neligan PC. Current concepts in the surgical management of lymphedema. Plast Reconstr Surg. 2017;139(4):1003e–13e. https://doi.org/10.1097/PRS.0000000000003218. PMID: 28350684.
21. van Heumen S, Riksen JJM, Bramer WM, van Soest G, Vasilic D. Imaging of the lymphatic vessels for surgical planning: a systematic review. Ann Surg Oncol. 2023;30(1):462–79. https://doi.org/10.1245/s10434-022-12552-7. Epub 2022 Sep 28. Erratum in: Ann Surg Oncol. 2022 Dec;29(Suppl 3):628. PMID: 36171528; PMCID: PMC9726677.
22. Singhal D, Tran BN, Angelo JP, e al. Technological advances in lymphatic surgery: bringing to light the invisible. Plast Reconstr Surg. 2019;143(1):283–93.
23. Tartaglione G, Pagan M, Morese R, et al. Intradermal lymphoscintigraphy at rest and after exercise: a new technique for the functional assessment of the lymphatic system in patients with lymphedema. Nucl Med Commun. 2010;31(6):547–51.
24. Allen RJ Jr, Cheng M-H. Lymphedema surgery: patient selection and an overview of surgical techniques. J Surg Oncol. 2016;113(8):923–31.
25. Maclellan RA, Zurakowski D, Voss S, Greene AK. Correlation between lymphedema disease severity and lymphoscintigraphic findings: a clinical-radiologic study. J Am Coll Surg. 2017;225(3):366–70.
26. Visconti G, Hayashi A, Tartaglione G, Yamamoto T, Bianchi A, Salgarello M. Preoperative planning of lymphaticovenular anastomosis in patients with iodine allergy: a multicentric experience. J Plast Reconstr Aesthet Surg. 2020;73(4):783–808. https://doi.org/10.1016/j.bjps.2019.11.020. Epub 2019 Nov 29. PMID: 31813793.
27. Narushima M, Yamamoto T, Ogara F, et al. Indocyanine green lymphography findings in limb lymphedema. J Reconstr Microsurg. 2016;32:72–9.
28. Pons G, Clavero JA, Alomar X, Rodríguez-Bauza E, Tom LK, Masia J. Preoperative planning of lymphaticovenous anastomosis: the use of magnetic

resonance lymphangiography as a complement to indocyanine green lymphography. J Plast Reconstr Aesthet Surg. 2019;72(6):884–91. https://doi.org/10.1016/j.bjps.2019.02.024. Epub 2019 Mar 2. PMID: 30944074.
29. Zeltzer AA, Brussaard C, Koning M, De Baerdemaeker R, Hendrickx B, Hamdi M, de Mey J. MR lymphography in patients with upper limb lymphedema: the GPS for feasibility and surgical planning for lympho-venous bypass. J Surg Oncol. 2018;118(3):407–15. https://doi.org/10.1002/jso.25145. Epub 2018 Aug 16. PMID: 30114316.
30. Bianchi A, Salgarello M, Hayashi A, Yang JC, Visconti G. Recipient venule selection and anastomosis configuration for lymphaticovenular anastomosis in extremity lymphedema: algorithm based on 1,000 lymphaticovenular anastomosis. J Reconstr Microsurg. 2022;38(6):472–80. https://doi.org/10.1055/s-0041-1735836. Epub 2021 Sep 28. PMID: 34583393.
31. Hayashi A, Hayashi N, Yoshimatsu H, et al. Effective and efficient lymphaticovenular anastomosis using preoperative ultrasound detection technique of lymphatic vessels in lower extremity lymphedema. J Surg Oncol. 2018;117:290–8.
32. Hayashi A, Yamamoto T, Yoshimatsu H, et al. Ultrasound visualization of the lymphatic vessels in the lower leg. Microsurgery. 2016;36:397–401.
33. Hayashi A, Giacalone G, Yamamoto T, et al. Ultra high-frequency ultrasonographic imaging with 70 MHz scanner for visualization of the lymphatic vessels. Plast Reconstr Surg Glob Open. 2019;7(1):e2086.
34. Visconti G, Hayashi A, Bianchi A, et al. Technological advances in lymphatic surgery: bringing to light the invisible. Plast Reconstr Surg. 2019;144(9):734–41.
35. Bianchi A, Visconti G, Hayashi A, Santoro A, Longo V, Salgarello M. Ultra-high frequency ultrasound imaging of lymphatic channels correlates with their histological features: a step forward in lymphatic surgery. J Plast Reconstr Aesthet Surg. 2020;73(9):1622–9. https://doi.org/10.1016/j.bjps.2020.05.053. Epub 2020 May 25. PMID: 32591265.

Finding the Ideal Vein in Lymphaticovenular Anastomosis

21

Giuseppe Visconti

21.1 Introduction

Lymphaticovenular anastomosis (LVA) is nowadays considered a minimally invasive and effective treatment of peripheral lymphedema [1–9].

It is nowadays clear that efficient and effective LVAs are possible when overloaded yet functional lymphatic channels are bypassed [8]. Those lymphatic channels are usually classified as ectatic type according to the Mihara classification or S1 according to the Yamamoto classification [10, 11]. Both classifications are based on the natural involution of lymphatic channels in obstructive lymphedema that become sclerotic over time after lymph flow obstruction and lose their function to drain lymph flow from the affected limb. Bypassing sclerotic lymphatic vessels leads to minimal or no therapeutic effect, and therefore the identification of ectasis or s1 lymphatic channels has crucial importance in planning LVA surgery as described in the other dedicated chapters of this textbook [11].

However, lymphatic channels are only one side of the coin as the other side is represented by the recipient venule, although this topic has been usually neglected in literature. In 2018, we demonstrated that recipient venules have an independent impact on the outcomes of patients undergoing LVA [9].

So far, preoperative selection of the adequate recipient venules is of paramount importance as for finding the right lymphatic channels to be anastomosed.

In our experience, the use of ultrasound in preoperative planning allows to evaluate both lymphatic channels and recipient venule in order to perform preoperatively the best vessels. We found this approach very effective as we experienced a corresponding increasing clinical positive effect in terms of predictability and improvement.

21.2 Recipient Venule: Hemodynamics

The venous system allows to bring the blood from periphery back to the heart. This flow is possible because the venous pressure is higher than atrial pressure, thanks to the three main factors:

(a) Skeletal muscle pump
(b) Respiratory pump
(c) The structure of venous system tree itself
    - The progressive increase of vessel diameter from small peripheral venule to the larger veins with a progressive decrease in total cross-sectional area allows a pro-

G. Visconti (✉)
UO Chirurgia Plastica, Dipartimento Scienze Salute della Donna, del Bambino e Sanità Pubblica—Fondazione Policlinico Gemelli IRCCS—Largo Agostino Gemelli, Rome, Italy

J. P. Hong et al. (eds.), *Imaging for Reconstructive Microsurgery*,
https://doi.org/10.1007/978-981-97-7278-0_21

gressive drop on blood pressure from peripheral to central veins and an increased velocity.

- The presence of one-way valves helps this system to keep the flow forward.
- Venoconstriction.

Peripheral venule pressure has been demonstrated to be higher than central venule pressure of around 3–5 mmHg. Data on peripheral venule pressure are available for large peripheral veins rather than for the small venule used in LVA surgery. However, the more peripheral the venule is, the larger is its intraluminal pressure [8].

21.3 Recipient Venule: Pressure Gradient

To perform an effective and efficient LVA, a favorable pressure gradient from lymphatic collector to venule must be established, in order to allow the lymph to flow successfully into venule, thus downloading the increased lymphatic intraluminal pressure.

As the lymphatic channels of lymphedematous limbs show an increased intraluminal pressure, a venule with lower intraluminal pressure should be used as recipient in order to establish a favorable pressure gradient. As for now, it is technically not possible to precisely calculate the pressure within the single peripheral venule used for LVA.

However, by using intraoperative ICG camera, we can appreciate the lymph flow at the anastomosis interface, and thus we can indirectly evaluate the pressure gradient between the lymphatic collector used for the LVA and the recipient venule.

According to this method, we classified four subtypes of venules such as "backflow" venule, when the pressure gradient was not favorable and the blood flows into lymphatic channel, "slack" venule when the pressure gradient was slightly favorable, "outlet" venule when the pressure gradient was highly favorable, and "hydropower" venule when there is a kind of sucking effect of the vein [8, 9, 12] (Fig. 21.1).

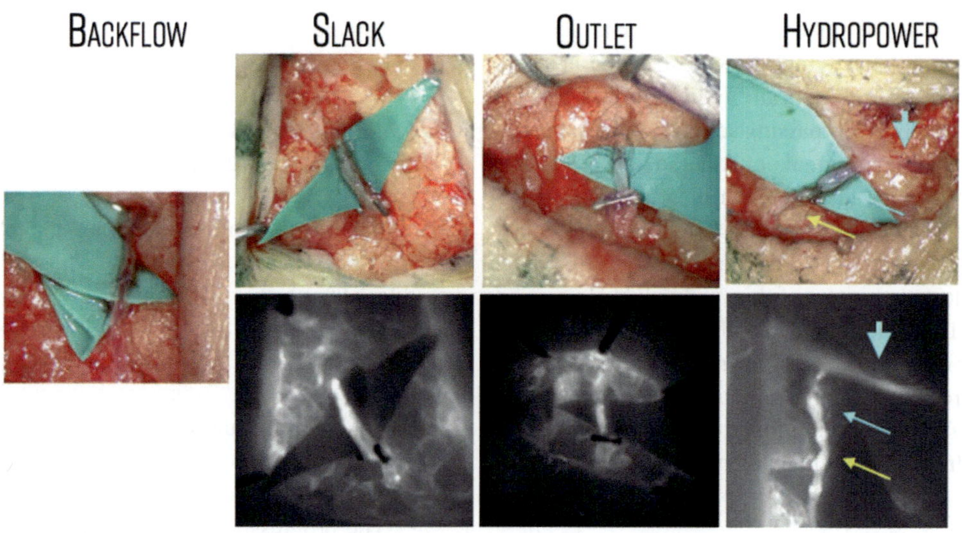

Fig. 21.1 BSOH classification. (With permission, from Hayashi and Visconti [8]. ISBN 9781304945730)

21.4 BSOH Classification

Once the LVA is established, the anastomosis is evaluated both clinically under the operating microscope and by turning on the fluorescence mode. The anastomosis can be classified according to the flow dynamics observed, and the venules can be classified in four patterns: backflow, slack, outlet, and outlet hydropower [8, 9, 12].

- ***Backflow***: We can appreciate clinically that the blood enters the lymphatic channels that became reddish, losing its transparent color or the blood is being blocked at the anastomosis level. On the intraoperative fluorescence, the venule showed lower fluorescence signal than lymphatic, highlighting an unfavorable pressure gradient (blood to lymph), thus suggesting an intraluminal venule pressure higher than the lymphatic one.
- ***Slack***: Clinically, we can observe that the lymph flow passed into the venule. At a continuous observation of 15 s, some blood passed into lymphatic and then was cleared by the lymph flow. On the intraoperative fluorescence, the venule and the lymphatic vessel showed the same fluorescence signal, suggesting a low but still favorable pressure gradient from the lymphatic to the venule.
- ***Outlet***: At clinical observation, we can see that the venule is cleared by the lymph and no blood can be seen into the venule. The lymph flow successfully passes into the venule with no blood detected in the venule at a continuous observation of 15 s. On the intraoperative fluorescence, the venule results more fluorescent than lymphatic, highlighting a favorable pressure gradient (lymph to blood), thus suggesting that the venule had a lower intraluminal pressure than lymphatic.
- ***Hydropower***: This is a subtype of "outlet" venule with specific clinical features. At clinical observation, we can see that the venule is cleared by the lymph and no blood can be seen into the venule, similarly to outlet venule. On the intraoperative fluorescence, we can appreciate a continuous flow from lymphatic channel to recipient venule, as there is a kind of "aspirating" effect from the venule.

According to two studies that we published in 2018 and 2022, backflow anastomosis is associated with poor composite outcome and should be avoided. Slack anastomosis is associated with good composite outcomes but indicates that the patient will need compression bandages in the postoperative period to favor a positive lymph progression. Outlet and outlet hydropower anastomosis are the most effective ones with the best composite outcomes [8, 9, 12].

So far, the recipient venule has an independent influence on the effectiveness of LVA and should be considered with the same importance given to lymphatic channels. Moreover, the lymphatic channel is what we have, and the recipient venule is what we select.

21.5 Algorithm for Venule Selection

In a recent study published in 2022, we reviewed 1000 LVAs that differ only for recipient venule characteristics, and we developed an algorithm for venule selection [12]. This algorithm might aid microsurgeons in the clinical decision-making process during LVA, in choosing the anastomosis configuration, with the best dynamics in every clinical scenario. The algorithm is based on the analysis of three components: the caliber match, the location, and the presence of blood backflow (Fig. 21.2).

The use of preoperative ultrahigh-frequency ultrasound allows to clearly evaluate lymphatic channels, including measuring the caliber [13, 14]. The ideal scenario would be to have a nearby ideal recipient venule where a good lymphatic channel has been located.

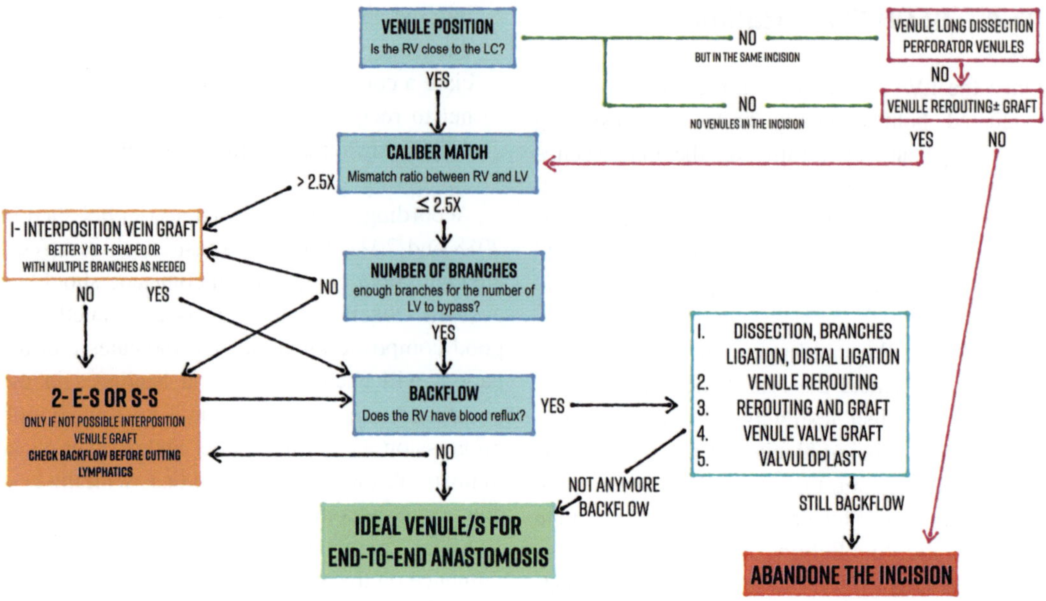

Fig. 21.2 Our algorithm for venule selection in LVA (with permission, From Bianchi A, Salgarello M, Hayashi A, Yang JC, Visconti G. Recipient Venule Selection and Anastomosis Configuration for Lymphaticovenular Anastomosis in Extremity Lymphedema: Algorithm Based on 1,000 Lymphaticovenular Anastomosis. J Reconstr Microsurg. 2022 Jul;38(6):472–480. https://doi.org/10.1055/s-0041-1735836. Epub 2021 Sep 28. PMID: 34583393).

The ideal recipient venule should have a similar caliber match to that of lymphatic channel, being close to the lymphatic and without blood backflow.

Ultrahigh-frequency ultrasound has revolutionized the lymphatic supermicrosurgery as this technology allows to anticipate the very superficial anatomy, provide a "histological"-like quality imaging of the lymphatic channels and found the recipient venule [14].

Both 48 and 70 MhZ probes are valid for the preoperative study of the recipient venule. In some cases, high-frequency ultrasound may also be enough in doing so [15].

The venules are initially identified using the B-mode. This modality allows to delineate the venous tree, measure the venule caliber and seeing valves. A clear three-dimensional planning can be done in surgeon's mind, by evaluating the position of the venous tree with that of the lymphatic channels. The selected recipient venule is then evaluated hemodynamically by switching to the color-coded modality. The push and release technique allows to understand if the selected venule is interested by the blood backflow or it has a protective valve that avoids such phenomenon (Figs. 21.3 and 21.4).

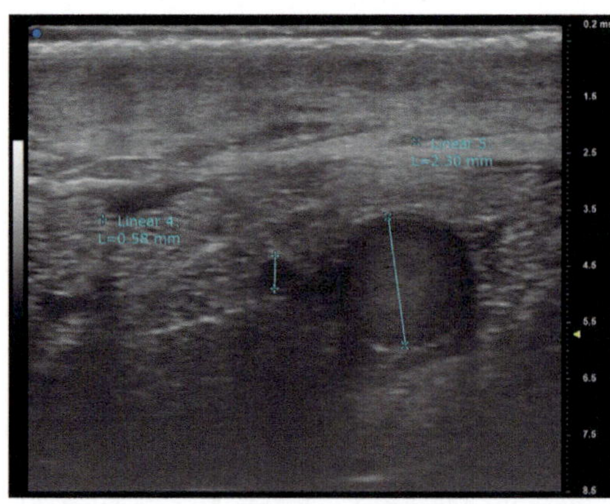

Fig. 21.3 Ultrahigh-frequency ultrasound visualization of favorable recipient venule in B-mode. The linear measurement tool (blue dots) has been used to precisely establish the caliber of recipient venule to choose the best match with that of lymphatic channels

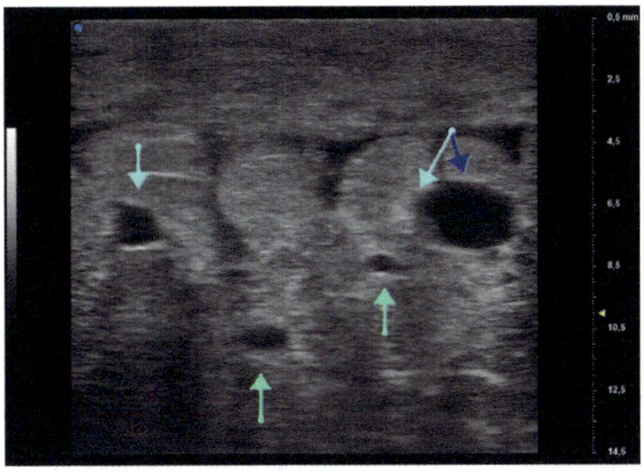

Fig. 21.4 Ultrahigh-frequency ultrasound visualization of an incision site for LVA. Two ectasis, high-flow lymphatic channels have been found (green arrow) and two nearby favorable recipient venules with good caliber match and no backflow (light blue). One recipient venule is a direct branch of a larger subcutaneous vein (deep blue arrow)

In cases where no ideal recipient venule is found nearby the lymphatic channels, further strategy should be adopted to be able to perform an effective anastomosis in the operating room [12].

According to our clinical experience, there are some key rules to follow to enhance the feasibility of an effective LVA:

- **Rule #1: Venule First**

  Our rule number one is to never cut the lymphatic channel(s), until we are sure of having favorable recipient venule(s) to which we will perform the bypass. In the worst scenario (refractory high-flow blood backflow), we do not proceed with lymphatic channel division and anastomosis; rather, we close the incision and move to the next planned site.
- **Caliber Match**

  The use of preoperative ultrahigh-frequency ultrasound allows to clearly evaluate lymphatic channels, including measuring the caliber. The ideal scenario would be to have two nearby venules with the same caliber match with that of the lymphatic channel. This will allow to perform one or two E-E anastomoses, based on lymphatic dynamics. In cases of caliber mismatch or presence of one venule only, other techniques should be carried out including interposition vein graft or E-S and S-S anastomosis (Fig. 21.5).
- **Location**

  The recipient venule should ideally be located nearby the lymphatic channel, and the short distance between the two also favors an easier inset and a shorter scar.

  If venules with good flow dynamics cannot be preoperatively identified, other adequate venules must be carried at the anastomotic site, as venule with poor dynamics compromises the outcome of the LVA. The alternative options are venule rerouting method and venule graft (Figs. 21.6 and 21.7).
- **Venous Backflow**

  The color-coded mode on ultrasound usually allows to evaluate the presence of blood reflux preoperatively. However, in some case, this may be not clear, so the surgeon should consider other plans in case high-reflux blood backflow is found. In the absence of other favorable recipient venules, we advise to not proceed with LVA; rather, close the incision and move to the next one.

  The strategies to be considered preoperatively in case of doubtful venule for backflow are the following: venule rerouting, venule rerouting and graft, and venule valve graft [16–18]. Intraoperatively, dissection and branch ligation along with valvuloplasty may be employed to manage a high-reflux venule [19].

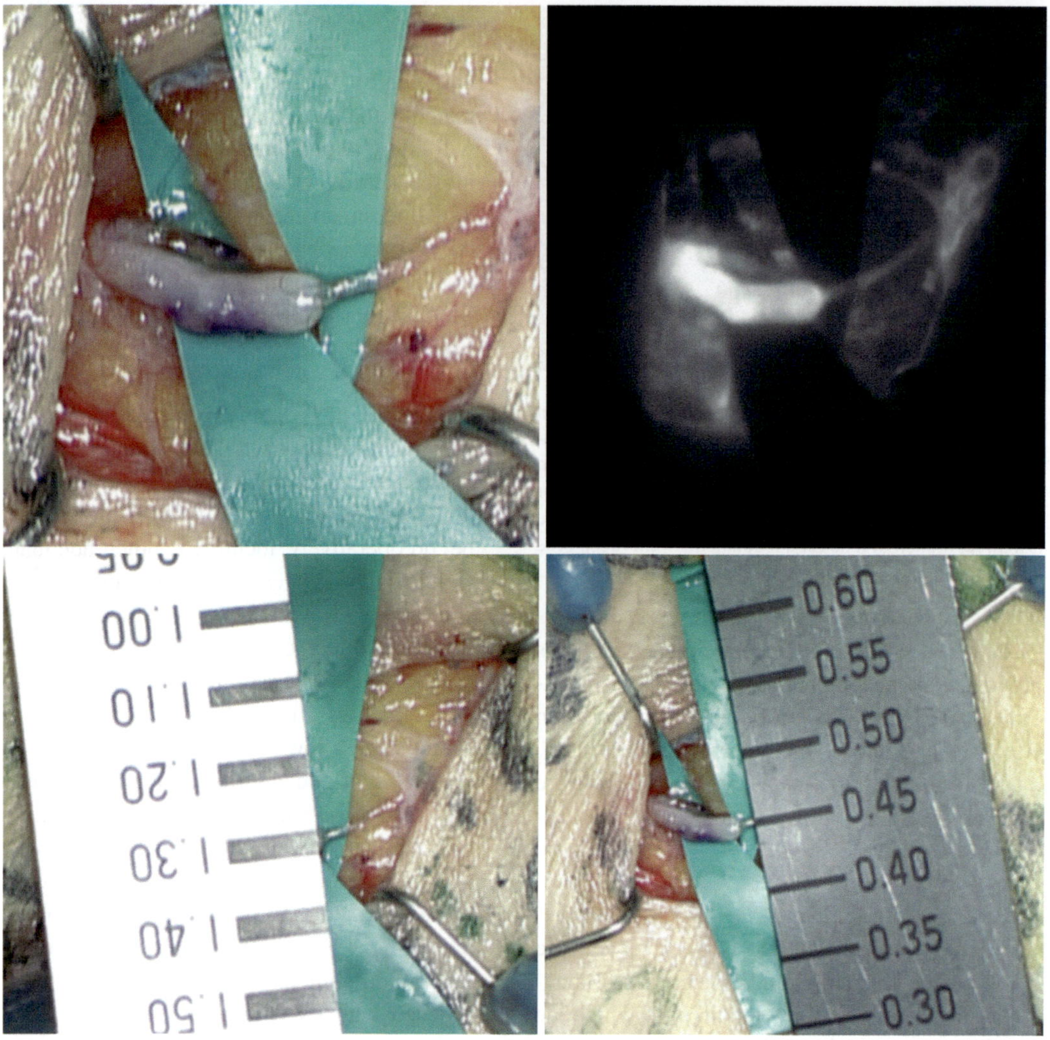

Fig. 21.5 (Above, left) Intraoperative picture showing a large recipient venule with no backflow and high caliber mismatch with that of the lymphatic channel with good E-E anastomosis. (Above, right) The intraoperative infrared fluorescence showed outlet anastomosis. (Below, left) The caliber of recipient venule was 1.3 mm, and that of lymphatic channel (below, right) was 0.45 mm with a corresponding ratio of 2.8×. This extreme example shows that up to 2.5× ratio is possible to perform a safe and effective E-E anastomosis. (with permission, from Bianchi A, Salgarello M, Hayashi A, Yang JCS, Visconti G. Recipient venule selection and anastomosis configuration for lymphaticovenular anastomosis in extremity lymphedema: algorithm-based on 1000 lymphaticovenular anastomosis. J Reconstr Microsurg. 2022 Jul; 38(6):472–480.)

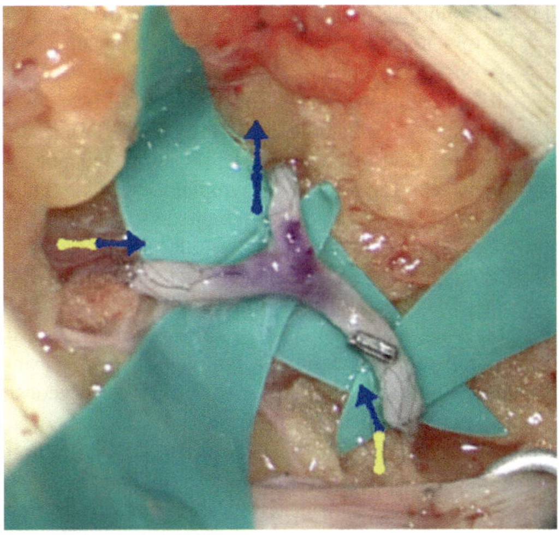

Fig. 21.6 A venule valve graft for harvested for elsewhere to be anastomosed to antegrade and retrograde lymphatic channel and then to the recipient venule located in the incision showing backflow. After the venule valve graft, a correct lymph-to-blood flow is established. Notice the graft is lymph-expanded and no sign of blood can be seen. The valve in the central portion of the graft (in blue ink) is protective. In yellow lymphatic channel and in blue venule. The arrow shows the direction of flow (With permission, from Hayashi and Visconti [8]. ISBN 9781304945730)

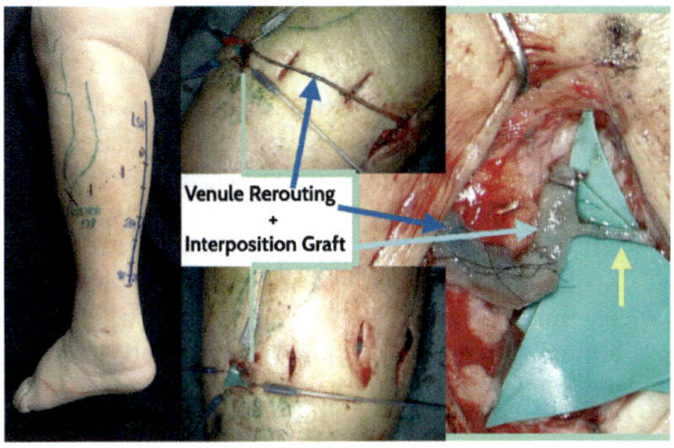

Fig. 21.7 (Left) Preoperative picture showing the preoperative planning using ICG-L and UHFUS of a patient affected by LLL with severe vein insufficiency and previous saphenectomy. Anterolateral lymphatics were found preoperatively with ICG-L and verified with UHFUS. No nearby favorable venule was available (high reflux at color Doppler examination). The lesser saphenous vein was found competent and with no reflux at color Doppler ultrasound with UHFUS. A long venule rerouting was planned including a venule interposition graft from the LSV itself to match the caliber at the anastomotic point. (Center, above, and below). These figures show the harvest of LSV and its transposition toward the lymphatic channels via subcutaneous tunnels. (Right) Venule interposition graft (light blue arrow) sutured to the transposed LSV (blue arrow) with nylon 11/0. The interposition graft was planned having a small branch that can match with the lymphatic channel (yellow arrow), as it was. *LV* lymphatic vessels, *RV* recipient venules, *UHFUS* ultrahigh-frequency ultrasound, *LSV* lesser saphenous vein. (With permission, from Bianchi et al. [12])

21.6 Conclusion

Recipient venules represent the exit point of the lymph from the affected limb and have an independent impact on the clinical outcome of LVA. Ultrasound technology allows to precisely study the venous tree and identify ideal recipient venule for LVA. It also allows to plan alternative options before surgery, in case an ideal recipient venule cannot be found. If the venule does not let the lymph flow into the venous system, the LVA is not just ineffective but represents another obstruction in the lymphatic system. Based on 1000 LVAs with similar lymphatic characteristics, we proposed our algorithm that may aid the lymphatic microsurgeon in the selection of recipient venule and the consequent anastomosis configuration, in order to obtain the best flow dynamics through the LVA.

References

1. Basta MN, Gao LL, Wu LC. Operative treatment of peripheral lymphedema: a systematic meta-analysis of the efficacy and safety of lymphovenous microsurgery and tissue transplantation. Plast Reconstr Surg. 2014;133(4):905–13.
2. Koshima I, Inagawa K, Urushibara K, Moriguchi T. Supermicrosurgical lymphaticovenular anastomosis for the treatment of lymphedema in the upper extremities. J Reconstr Microsurg. 2000;16:437–42.
3. Chang DW, Suami H, Skoracki R. A prospective analysis of 100 consecutive lymphovenous bypass cases for treatment of extremity lymphedema. Plast Reconstr Surg. 2013;132(5):1305–14.
4. Mihara M, Hara H, Tange S, Zhou HP, Kawahara M, Shimizu Y, Murai N. Multisite lymphaticovenular bypass using supermicrosurgery technique for lymphedema management in lower lymphedema cases. Plast Reconstr Surg. 2016;138(1):262–72.
5. Scaglioni M, Fontein DB, Arvanitakis M, et al. Systematic review of lymphaticovenous anastomosis (LVA) for the treatment of lymphedema. Microsurgery. 2017;37:947–53.
6. Aljindan FK, Lin CY, Cheng MH. Comparison of outcomes between side-to-end and end-to-end lymphovenous anastomoses for early-grade extremity lymphedema. Plast Reconstr Surg. 2019;144(2):486–96.
7. Tsai PL, Wu SC, Lin WC, et al. Determining factors in relation to lymphovascular characteristics and anastomotic configuration in supermicrosurgical lymphaticovenous anastomosis—a retrospective cohort study. Int J Surg. 2020;81:39–46.
8. Hayashi A, Visconti G. Supermicrosurgical lymphaticovenular anastomosis: a practical textbook. HV Projects; 2020.
9. Visconti G, Salgarello M, Hayashi A. The recipient venule in supermicrosurgical lymphaticovenular anastomosis: flow dynamic classification and correlation with surgical outcomes. J Reconstr Microsurg. 2018;34(8):581–9.
10. Mihara M, Hara H, Hayashi Y, et al. Pathological steps of cancer-related lymphedema: histological changes in the collecting lymphatic vessels after lymphadenectomy. PLoS One. 2012;7(7):e41126.
11. Yamamoto T, Yamamoto N, Yoshimatsu H, et al. Factors associated with lymphosclerosis: an analysis on 962 lymphatic vessels. Plast Reconstr Surg. 2017;140:734–41.
12. Bianchi A, Salgarello M, Hayashi A, Yang JC, Visconti G. Recipient venule selection and anastomosis configuration for lymphaticovenular anastomosis in extremity lymphedema: algorithm based on 1,000 lymphaticovenular anastomosis. J Reconstr Microsurg. 2022;38(6):472–80. https://doi.org/10.1055/s-0041-1735836.
13. Hayashi A, Visconti G, Yamamoto T, et al. Intraoperative imaging of lymphatic vessels using ultra high-frequency ultrasound. J Plast Reconstr Aesthet Surg. 2018;71(5):778–80.
14. Bianchi A, Visconti G, Hayashi A, et al. Ultra-high frequency ultrasound imaging of lymphatic channels correlates with their histological features: a step forward in lymphatic surgery. J Plast Reconstr Aesthet Surg. 2020;73(9):1622–9.
15. Visconti G, Yamamoto T, Hayashi N, et al. Ultrasound-assisted lymphaticovenular anastomosis for the treatment of peripheral lymphedema. Plast Reconstr Surg. 2017;139:1380e–1e.
16. Visconti G, Salgarello M. Venule valve graft in lymphatic supermicrosurgery: a novel strategy for managing blood backflow. Microsurgery. 2017;37(8):958–9. https://doi.org/10.1002/micr.30242.
17. Visconti G, Salgarello M. Supermicrosurgical lymphatico comitantes perforator venule anastomosis for the treatment of peripheral lymphedema: a new configuration for patients with superficial vein insufficiency? Microsurgery. 2017;37(6):719–20. https://doi.org/10.1002/micr.30117.
18. Visconti G, Bianchi A, Hayashi A, Salgarello M. Ultra-high frequency ultrasound preoperative planning of the rerouting method for lymphaticovenular anastomosis in incisions devoid of vein. Microsurgery. 2020;40(6):717–8. https://doi.org/10.1002/micr.30600.
19. Akita S, Mitsukawa N, Kuriyama M, Hasegawa M, Kubota Y, Koizumi T, Ishigaki T, Tokumoto H, Satoh K. External valvuloplasty for subcutaneous small veins to prevent venous reflux in lymphaticovenular anastomosis for lower extremity lymphedema. Plast Reconstr Surg. 2013;132(4):1008–14. https://doi.org/10.1097/PRS.0b013e31829fe12f.

---

22 Patency Evaluation of Lymphovenous Anastomosis

Takumi Yamamoto

22.1 Lymph Flow Evaluation

There are various modalities for lymph flow visualization. Most lymph flow imaging modalities require intradermal or subcutaneous injection of contrast or radioactive agent for visualization [1–10]. Lymphoscintigraphy (LSG) is a gold standard for lymphedema evaluation, which can visualize superficial and lymph flows of the whole body (Fig. 22.1) [1, 11–13]. Disadvantages of LSG include a risk of ionized radiation exposure and obscure images of lymph flows. Single-photon emission computed tomography-computed tomography (SPECT-CT) allows three-dimensional lymph flow imaging based on LSG, but obtained images are still obscure compared with magnetic resonance lymphography (MRL), computed tomography lymphography (CTL), indocyanine green lymphography (ICGL), and photoacoustic lymphography (PAL) (Figs. 22.2 and 22.3) [1–10]. MRL, CTL, and PAL allows three-dimensional clear lymph flow imaging but requires special instruments/facilities and some time to obtain images [3, 4, 10]. On the other hand, ICGL visualized two-dimensional clear lymph flow imaging on the skin surface in real time [5–9, 11–17]. As injection of contrast agents has a risk of severe adverse events such as skin necrosis, MRL and CTL cannot be performed in some institutions due to restriction in terms of ethics [3, 4, 11, 12]. Lymphatic ultrasound (LUS) is reported to be useful for visualization of the collecting lymph vessels, but its quality largely depends on an examiner's skill and experience (Fig. 22.4) [18, 19].

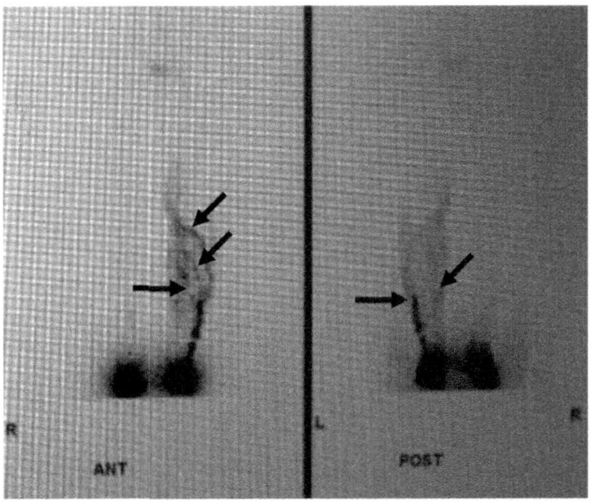

Fig. 22.1 Lymph vessels (arrow) visualized on LSG

T. Yamamoto (✉)
Department of Plastic and Reconstructive Surgery, Center Hospital of National Center for Global Health and Medicine, Tokyo, Japan
e-mail: tyamamoto-tky@umin.ac.jp

J. P. Hong et al. (eds.), *Imaging for Reconstructive Microsurgery*,
https://doi.org/10.1007/978-981-97-7278-0_22

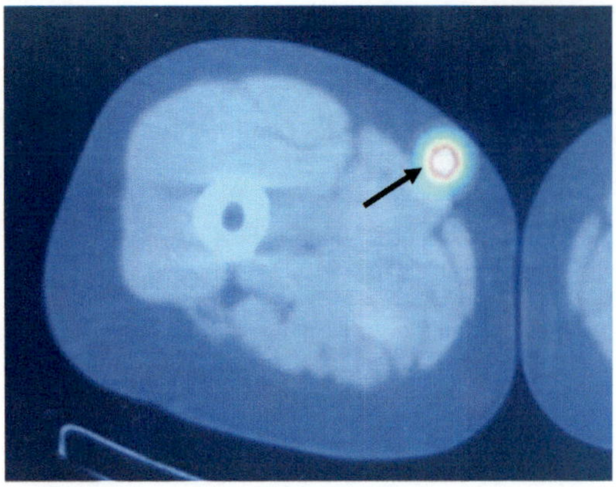

Fig. 22.2 Lymph vessels (arrow) visualized on SPECT-CT

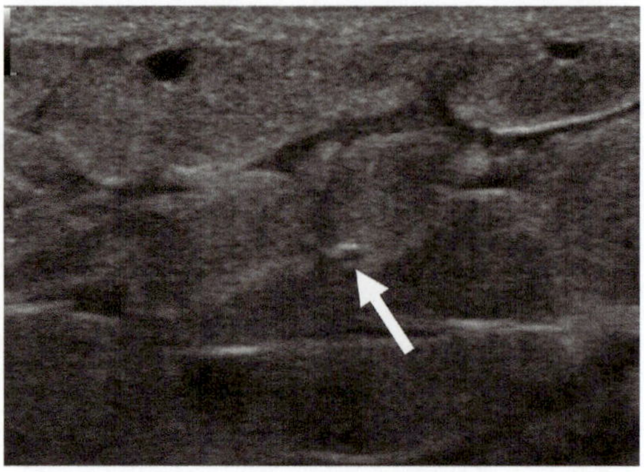

Fig. 22.4 Lymph vessel (arrow) visualized on LUS

Fig. 22.3 Lymph vessels (arrows) visualized on ICGL

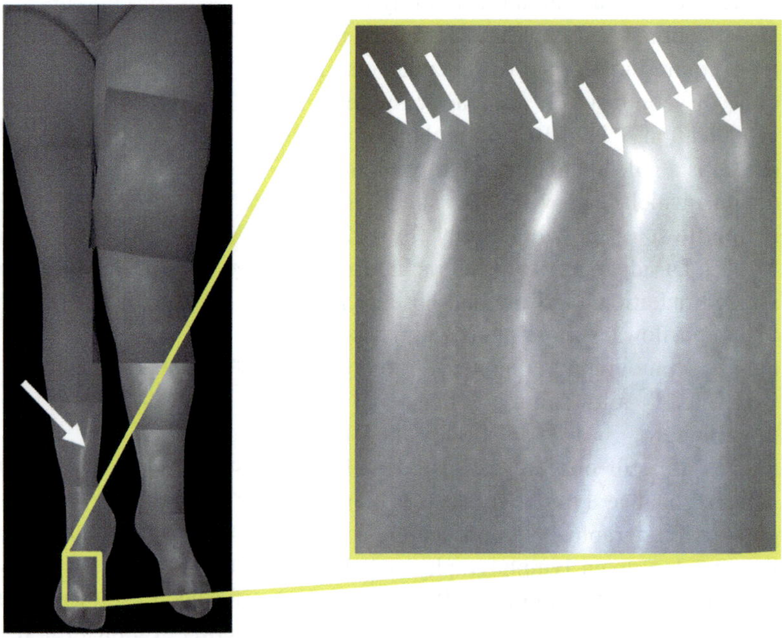

22.2 Characteristics of Lymphovenous Anastomosis

Lymphovenous shunt operations are performed for lymphedema treatment, which addresses pathophysiology of obstructive lymphedema [11, 12, 17, 20–25]. There are several methods of lymphovenous shunt, and lymphovenous implantation (LVI) and supermicrosurgical lymphovenous anastomosis (LVA) are widely applied methods [11, 12, 20–27]. In LVI, the collecting lymph vessels are inserted into a relatively large vein, whereas the collecting vessel is anastomosed to a similar-sized vein in an intima-to-intima coaptation in LVA (Fig. 22.5). There are various configurations of lymphovenous shunts, and end-to-end (EE) configuration is commonly applied in LVI, and other configurations such as end-to-side (ES), side-to-end (SE), and side-to-

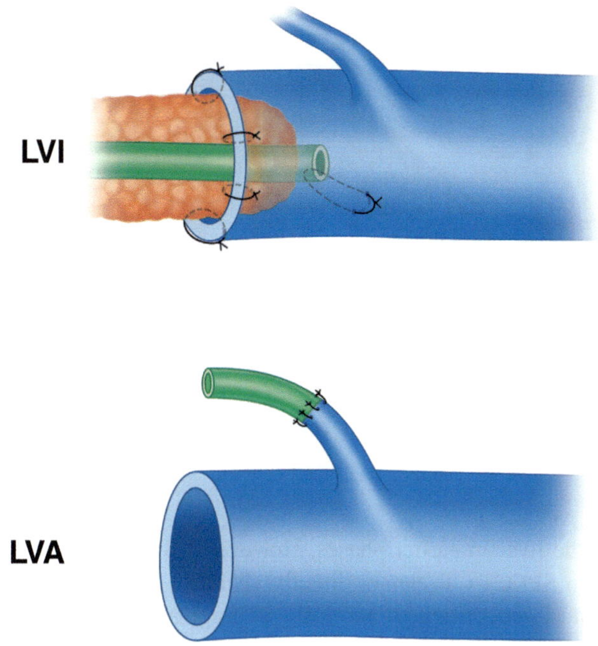

Fig. 22.5 LVI and LVA

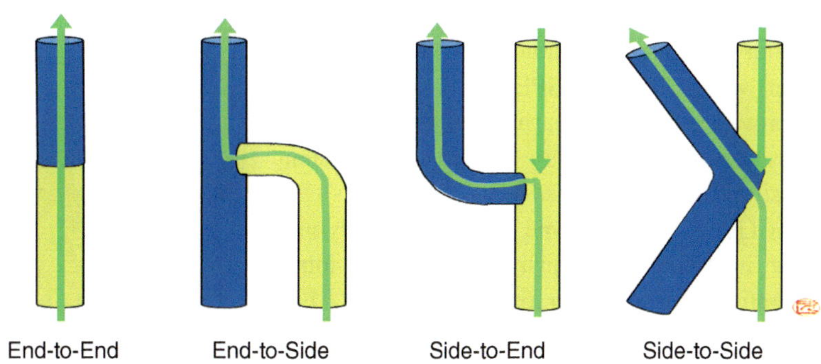

Fig. 22.6 Anastomosis configurations in LVA

side (SS) are also used in LVA (Fig. 22.6) [11, 12, 20, 22, 27]. As a submillimeter vein is used in LVA, precise lymph flow imaging is required to evaluate postoperative patency. As it is well known that clinical conditions and lymph circulation can be improved without patent anastomosis, it is mandatory to confirm anastomosis patency for proof of LVI or LVA efficacy, from the scientific point of view [12, 16, 28, 29].

22.3 Postoperative Evaluation of Patency

LSG allows qualitative and quantitative evaluation of lymph circulation, and postoperative patency can be assessed by comparing perioperative findings [1, 2, 11]. After successful lymphovenous shunt, injected radioactive agent is drained into venous circulation and accumulated

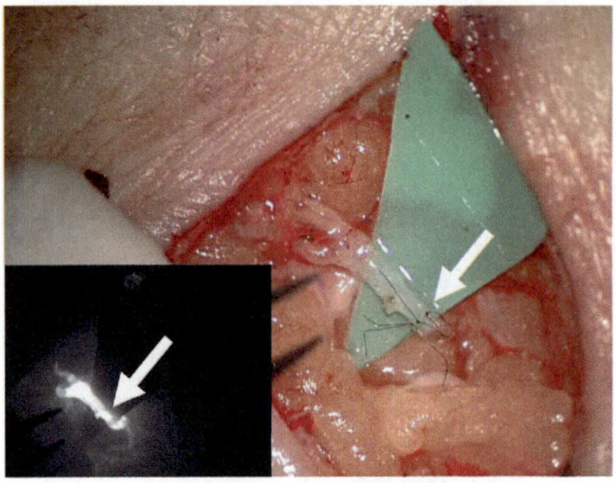

Fig. 22.7 Intraoperative ICGL showing patency of LVA (arrows)

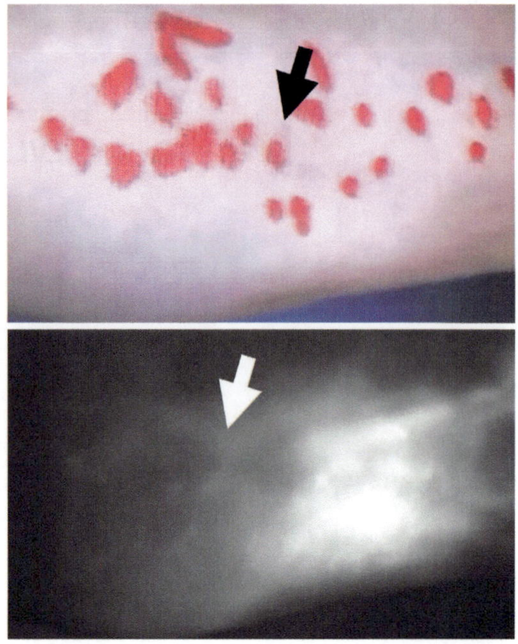

Fig. 22.8 Patent anastomosis shown on ICGL after successful LVA. Postoperative ICGL directly visualizes patency of LVA (arrows); lymph flows from the right side (lymph vessel) to the left side (vein) through the anastomosis

in the liver in earlier phases. However, LSG, or even SPECT-CT, cannot directly visualize anastomosis site patency, and only indirect assessment is possible. On cases where multiple lymphovenous shunts are created, LSG only indicates total effect of created shunts; each patency cannot be assessed separately [1, 11]. Therefore, even when LSG or SPECT-CT findings are improved and indicate earlier venous drainage, it does not necessarily represent patent anastomosis.

ICGL allows real-time evaluation of lymph flows including anastomosis site (Fig. 22.7) intraoperatively or postoperatively [5–10, 16, 17]. Unlike other lymph flow imaging modalities, ICGL directly visualizes anastomosis sites with clear images, and each anastomosis site patency can be assessed (Fig. 22.8). Thus, ICGL is presently the most common method for direct evaluation of anastomosis patency [11, 16, 17, 29]. As ICG fluorescent images are most clear immediately after injection, anastomosis patency should be evaluated immediately after ICG injection. Characteristics of fluorescent images are different between lymph vessels and veins; fluorescent enhancement remains in lymph vessels after squeezing along the vessel, whereas venous fluorescent enhancement is transient and easily washed out with squeezing along the vein (Figs. 22.9 and 22.10). Anastomosis is evaluated as patent, when ICGL shows enhancement flowing from a lymph vessel to a vein, where an anastomosis is created. It is difficult to assess anastomosis patency, where dermal backflow

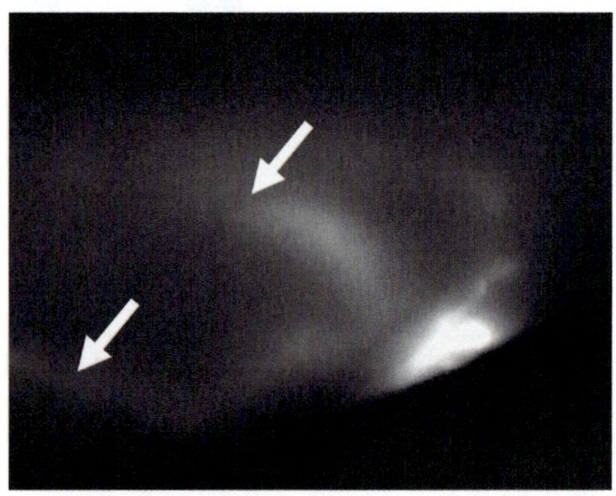

Fig. 22.9 Typical enhanced image of the lymph vessel on ICGL. Lymph vessels are visualized as slightly wider lines (arrows) on ICGL in most body parts except for very thin skin regions such as hand/foot. Enhancement can hardly be washed out by squeezing the vessels

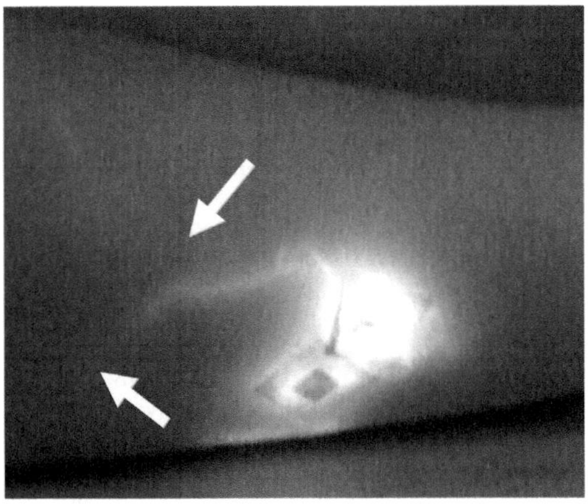

Fig. 22.10 Typical enhanced image of the vein on ICGL. Veins are visualized as narrow sharp lines on ICGL, and some branches without enhancement are shown as black lines (arrows). Enhancement can be easily washed out by squeezing the vessels

extends or lymph vessels exist 2 cm or deeper from the skin surface; linear pattern visualization is required for patency assessment with ICGL.

MRL, CTL, and PAL allow three-dimensional clear imaging of lymph flows, which is useful to evaluate anastomosis patency [3, 4, 10–12]. Although not suitable for real-time evaluation, their clear three-dimensional images are precise enough to evaluate anastomosis patency. Differentiation of lymph vessel and vein and precise localization of anastomosis sites are critical to evaluate patency using MRL, CTL, and PAL; when images show enhancement of vessels continuously flowing from a lymph vessel to a vein, anastomosis can be evaluated as patent. Unlike ICGL, anastomosis site can be visualized even in regions with dermal backflow, if dermal backflow is limited in the superficial region above the anastomosis site. As in ICGL, multisite injection would be required for evaluation of multiple anastomosis sites; as contrast agent may be drained in the most distal anastomosis and the remaining proximal anastomoses may not be enhanced, additional injection would be needed distal to the remaining proximal anastomosis sites. Although PAL's images are clearer than MRL and CTL, PAL can visualize only superficial flows as in ICGL [3–10].

LUS can be used to assess anastomosis patency. Although contrast-enhanced LUS is possible, enhancement duration after contrast agent injection is as short as few seconds to minutes, and patency evaluation based on real-time flow imaging is technically difficult and impractical [11, 12, 18, 19]. Therefore, patency evaluation using LUS is basically based on non-contrast images; anastomosis site should be directly visualized on LUS for patency evaluation. As imaging resolution is critical for patency evaluation using LUS, ultrahigh-frequency ultrasound is recommended, although it is possible to evaluate patency using conventional high-frequency ultrasound. Anastomosis site should be visualized longitudinally with an image showing a lymph vessel, anastomosis site, and a recipient vein continuously.

22.4 Future Perspective

With advancement of lymph flow imaging technology, patency of small vessel anastomosis such as LVA can be assessed. However, none of presently applied imaging modality allows 100% evaluation of multiple anastomosis patency within a short time as feasible and practical for usual clinical evaluation. Clinically needed qualities include clear images; visualization of deep flows; visualization of lymphatics even in dermal backflow region; real-time imaging, if possible; whole limb scan at once within a short time; and absence of significant adverse effects. Presently, it is better to utilize multiple modalities for maximization of efficacy of patency evaluation. Even with all presently available lymph flow imaging modalities, it is impossible to assess all anastomosis sites, especially due to limitations of visualization of deep flow or flow in dermal backflow area. Further technical advancement and clinical studies are warranted to clarify an optimal way of patency evaluation following lymphovenous anastomosis operation.

Disclaimers and Disclosure of Conflicts of Interest None.

Prior Presentations None.

Sources of Support that Require Acknowledgement None.

References

1. Boccardo F, Casabona F, De Cian F, Friedman D, Murelli F, Puglisi M, Campisi CC, Molinari L, Spinaci S, Dessalvi S, Campisi C. Lymphatic microsurgical preventing healing approach (LYMPHA) for primary surgical prevention of breast cancer-related lymphedema: over 4 years follow-up. Microsurgery. 2014;34(6):421–4.
2. Gentileschi S, Albanese R, Pino V, Stefanizzi G, Fragomeni S, Zagaria L, Ieria FP, Salgarello M, Scambia G, Garganese G. SPECT/CT and fusion ultrasound to target the efferent groin lymph node for lymphatic surgery. Microsurgery. 2019;39(7):605–12.
3. Baumeister RG, Mayo W, Notohamiprodjo M, Wallmichrath J, Springer S, Frick A. Microsurgical lymphatic vessel transplantation. J Reconstr Microsurg. 2016;32(1):34–41.
4. Almujally A, Sulieman A, Calliada F. Patients radiation risks from computed tomography lymphography. J Clin Imaging Sci. 2020;10:46.
5. Yamamoto T, Narushima M, Doi K, Oshima A, Ogata F, Mihara M, Koshima I, Mundinger GS. Characteristic indocyanine green lymphography findings in lower extremity lymphedema: the generation of a novel lymphedema severity staging system using dermal backflow patterns. Plast Reconstr Surg. 2011;127(5):1979–86.
6. Yamamoto T, Yamamoto N, Doi K, Oshima A, Yoshimatsu H, Todokoro T, Ogata F, Mihara M, Narushima M, Iida T, Koshima I. Indocyanine green (ICG)-enhanced lymphography for upper extremity lymphedema: a novel severity staging system using dermal backflow (DB) patterns. Plast Reconstr Surg. 2011;128(4):941–7.
7. Yamamoto T, Yamamoto N, Yoshimatsu H, Hayami S, Narushima M, Koshima I. Indocyanine green lymphography for evaluation of genital lymphedema in secondary lower extremity lymphedema patients. J Vasc Surg Venous Lymphat Disord. 2013;1(4):400–5.
8. Yamamoto T, Iida T, Matsuda N, Kikuchi K, Yoshimatsu H, Mihara M, Narushima M, Koshima I. Indocyanine green (ICG)-enhanced lymphography for evaluation of facial lymphoedema. J Plast Reconstr Aesthet Surg. 2011;64(11):1541–4.
9. Yamamoto T, Yamamoto N. Indocyanine green lymphography for evaluation of breast lymphedema secondary to breast cancer treatments. J Reconstr Microsurg. 2022. [Epub ahead of print].;38:630.
10. Suzuki Y, Kajita H, Watanabe S, Okabe K, Sakuma H, Imanishi N, Aiso S, Kishi K. Application of photoacoustic imaging for lymphedema treatment. J Reconstr Microsurg. 2022;38(3):254–62.
11. Brahma B, Yamamoto T. Breast cancer treatment-related lymphedema (BCRL): an overview of the literature and updates in microsurgery reconstruction. Eur J Surg Oncol. 2019;45(7):1138–45.
12. Yamamoto T, Yamamoto N, Kageyama T, Sakai H, Fuse Y, Tsuihiji K, Tsukuura R. Technical pearls in lymphatic supermicrosurgery. Glob Health Med. 2020;2(1):29–32.
13. Yamamoto T, Matsuda N, Doi K, Oshima A, Yoshimatsu H, Todokoro T, Ogata F, Mihara M, Narushima M, Iida T, Koshima I. The earliest finding of indocyanine green (ICG) lymphography in asymptomatic limbs of lower extremity lymphedema patients secondary to cancer treatment: the modified dermal backflow (DB) stage and concept of subclinical lymphedema. Plast Reconstr Surg. 2011;128(4):314e–21e.
14. Yamamoto T, Narushima M, Yoshimatsu H, Yamamoto N, Oka A, Seki Y, Todokoro T, Iida T, Koshima I. Indocyanine green velocity: lymph transportation capacity deterioration with progression of lymphedema. Ann Plast Surg. 2013;71(5):59–594.
15. Yamamoto T, Narushima M, Yoshimatsu H, Yamamoto N, Kikuchi K, Todokoro T, Iida T, Koshima I. Dynamic indocyanine green lymphography for breast cancer-related arm lymphedema. Ann Plast Surg. 2014;73(6):706–9.
16. Yamamoto T, Yoshimatsu H, Yamamoto N. Complete lymph flow reconstruction: a free vascularized lymph node true perforator flap transfer with efferent lymphaticolymphatic anastomosis. J Plast Reconstr Aesthet Surg. 2016;69(9):1227–33.
17. Yamamoto T, Yamamoto N, Azuma S, Yoshimatsu H, Seki Y, Narushima M, Koshima I. Near-infrared illumination system-integrated microscope for supermicrosurgical lymphaticovenular anastomosis. Microsurgery. 2014;34(1):23–7.
18. Hayashi A, Yamamoto T, Yoshimatsu H, Hayashi N, Furuya M, Harima M, Narushima M, Narushima M, Koshima I. Ultrasound visualization of the lymphatic vessels in the lower leg. Microsurgery. 2016;36(5):397–401.
19. Hayashi A, Hayashi N, Yoshimatsu H, Yamamoto T. Effective and efficient lymphaticovenular anastomosis using preoperative ultrasound detection technique of lymphatic vessels in lower extremity lymphedema. J Surg Oncol. 2018;117(2):290–8.
20. Yamamoto T, Narushima M, Kikuchi K, Yoshimatsu H, Todokoro T, Mihara M, Koshima I. Lambda-shaped anastomosis with intravascular stenting method for safe and effective lymphaticovenular anastomosis. Plast Reconstr Surg. 2011;127(5):1987–92.
21. Hong JPJ, Song S, Suh HSP. Supermicrosurgery: principles and applications. J Surg Oncol. 2018;118(5):832–9.
22. Yamamoto T, Yoshimatsu H, Narushima M, Seki Y, Yamamoto N, Shim TWH, Koshima I. A modified side-to-end lymphaticovenular anastomosis. Microsurgery. 2013;33(2):130–3.
23. Pak CS, Suh HP, Kwon JG, Cho MJ, Hong JP. Lymph node to vein anastomosis (LNVA) for lower extremity lymphedema. J Plast Reconstr Aesthet Surg. 2021;74(9):2059–67.
24. Visconti G, Hayashi A, Salgarello M, Narushima M, Koshima I, Yamamoto T. Supermicrosurgical T-shaped

lymphaticovenular anastomosis for the treatment of peripheral lymphedema: bypassing lymph fluid maximizing lymphatic collector continuity. Microsurgery. 2016;36. [Epub ahead of print].:714.

25. Yamamoto T, Narushima M, Yoshimatsu H, Seki Y, Yamamoto N, Oka A, Hara H, Koshima I. Minimally invasive lymphatic supermicrosurgery (MILS): indocyanine green lymphography-guided simultaneous multi-site lymphaticovenular anastomoses via millimeter skin incisions. Ann Plast Surg. 2014;72(1):67–70.
26. Friedman R, Bustos VP, Postian T, Pardo J, Hamaguchi R, Lee BT, James TA, Singhal D. Utilizing a lower extremity vein graft for immediate lymphatic reconstruction. J Plast Reconstr Aesthet Surg. 2022;75(8):2831–70.
27. Yamamoto T, Chen WF, Yamamoto N, Yoshimatsu H, Tashiro K, Koshima I. Technical simplification of the supermicrosurgical side-to-end lymphaticovenular anastomosis using the parachute technique. Microsurgery. 2015;35(2):129–34.
28. Yamamoto T, Yamamoto N. Possibility of new lymphatic pathway creation through neo-lymphangiogenesis induced by subdermal dissection. Lymphology. 2021;54(3):154–63.
29. Yamamoto T, Yoshimatsu H, Narushima M, Yamamoto N, Shim TWH, Seki Y, Kikuchi K, Karibe J, Azuma S, Koshima I. Sequential anastomosis for lymphatic supermicrosurgery: multiple lymphaticovenular anastomoses on one venule. Ann Plast Surg. 2014;73(1):46–9.

Part VI

Section F. Future modalities

23 Laser Tomography for Lymphatic Supermicrosurgery

Akitatsu Hayashi

23.1 Introduction

Lymphaticovenular anastomosis (LVA) is effective and minimally invasive treatment for refractory lymphedema [1–3]. The lymphatic vessels become sclerotic over time after lymph flow obstruction and lose their function to drain lymph fluid in peripheral lymphedema patient [2]. Anastomosing the severely sclerotic lymphatic vessels leads to minimum therapeutic effect in LVA. What defines a "functional" lymphatic vessel should be its ability to transport lymph. Therefore, identification of functional lymphatic vessels is important for LVA [3, 4]. For intraoperative identification of them, surgeons often use microscope-integrated indocyanine green (ICG) fluorescence imaging or other ICG florescence imaging tools. Although it has been thought that ICG-enhanced lymphatic vessels were considered "functional" for its capability to transport contrast-containing lymph and non-ICG-enhanced lymphatic vessels were regarded as "nonfunctional," it was found that lymphatic flow-positive but non-ICG-enhanced lymphatic vessels should also be considered functional [5]. Previous study reported noninvasive ultrasound visualization of lymphatic vessels in a region masked by dermal backflow pattern of ICG lymphography is useful for selecting appropriate lymphatic vessels for LVA not only preoperatively but also intraoperatively [3, 4, 6], but they have limitations.

From 2021, new capabilities of laser tomography which is optical coherence tomography (OCT) for imaging of the lymphatic vessels for intraoperative selection of appropriate lymphatic vessels [7]. It is reported that intraoperative laser tomography overcomes the weakness of the conventional techniques.

23.2 Laser Tomography: New Modality for Intraoperative Supervision

Laser tomography has significantly refined clinicians' approach to diagnosis, management, and surveillance of ophthalmic diseases [8, 9]. Laser tomography is an imaging modality that uses reflection of near-infrared light to generate images and provides high-resolution cross-sectional and optical coherence tomographic data. Using this technology, surgeons would potentially have immediate feedback on completion of surgical tasks or new understanding of the

Supplementary Information The online version contains supplementary material available at https://doi.org/10.1007/978-981-97-7278-0_23.

A. Hayashi (✉)
Lymphedema Center, Kameda General Hospital, Kamogawa, Japan

J. P. Hong et al. (eds.), *Imaging for Reconstructive Microsurgery*,
https://doi.org/10.1007/978-981-97-7278-0_23

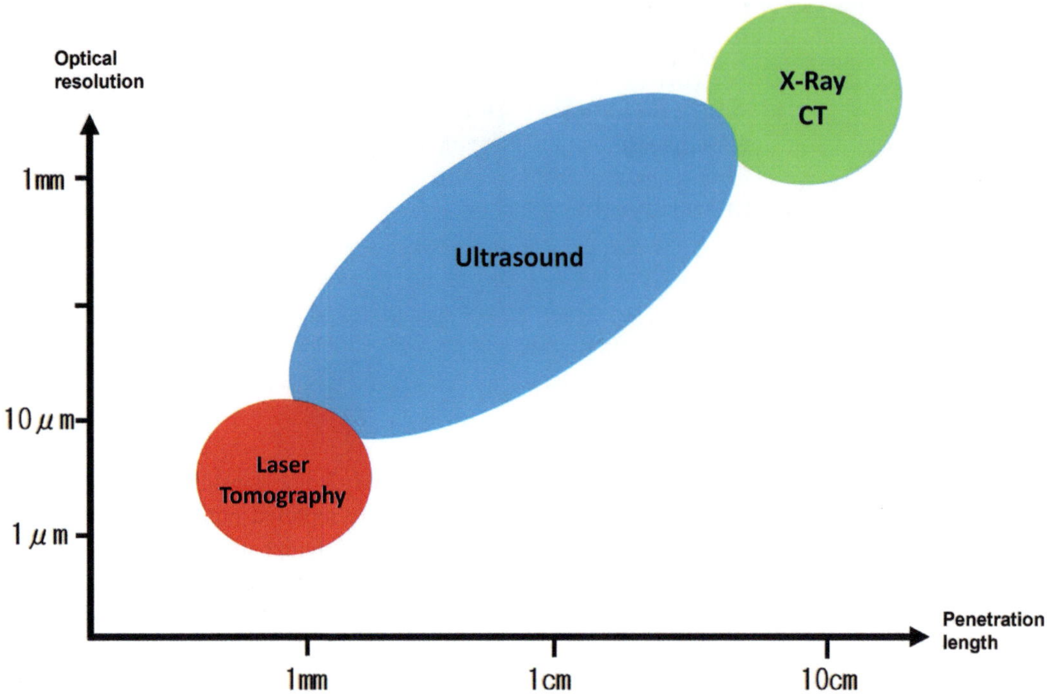

Fig. 23.1 Laser tomography is an imaging modality that uses reflection of near-infrared light to generate images and provides high-resolution cross-sectional and optical coherence tomographic data

anatomic configuration of the tissues. Laser tomography could provide specific real-time guidance for surgical manipulations and thus intraoperative selection of functional lymphatic vessels for LVA.

Surgeons need to use the microscope which installed laser tomography system, thus allowing intraoperative real-time laser tomographic imaging with immediate feedback. Black and white scales express the strength of the reflection of near-infrared light against subject objects in this system. White color represents the most intense reflection, and black color represents the weakest reflection. This system provides an imaging depth of 2.5 mm at an optical axial resolution of <4 μm. Images are acquired at 32,000 cross-sectional scans per second. It allows continuous visualization in a crosshair aiming mode or acquisition of volumes of up to 1000 × 1000 lateral pixels. The scan length is up to 16 mm (Fig. 23.1).

Dynamic scan is controlled via footswitch for swift adjustment of the scan angle to align with the lymphatic vessels. Imaging data is displayed on external screen-based display immediately after completion of scanning. A trained mechanical engineer or nurse can assist intraoperatively with laser tomographic image acquisition and collecting surgeon feedback and data (Fig. 23.2).

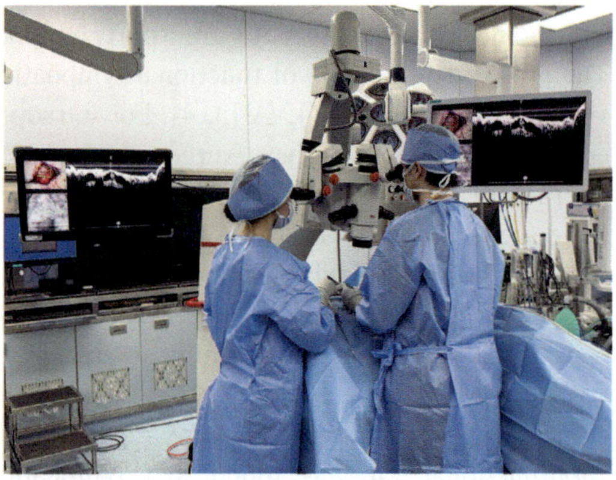

Fig. 23.2 Real-time microscope-integrated laser tomography imaging data is displayed on an external screen-based display immediately after completion of scanning of the lymphatic vessels

23.3 Intraoperative Selection of the Lymphatic Vessel Using Laser Tomography

The lymphatic vessel wall is demonstrated as white region, and the lumen of the lymphatic vessel is demonstrated as black region in laser tomography images (Fig. 23.3). If the lymphatic vessel has valves, it is found inside the lumen and is seen as white winding lines (Fig. 23.4). Also, if the lymphatic vessels converge or diverge again in proximal, laser tomography can detect exact conversing point (Video 23.1). This image information is extremely useful for achieving efficient LVA.

The lymphatic vessels become sclerotic over time after lymph flow obstruction and lose their function to drain lymph fluid. It is essential to select the best functional lymphatic vessels with less sclerosis in LVA for maximum therapeutic effects. Laser tomography can provide objective information regarding the thickness of lymphatic vessel wall, which correlated with histologically measured thickness (Fig. 23.5). Thus, using laser tomography, even surgeons with less experience can choose the most suitable lymphatic vessels, including those not highlighted with ICG, in the surgical field just by scanning the region.

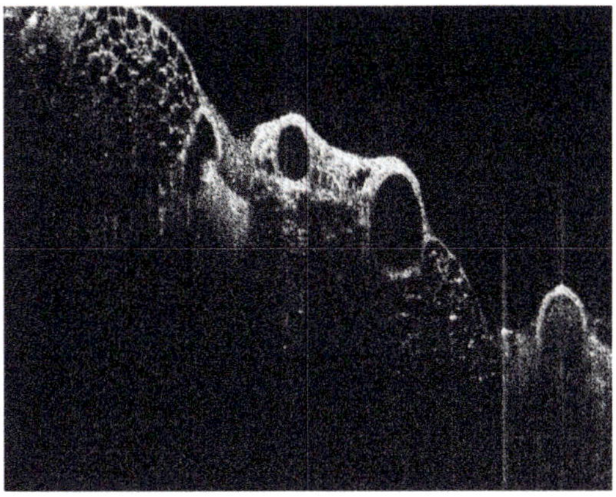

Fig. 23.3 The lymphatic vessel wall is demonstrated as white region, and the lumen of the lymphatic vessel is demonstrated as black region in laser tomography images

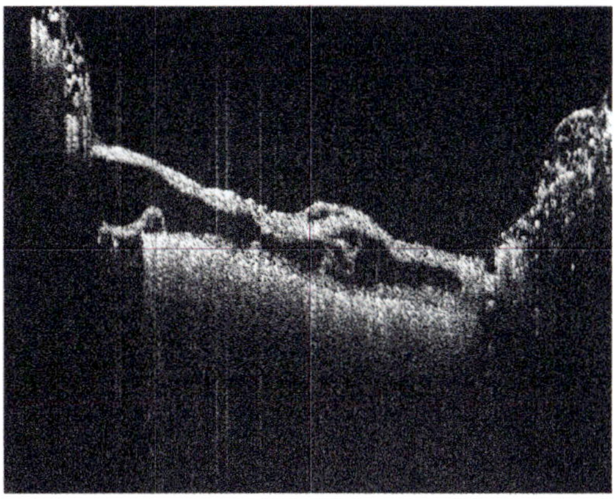

Fig. 23.4 Valves, which were seen as white winding lines, were found inside the lumen of the lymphatic vessels with the obtained cross-sectional images of the lymphatic vessels in microscope-integrated laser tomography

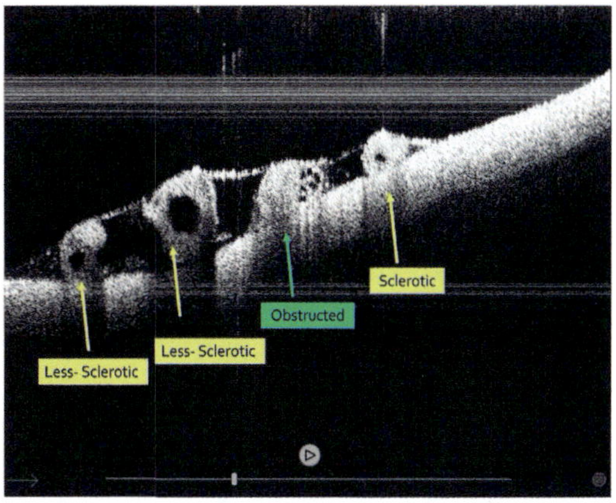

Fig. 23.5 Axial scans with laser tomography are performed intraoperatively on the dissected lymphatic vessels before LVA. Laser tomography can provide objective information regarding the thickness of lymphatic vessel wall

23.4 Patency Assessment of Anastomosis Sites Using Laser Tomography

As of now, in all previous reports, the patency of the anastomosis sites was evaluated via intraoperative ICG observation, where in most cases the

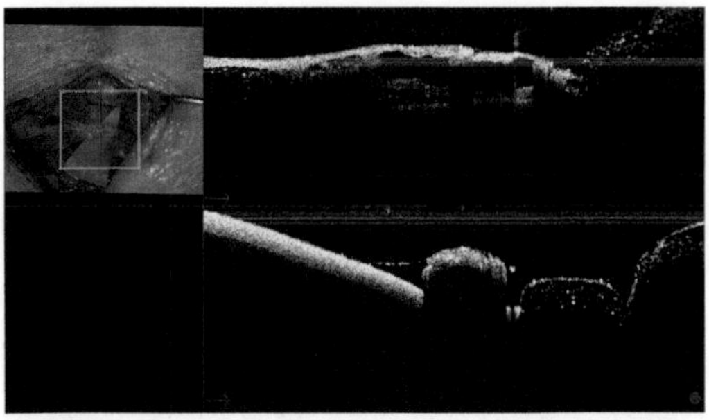

Fig. 23.6 Patency of the anastomosis sites was determined in end-to-end anastomosis between lymphatic vessel and vein using laser tomography scanning (above, sagittal plane; below, axial plane)

lymphatic vessel distal to the anastomosis site was "milked" to push the lymphatic fluid through the anastomosis site. While this procedure may be optimal for assessment of leakage in the anastomosis site, the patency will be determined as positive even in anastomoses with a minimum patent lumen. Due to extremely high resolution of the images that can be obtained with laser tomography, the patency of the anastomosis sites can be more precisely determined, thus possibly leading to higher efficacy of LVA (Fig. 23.6). Laser tomography is useful also for beginner of lymphatic surgery because it provides immediate feedback of the anastomosis status.

Laser tomography can detect anastomosis sites which demonstrated inverted edges of the vessels, which necessitated immediate reanastomosis even though the patency was confirmed with ICG observation. In our recent study, 200 anastomoses using laser tomography were compared with 150 anastomoses without using laser tomography; postoperative 1-year patent rate was increased by 13% with significant differences.

23.5 Limitation of Using Laser Tomography

A disadvantage of this new imaging modality is its limited reaching distance of near-infrared light. The deepest layer from which the device can obtain images is 2.5 mm from the superficial surface. This precludes its use in preoperative examination, but the reaching distance is sufficient for intraoperative use, where the lymphatic vessels are already dissected out.

23.6 Conclusion

This novel device provides real-time images of the lymphatic vessels in extremely high resolution and enables intraoperative evaluation of lymphatic degeneration status. In addition, patency of the anastomosis sites can be determined with extreme precision. This advanced technology for lymphedema may open new frontiers in understanding and treatment of this complex disease.

References

1. Koshima I, Inagawa K, Urushibara K, Moriguchi T. Supermicrosurgical lymphaticovenular anastomosis for the treatment of lymphedema in the upper extremities. J Reconstr Microsurg. 2000;16:437–42.
2. Yamamoto T, Yamamoto N, Yoshimatsu H, et al. Factors associated with lymphosclerosis: an analysis on 962 lymphatic vessels. Plast Reconstr Surg. 2017;140:734–41.
3. Hayashi A, Hayashi N, Yoshimatsu H, et al. Effective and efficient lymphaticovenular anastomosis using preoperative ultrasound detection technique of lymphatic vessels in lower extremity lymphedema. J Surg Oncol. 2018;117:290–8.
4. Hayashi A, Yamamoto T, Yoshimatsu H, et al. Ultrasound visualization of the lymphatic vessels in the lower leg. Microsurgery. 2016;36:397–401.
5. Yang JC, Wu SC, Chiang MH, et al. Intraoperative identification and definition of "functional" lymphatic collecting vessels for supermicrosurgical lymphaticovenous anastomosis in treating lymphedema patients. J Surg Oncol. 2018;117:94–1000.
6. Hayashi A, Visconti G, Yamamoto T, et al. Intraoperative imaging of lymphatic vessel using ultra high-frequency ultrasound. J Plast Reconstr Aesthet Surg. 2018;71:778–80.
7. Hayashi A, Yoshimatsu H, Visconti G, et al. Intraoperative real-time visualization of the lymphatic vessels using microscope-integrated laser tomography. J Reconstr Microsurg. 2021;37(5):427–35.
8. Chen TC, Cense B, Pierce MC, et al. Spectral domain optical coherence tomography: ultrahigh speed, ultra-high resolution ophthalmic imaging. Arch Ophthalmol. 2005;123:1715–20.
9. Hee MR, Izatt JA, Swanson EA, et al. Optical coherence tomography of the human retina. Arch Ophthalmol. 1995;113:325–32.

Photoacoustic

24

Yushi Suzuki

24.1 Background

Photoacoustic (PA) effect has been a known phenomenon since 1880. Photoacoustic imaging (PAI) is a technology to visualize an object by repeatedly irradiating pulsed laser to an object and detecting weak ultrasound waves generated when the volume of the object changes due to thermal expansion [1]. Recently, based on this principle, PAI systems have been developed. Although it is still an upcoming modality compared to conventional imaging, PAI has been reported to have been used in reconstructive surgery to clearly visualize blood vessels and lymphatic vessels [2–4].

In this chapter, we will discuss what can be visualized by using this new modality, as well as its future prospects.

24.2 Principle of Photoacoustic Imaging

First, the principle of photoacoustic imaging will be discussed as described in other published articles [5–7]. When a pulsed laser irradiates an object to be imaged, the object absorbs light energy according to its specific wavelength and converts it into thermal energy. The temperature rise during this process causes thermal expansion. This expansion generates weak photoacoustic ultrasonic waves that can be detected by an ultrasonic sensor outside the body to construct an image (Fig. 24.1).

Hemoglobin can act as the absorber to visualize blood vessels without the use of contrast agents. PAI system has been utilized in animal experiments to observe capillaries, lymph nodes, and so on [8–11]. In addition, some PAI devices have been approved for clinical use in some countries.

In practice, multispectral optoacoustic tomography (MSOT, iThera Medical GmbH, Germany) and PAI-05 (Luxonus Inc. Japan) have been reportedly used in reconstructive surgery. Among them, the MSOT has been used for preoperative assessment of lymphaticovenular anastomosis (LVA) [3], whereas the PAI-05 has been used for anterolateral thigh (ALT) flap elevation in head and neck cancer reconstruction and for LVA preoperatively and postoperatively [2, 4, 5].

Supplementary Information The online version contains supplementary material available at https://doi.org/10.1007/978-981-97-7278-0_24.

Y. Suzuki (✉)
Department of Plastic and Reconstructive Surgery, Keio University School of Medicine, Tokyo, Japan
e-mail: fi080150@keio.jp

J. P. Hong et al. (eds.), *Imaging for Reconstructive Microsurgery*,
https://doi.org/10.1007/978-981-97-7278-0_24

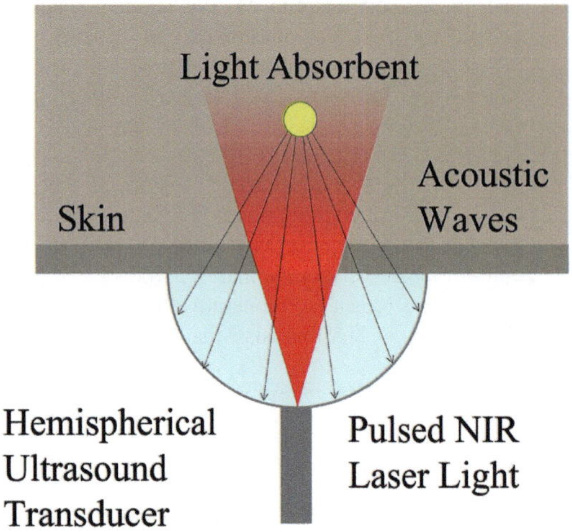

Fig. 24.1 Schematic of the mechanism of photoacoustic imaging. Photoacoustic waves generated by laser irradiation can be detected by ultrasonic sensors outside the body to construct images (Reprinted with permission from Kajita H, Suzuki Y, Sakuma Het al. Keio J Med. 2021;70:82-92)

MSOT utilizes a handheld device that can visualize where the examiner wants to observe. The device can penetrate 1–2 cm below the skin surface and take three-dimensional images. Light of several wavelengths (700–875 nm) emits to an optimal absorber. MSOT differentiates lymphatics and vessels by comparing the difference between two wavelengths. The handheld device is easy to handle and makes it easy to utilize MSOT for patients. However, the field of view during MSOT is narrow (15 × 15 mm), and MSOT image quality still has room for improvement.

On the other hand, the PAI-05, which is a prototype not available for clinical use, can capture a wide field of view (270 × 180 mm), and its use has been published extensively in the field of plastic and reconstructive surgery. This chapter specifically describes the clinical applications of this bed-shaped device.

This device has a scanning stage in the bed unit, which enables stable imaging over a wide range. Furthermore, since this device receives photoacoustic waves generated by the abovementioned principle at multiple points with a bowl-shaped sensor, it is also possible to evaluate the three-dimensional positioning of the light absorber. By sliding the sensor, the images can be superimposed, and the maximum area can be imaged in about 10 min. The sensor can also be fixed in place to capture moving images.

Furthermore, this device can irradiate any two wavelengths between 750 and 850 nm, and it is possible to color-code the optical absorber according to the difference in intensity of the PA wave obtained at each wavelength. For example, by selecting the two wavelengths distinguishing between reduced hemoglobin and oxidized hemoglobin as larger and smaller, it is possible to color-code the arteries and veins without using contrast agents [12].

We will describe the application of this device in the field of reconstructive surgery.

24.3 Application to Preoperative Planning of Flap Surgeries

As mentioned above, this device can be used to identify the three-dimensional vascular course of vessels without the use of contrast agents. Until now, preoperative planning of flap surgeries has been performed using computed tomography angiography and ultrasonography (US), but the superficial layers of the subcutaneous tissue, especially above the fascia, were difficult to visualize, and ultrasound was dependent on the skill of the surgeon. However, this device can clearly delineate superficial blood vessels running above the fascia (Figs. 24.2 and 24.3) [4, 5, 13].

For example, it not only depicts how the perforating arteries rising from the fascia spread above the fascia, but also, by taking videos, it can show that the perforating arteries are pulsating (Video 24.1).

The ability to color-code the images also shows the depth to which the vessels run after penetrating the fascia, allowing the intuitive understanding of how the vessels run within the flap. This vascular depth information is useful for

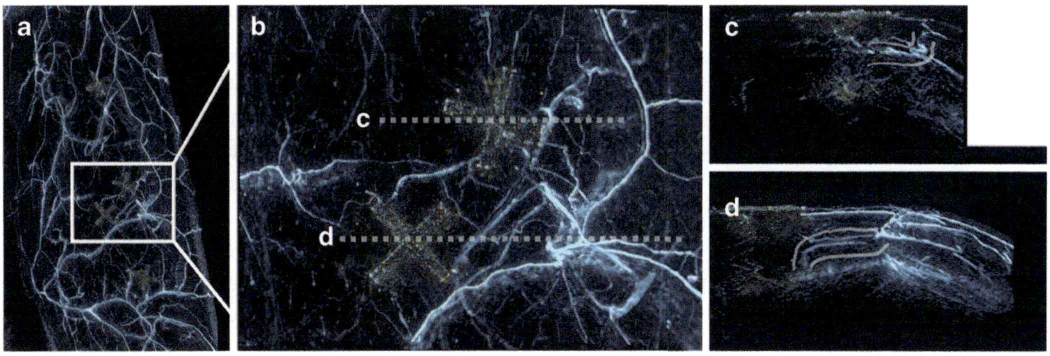

Fig. 24.2 Images of healthy volunteer of the left thigh: X marker is set on the place where the perforator artery is detected by ultrasonography. (**a**) Vascular imaging of left anterolateral thigh area. (**b**) Zoomed-in image of the squared portion in Fig. 24.2a. Two perforator arteries can be seen. (**c**) Cross-sectional view of Fig. 24.2b. Perforator artery is outlined by translucent white line. (**d**) Cross-sectional view of Fig. 24.2b. Translucent white line shows perforator artery initially rises vertically and runs horizontally unlike Fig. 24.2c

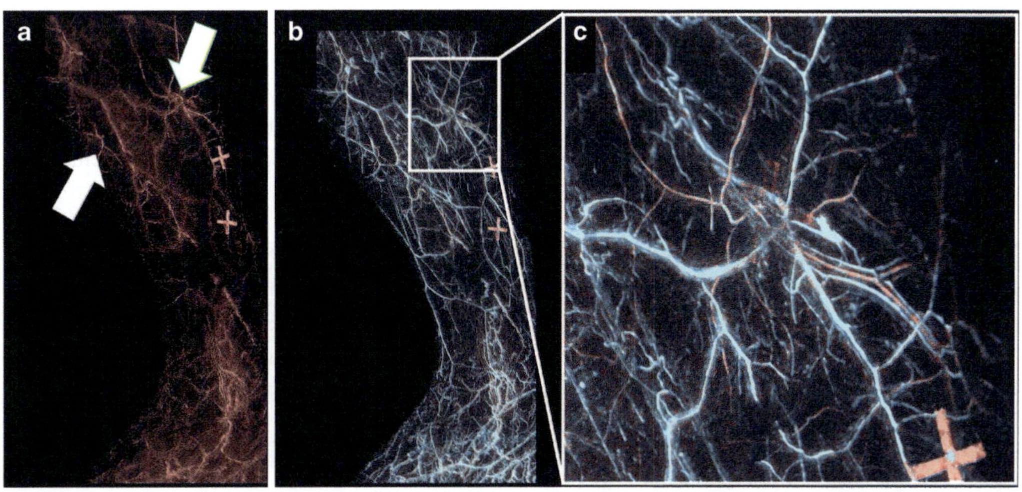

Fig. 24.3 Images of a healthy volunteer of the left lower leg: the red coloration signifies the artery, whereas the blue coloration signifies the vein (Reprinted with permission from Suzuki Y, Kajita H, Watanabe S et al. J Reconstr Microsurg. 2022; 38(3):254–262). (**a**) Arterial imaging of the lateral side of the lower leg. The arrow points to the perforator artery. The vein signal remained slightly indistinct. (**b**) Photoacoustic image of the artery and vein. (**c**) Zoomed-in image of the squared portion in Fig. 24.3b. One running artery and two running veins can be seen

flap thinning. In particular, ALT has variations in the vascular run above the fascia, but this information allows surgeons to elevate thin ALT safely [4].

Although the PAI-05 can theoretically confirm a depth of about 2 cm [12], the ultrasound generated by the PA effect cannot exceed the thick fascia of the thigh and other areas, so only the superficial area above the fascia can be evaluated. In the back, however, the fascia is thin, so subcutaneous blood perfusion can be evaluated in real time, even in the region below the latissimus dorsi muscle, and the knowledge of vascular anatomy of the flap can be further developed [14].

24.4 Application to Lymphedema Treatment

This technology can also be used to delineate lymphatic vessels. Lymphatic vessel delineation by PAI is called photoacoustic lymphangiography [2, 5, 6, 15, 16]. Since lymph fluid is transparent, there is no light absorber necessary for the PA effect to occur, and therefore it is impossible to delineate the lymphatic vessels in their original condition. Hence, contrast agents must be used to observe the lymphatic system using photoacoustic technology. The commonly used contrast agent is indocyanine green (ICG), which is also used in the near-infrared fluorescent (NIRF) lymphography. The maximum absorbance of ICG reaches at around 797 nm and decreases significantly at 835 nm. On the other hand, the absorbance of hemoglobin does not change dramatically between these two wavelengths. Therefore, PAI-05 color-codes lymphatic vessels and blood vessels by taking the difference between the two wavelengths of 797 nm and 835 nm. If only the larger difference between the two wavelengths is displayed, only lymphatic vessels can be displayed, while, on the other hand, only blood vessels can be depicted if you select the one with the smallest difference (Fig. 24.4).

On the other hand, there are reports of lymphatic vessels being imaged by MSOT, which also evaluates ICG in lymphatic vessels and hemoglobin in blood vessels [3, 17] and can intuitively assess the depth of both lymphatic vessels and veins. Because MSOT is a handheld device, it allows real-time imaging during the operation and can obtain tomographic images at any position, allowing intuitive assessment of the depth of both lymphatic vessels and veins.

Meanwhile, PAI-05 can create three-dimensional images using sensors placed at multiple points, but the bed-shaped configuration makes intraoperative use difficult. It can however depict the three-dimensional relationship

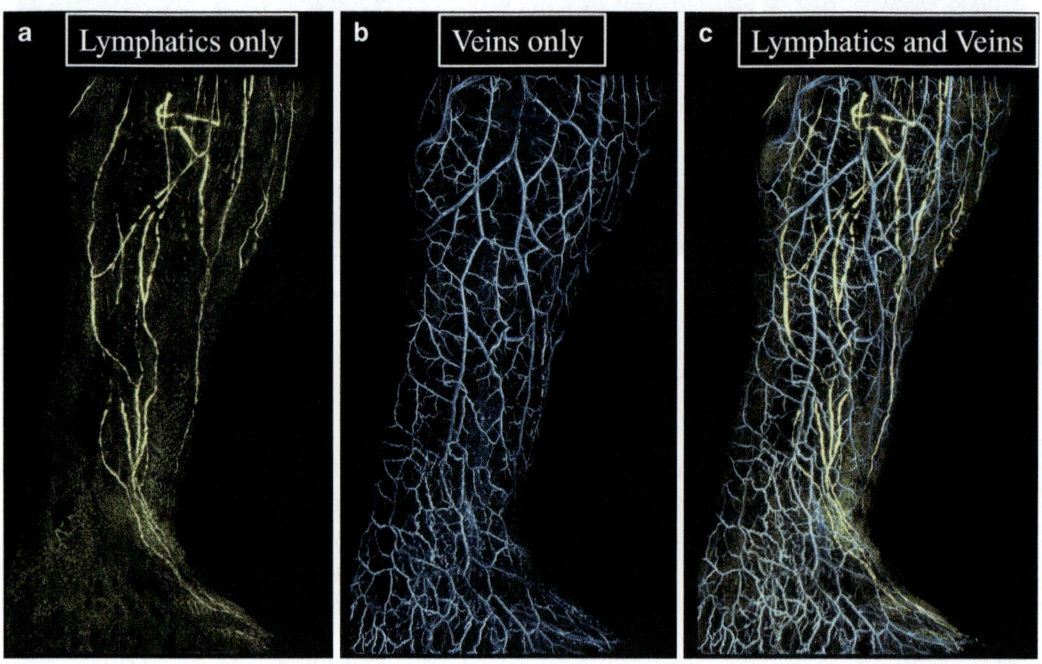

Fig. 24.4 Images of a healthy volunteer of medial side of lower leg. PAI-05 color-codes lymphatic vessels and blood vessels by taking the difference between the two wavelengths of 797 nm and 835 nm (Reprinted with permission from Suzuki Y, Kajita H, Konishi N et al. Radiology 2020; 95(2):469–474). (**a**) Only lymphatic vessels are visualized by displaying a larger difference. (**b**) Only blood vessels are also depicted. (**c**) The lymphatic vessels and veins are displayed at the same time revealing their mutual location

between lymphatic vessels and veins over a wide area, making it easy to intuitively identify areas where they run in close proximity to each other. The captured images are retrieved as DICOM data and analyzed with the Kyoto University Rapid and Universal MIP Imager (KURUMI), a 3D image viewer suitable for displaying photoacoustic images. The KURUMI allows free rotation of visualized vessels in 3D and trimming of obstructing areas to analyze the running of the vessels [2, 5, 6, 15, 16].

In healthy individuals, good lymphatic vessels toward the cranial side are depicted, reflecting good functionality (Fig. 24.5; Video 24.2), but when lymphedema occurs, lymphatic backflow into the lymphatic precollector, called dermal backflow, occurs. The wide imaging range and high resolution of the PAI-05 also allow observation of dermal backflow [2, 5, 16, 18], suggesting that it may lead to the diagnosis of lymphedema (Fig. 24.6).

24.4.1 Comparison of Each Imaging Modality (Table 24.1)

Lymphedema is symptomatic because of backflow of congested lymph causing edema. The imaging modalities known to evaluate lymphedema include lymphoscintigraphy [19], NIRF [20–22], magnetic resonance lymphangiography (MRL) [23–26], and US [27, 28]. Lymphoscintigraphy can evaluate the entire lower extremity, while detailed evaluation of each lymphatic vessel is difficult. NIRF is widely used for lymphedema treatment and is presently

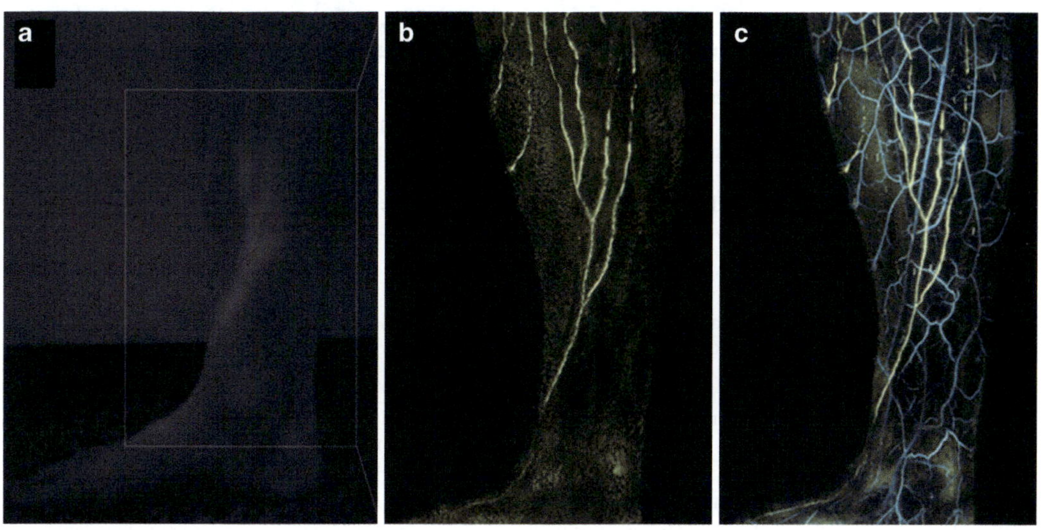

Fig. 24.5 The medial side of the right lower leg of the healthy young woman imaged. In healthy individuals, good lymphatic vessels toward the cranial side are depicted, reflecting good functionality (Reprinted with permission from Kajita H, Suzuki Y, Sakuma H et al. Keio J Med. 2021;70:82-92). (**a**) Near-infrared fluorescence lymphography showing the lymphatic vessels with a linear pattern. The rectangle corresponds to the area covered by panels B and C. (**b**) Photoacoustic lymphangiography (PAL) showing the lymphatic vessels (yellow lines) filled with ICG. (**c**) PAL showing the lymphatic vessels (yellow lines) and veins (blue lines)

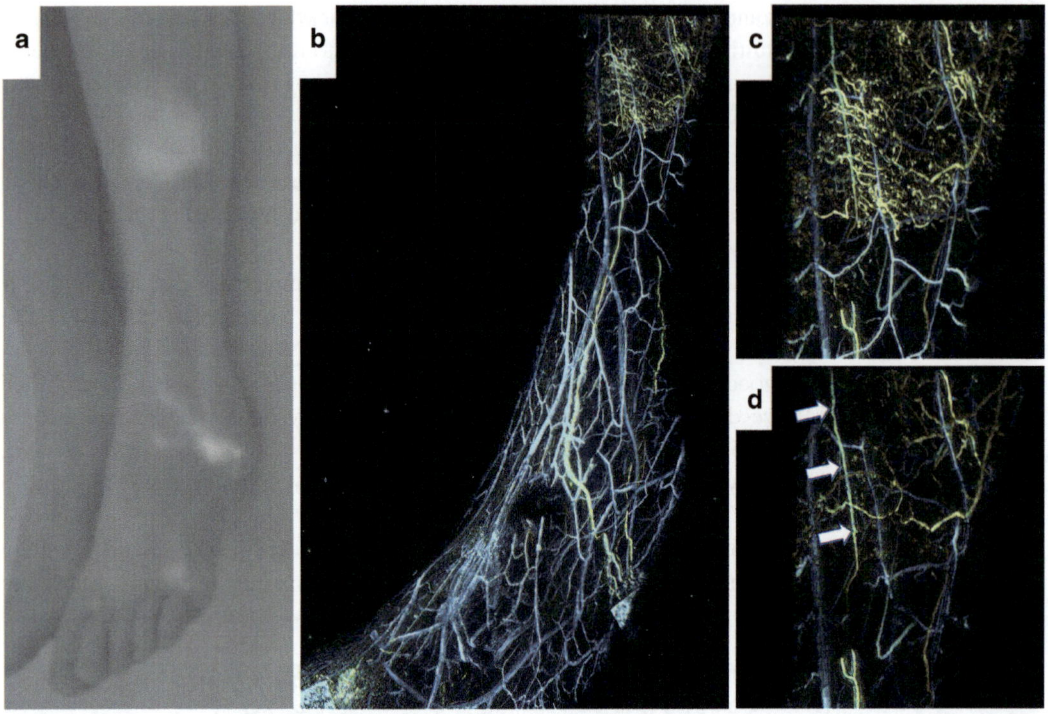

Fig. 24.6 The lateral side of lower leg of the lymphedema patient. Dermal backflow is observed in cranial side (Reprinted with permission from Suzuki Y, Kajita H, Imanishi N et al. Plast Reconstr Surg Glob Open. 2020;8(6):e2914). (**a**) Near-infrared fluorescence lymphography showing the collective lymphatic vessels and dermal backflow. (**b**) Photoacoustic lymphangiography (PAL) showing the lymphatic vessels (yellow lines) and veins (blue lines). We can observe dermal backflow on cranial side. (**c**) Enlarged dermal backflow area. (**d**) Erasing the dermal backflow digitally, we can find collective lymphatic vessels on deep side

Table 24.1 Comparison of each imaging modality (Reprinted with permission from Suzuki Y, Kajita H, Watanabe S et al. J Reconstr Microsurg. 2022; 38(3):254–262)

	Pros	Cons
LS	Enables complete evaluation of the lower extremities	Difficult to identify details of individual lymphatic vessels
NIRF	Real-time imaging Widely used in lymphatic surgery	Provides only two-dimensional information
MRL	Detailed resolution and wide imaging range in three dimensions	Smaller lymphatic vessels are not evident at early lymphedema stages Venous contamination may lead to misidentification of lymphatics
US	Simultaneous identification of lymphatics and veins No contrast agent required	Reproducibility issues because accuracy of image rendition depends on the skill of practitioner
PAL	High-definition images with a resolution of 0.2 mm enable simultaneous identification of lymphatics and veins three-dimensionally Video recording is possible	Imaging range is limited The device is still in its development stage

LS lymphoscintigraphy, *NIRF* near-infrared fluorescence lymphangiography, *MRL* magnetic resonance lymphangiography, *US* ultrasonography, *PAL* photoacoustic lymphangiography accumulating a large amount of evidence but does not provide depth information. MRL can evaluate a wide range of lymphatic vessels in three dimensions, but presently it is difficult to evaluate only dilated lymphatic vessels, and venous contamination can cause misidentification of lymphatic vessels in beginners. US is a very promising modality because it does not require contrast agents and allows simultaneous evaluation of lymphatic vessels and veins, but it is operator-dependent, which raises the issue of reproducibility. Compared to these conventional modalities, PAL has a limited imaging range and is still in its developing stage, but it can intuitively evaluate lymphatic vessels and veins with a resolution of 0.2 mm. Therefore, future development is expected. Comparison of dermal backflow in lymphedema patients with lymphoscintigraphy [29] and NIRF [7] has already suggested the usefulness of PAL in lymphedema treatment.

24.4.2 Preoperative Evaluation of LVA

As mentioned above, simultaneous evaluation of the lymphatic vessels and veins to depict their three-dimensional relationship is extremely useful for preoperative planning of LVA. It is possible to intuitively locate the crossing of lymphatic vessels and veins and the depth evaluation of each. In addition, there are often cases in which the dermal backflow spreads early and the collecting lymphatics are hidden beneath it by NIRF, but with PAL the superficial dermal backflow can be removed and the deeper lymphatics can be evaluated. Therefore, PAL has the potential to utilize lymphatic vessels that could not be anastomosed before. Although PAL has a lower sensitivity for ICG than NIRF, it can evaluate well-functioning lymphatic vessels that are stained by ICG without being disturbed by dermal backflow in the interstitium. This may allow for the identification of more functional lymphatic vessels compared to NIRF. In addition, there are reports that the images obtained in this way are reflected in the actual surgical field by methods such as superimposing multiple markings [4] or using augmented reality [30], and these methods can obtain the target vessels without discrepancy.

24.4.3 Postoperative Evaluation of LVA

Lymphedema is caused by lymphatic congestion due to impaired lymphatic transport capacity. LVA is a surgical procedure in which the lymphatic vessels are bypassed and drained into veins to relieve congestion. Therefore, postoperative evaluation should not only be based on circumferential diameter, such as LEL index or UEL index [31, 32], but also on the patency of the bypass created by anastomosis after surgery, which is regarded as the essence of the procedure. However, with conventional modalities, it is difficult to evaluate all anastomotic sites because it is difficult to visualize deep subcutaneous regions covered by dermal backflow. The PAI-05 can digitally process and erase the dermal backflow, making it possible to evaluate the patency of the anastomosis [33]. We would like to introduce these preoperative and postoperative procedures based on actual cases.

24.4.4 Case Presentation (48-Year-Old Female Patient with Secondary Lymphedema)

PAL was performed, and lymphatic vessels and veins could be visualized at the medial side of the ankle joint. An incision was made at the same site, and the lymphatic vessels and veins were identified and anastomosed smoothly (Fig. 24.7). At 1 month after surgery, the anastomosis was visualized, and the lymphatic vessels and veins were found to be in contact with each other, suggesting patency of the anastomosis (Fig. 24.8).

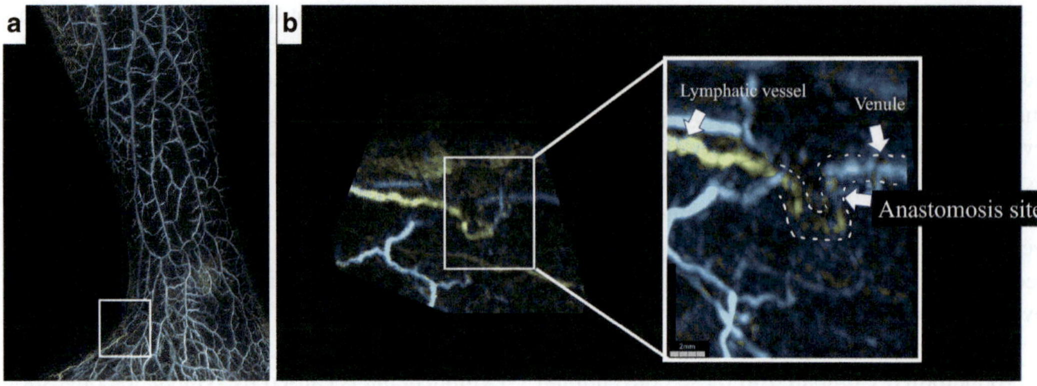

Fig. 24.8 The medial side of the lower leg of the same lymphedema patient as in Fig. 24.7. Photoacoustic lymphangiography (PAL) is performed at 1 month after lymphaticovenular anastomosis surgery (Reprinted with permission from Suzuki Y, Kajita H, Kono H et al. Plast Reconstr Surg Glob Open. 2021;9(1):e3348). (**a**) The anastomosis site is observed by PAL. (**b**) Enlarged anastomosis site. Lymphatic vessels and veins were found to be in contact with each other, suggesting patency of the anastomosis

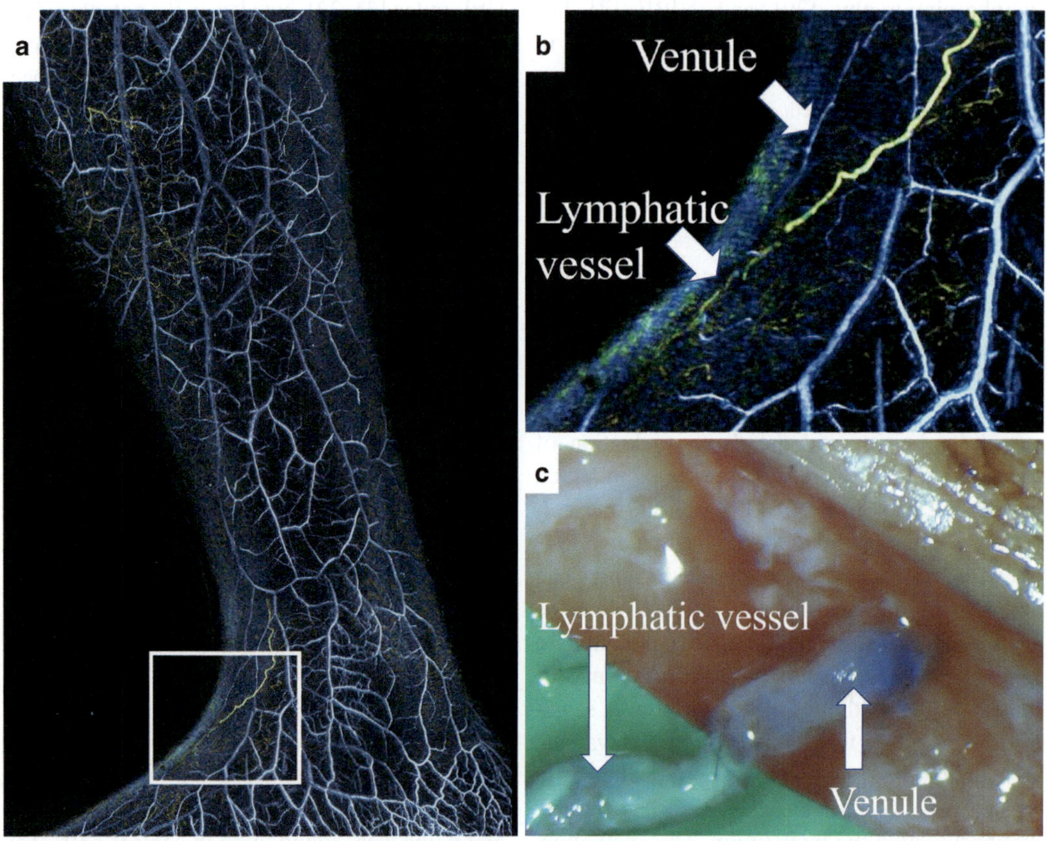

Fig. 24.7 The medial side of the lower leg of the lymphedema patient. There is a good collective lymphatic vessel on ankle area; thus, lymphaticovenular anastomosis is performed (Reprinted with permission from Suzuki Y, Kajita H, Kono Het al. Plast Reconstr Surg Glob Open. 2021;9(1):e3348). (**a**) Photoacoustic lymphangiography shows collective lymphatic vessel is running around ankle area. (**b**) Enlarged ankle area. (**c**) Lymphaticovenular end-to-end anastomosis is performed

24.5 Conclusion

PAI can produce very high-definition images of blood vessels without the use of contrast agents, and the use of ICG enables the delineation of lymphatic vessels. The ability to image blood and lymphatic vessels, both of which are crucial for reconstructive surgeons, is a promising feature of PAI. However, some issues remain to be resolved, such as the limited imaging range due to the need to be in contact with a water-filled tray, the inability to capture the entire limb, and the inability of the PAI-05 to perform real-time visualization during surgery. Further development toward better clinical applications is expected.

This work was supported by AMED under proposal number JP19he2302002.

References

1. Bell AG. On the production and reproduction of sound by light. Am J Sci. 1880;s3–20(118):305–24.
2. Oh A, Kajita H, Matoba E, Okabe K, Sakuma H, Imanishi N, Takatsume Y, Kono H, Asao Y, Yagi T, Aiso S, Kishi K. Photoacoustic lymphangiography before and after lymphaticovenular anastomosis. Arch Plast Surg. 2021;48(3):323–8.
3. Giacalone G, Yamamoto T, Belva F, Hayashi A. Bedside 3D visualization of lymphatic vessels with a handheld multispectral optoacoustic tomography device. J Clin Med. 2020;9(3):815.
4. Tsuge I, Saito S, Yamamoto G, Sekiguchi H, Yoshikawa A, Matsumoto Y, Suzuki S, Toi M. Preoperative vascular mapping for anterolateral thigh flap surgeries: a clinical trial of photoacoustic tomography imaging. Microsurgery. 2020;40(3):324–30.
5. Suzuki Y, Kajita H, Watanabe S, Okabe K, Sakuma H, Imanishi N, Aiso S, Kishi K. Application of photoacoustic imaging for lymphedema treatment. J Reconstr Microsurg. 2022;38(3):254–62.
6. Suzuki Y, Kajita H, Konishi N, Oh A, Urano M, Watanabe S, Asao Y, Imanishi N, Tsuji T, Jinzaki M, Aiso S, Kishi K. Radiology. 2020;295(2):469–74.
7. Suzuki Y, Kajita H, Oh A, Urano M, Watanabe S, Sakuma H, Imanishi N, Tsuji T, Jinzaki M, Kishi K. Photoacoustic lymphangiography exhibits advantages over near-infrared fluorescence lymphangiography as a diagnostic tool in patients with lymphedema. J Vasc Surg Venous Lymphat Disord. 2022;10(2):454–462.e1.
8. Wang LV, Hu S. Photoacoustic tomography: in vivo imaging from organelles to organs. Science. 2012;335(6075):1458–62.
9. Zackrisson S, van de Ven SMWY, Gambhir SS. Light in and sound out: emerging translational strategies for photoacoustic imaging. Cancer Res. 2014;74(4):979–1004.
10. Zhu Y, Feng T, Cheng Q, Wang X, Du S, Sato N, Kuniyil Ajith Singh M, Yuan J. Towards clinical translation of LED-based photoacoustic imaging: a review. Sensors (Basel). 2020;20(9):2484.
11. Song KH, Stein EW, Margenthaler JA, Wang LV. Noninvasive photoacoustic identification of sentinel lymph nodes containing methylene blue in vivo in a rat model. J Biomed Opt. 2008;13(5):054033.
12. Nagae K, Asao Y, Sudo Y, Murayama N, Tanaka Y, Ohira K, Ishida Y, Otsuka A, Matsumoto Y, Saito S, Furu M, Murata K, Sekiguchi H, Kataoka M, Yoshikawa A, Ishii T, Togashi K, Shiina T, Kabashima K, Toi M, Yagi T. Real-time 3D photoacoustic visualization system with a wide field of view for imaging human limbs. F1000Res. 2018;7:1813.
13. Tsuge I, Saito S, Sekiguchi H, Yoshikawa A, Matsumoto Y, Toi M, Suzuki S. Photoacoustic tomography shows the branching pattern of anterolateral thigh perforators in vivo. Plast Reconstr Surg. 2018;141(5):1288–92.
14. Shimizu H, Saito S, Yoshikawa A, Sekiguchi H, Tsuge I, Morimoto N, Toi M. Three-dimensional visualization of thoracodorsal artery perforators using photoacoustic imaging. J Plast Reconstr Aesthet Surg. 2022;75(9):3166–73.
15. Kajita H, Kishi K. High-resolution imaging of lymphatic vessels with photoacoustic lymphangiography. Radiology. 2019;292(1):35.
16. Kajita H, Oh A, Urano M, et al. Photoacoustic lymphangiography. J Surg Oncol. 2020;121(1):48–50.
17. Grünherz L, Gousopoulos E, Barbon C, Uyulmaz S, Lafci B, Razansky D, Boss A, Giovanoli P, Lindenblatt N. Preoperative mapping of lymphatic vessels by multispectral optoacoustic tomography. Lymphat Res Biol. (In Press). 2022;20:659.
18. Oh A, Kajita H, Imanishi N, Sakuma H, Takatsume Y, Okabe K, Aiso S, Kishi K. Three-dimensional analysis of dermal backflow in cancer-related lymphedema using photoacoustic lymphangiography. Arch Plast Surg. 2022;49(1):99–107.
19. Maegawa J, Mikami T, Yamamoto Y, et al. Types of lymphoscintigraphy and indications for lymphaticovenous anastomosis. Microsurgery. 2010;30(6):437–42.
20. Yamamoto T, Narushima M, Doi K, et al. Characteristic indocyanine green lymphography findings in lower extremity lymphedema: the generation of a novel lymphedema severity staging system using dermal backflow patterns. Plast Reconstr Surg. 2011;127(5):1979–86.
21. Hara H, Mihara M, Seki Y, Todokoro T, Iida T, Koshima I. Comparison of indocyanine green lymphographic findings with the conditions of collecting lymphatic vessels of limbs in patients with lymphedema. Plast Reconstr Surg. 2013;132(6):1612–8.

22. Narushima M, Yamamoto T, Ogata F, et al. Indocyanine green lymphography findings in limb lymphedema. J Reconstr Microsurg. 2016;32(1):72–9.
23. Notohamiprodjo M, Weiss M, Baumeister RG, et al. MR lymphangiography at 3.0 T: correlation with lymphoscintigraphy. Radiology. 2012;264(1):78–87.
24. Ruehm SG, Schroeder T, Debatin JF. Interstitial MR lymphography with gadoterate meglumine: initial experience in humans. Radiology. 2001;220(3):816–21.
25. Neligan PC, et al. MR lymphangiography in the treatment of lymphedema. J Surg Oncol. 2017;115(1):18–22.
26. Yasunaga Y, Nakajima Y, Mimura S, et al. Magnetic resonance lymphography as three-dimensional navigation for lymphaticovenular anastomosis in patients with leg lymphedema. J Plast Reconstr Aesthet Surg. 2021;74(6):1253–60.
27. Mihara M, Hara H, Kawakami Y. Ultrasonography for classifying lymphatic sclerosis types and deciding optimal sites for lymphatic-venous anastomosis in patients with lymphoedema. J Plast Reconstr Aesthet Surg. 2018;71(9):1274–81.
28. Hayashi A, Hayashi N, Yoshimatsu H, et al. Effective and efficient lymphaticovenular anastomosis using preoperative ultrasound detection technique of lymphatic vessels in lower extremity lymphedema. J Surg Oncol. 2018;117(2):290–8.
29. Watanabe S, Kajita H, Suzuki Y, Urano M, Otaki M, Sakuma H, Imanishi N, Tsuji T, Jinzaki M, Kishi K. Photoacoustic lymphangiography is a possible alternative for lymphedema staging. J Vasc Surg Venous Lymphat Disord. 2022;10(6):1318–1324.e2.
30. Suzuki Y, Kajita H, Watanabe S, Otaki M, Okabe K, Sakuma H, Takatsume Y, Imanishi N, Aiso S, Kishi K. Surgical applications of lymphatic vessel visualization using photoacoustic imaging and augmented reality. J Clin Med. 2022;11(1):194.
31. Yamamoto T, Matsuda N, Todokoro T, Yoshimatsu H, Narushima M, Mihara M, Uchida G, Koshima I. Lower extremity lymphedema index: a simple method for severity evaluation of lower extremity lymphedema. Ann Plast Surg. 2011;67(6):637–40.
32. Yamamoto T, Yamamoto N, Hara H, Mihara M, Narushima M, Koshima I. Upper extremity lymphedema index: a simple method for severity evaluation of upper extremity lymphedema. Ann Plast Surg. 2013;70(1):47–9.
33. Suzuki Y, Kajita H, Kono H, et al. The direct observation of lymphaticovenular anastomosis patency with photoacoustic lymphangiography. Plast Reconstr Surg Glob Open. 2021;9(1):e3348.

GPSR Compliance

The European Union's (EU) General Product Safety Regulation (GPSR) is a set of rules that requires consumer products to be safe and our obligations to ensure this.

If you have any concerns about our products, you can contact us on ProductSafety@springernature.com

In case Publisher is established outside the EU, the EU authorized representative is:

Springer Nature Customer Service Center GmbH
Europaplatz 3
69115 Heidelberg, Germany

Batch number: 10732801

Printed by Printforce, the Netherlands